WHY ARE SOME PEOPLE HEALTHY AND OTHERS NOT?

SOCIAL INSTITUTIONS AND SOCIAL CHANGE

An Aldine de Gruyter Series of Texts and Monographs

EDITED BY

Michael Useem • James D. Wright

Larry Barnett, **Legal Construct, Social Concept: A Macrosociological Perspective on Law**

Vern L. Bengtson and W. Andrew Achenbaum. **The Changing Contract Across Generations**

Remi Clignet, **Death, Deeds, and Descendants: Inheritance in Modern America**

Mary Ellen Colten and Susan Gore (eds.), **Adolescent Stress: Causes and Consequences**

Rand D. Conger and Glen H. Elder, Jr., **Families in Troubled Times: Adapting to Change in Rural America**

Joel A. Devine and James D. Wright, **The Greatest of Evils: Urban Poverty and the American Underclass**

G. William Domhoff, **The Power Elite and the State: How Policy is Made in America**

Paula S. England, **Comparable Worth: Theories and Evidence**

Paula S. England, **Theory on Gender/Feminism on Theory**

R. G. Evans, M. L. Barer, and T. R. Marmor, **Why Are Some People Healthy and Others Not? The Determinants of Health of Populations**

J. Rogers Hollingsworth and Ellen Jane Hollingsworth (eds.), **Care of the Chronically and Severely Ill: Comparative Social Policies**

Gary Kleck, **Point Blank: Guns and Violence in America**

Dean Knudsen and JoAnn L. Miller (eds.), **Abused and Battered: Social and Legal Responses to Family Violence**

Theodore R. Marmor, **The Politics of Medicare** (*Second Edition*)

Clark McPahil, **The Myth of the Madding Crowd**

John Mirowsky and Catherine E. Ross, **Social Causes of Psychological Distress**

Steven L. Nock, **The Costs of Privacy: Surveillance and Reputation in America**

Talcott Parsons on National Socialism (*Edited and with an Introduction by Uta Gerhardt*)

Carolyn C. and Robert Perrucci, Dena B. and Harry R. Targ, **Plant Closings: International Context and Social Costs**

Robert Perrucci and Harry R. Potter (eds.), **Networks of Power: Organizational Actors at the National, Corporate, and Community Levels**

Robert Perrucci, **Japanese Auto Transplants in the Heartland: Corporatism and Community**

James T. Richardson, Joel Best, and David G. Bromley (eds.), **The Satanism Scare**

Alice S. Rossi and Peter H. Rossi, **Of Human Bonding: Parent-Child Relations Across the Life Course**

David G. Smith, **Paying for Medicare: The Politics of Reform**

James D. Wright, **Address Unknown: The Homeless in America**

James D. Wright and Peter H. Rossi, **Armed and Considered Dangerous: A Survey of Felons and Their Firearms** (Expanded Edition)

James D. Wright, Peter H. Rossi, and Kathleen Daly, **Under the Gun: Weapons, Crime, and Violence in America**

Mary Zey, **Banking on Fraud: Drexel, Junk Bonds, and Buyouts**

WHY ARE SOME PEOPLE HEALTHY AND OTHERS NOT?

The Determinants of Health of Populations

Robert G. Evans, Morris L. Barer, and Theodore R. Marmor
EDITORS

Walter de Gruyter
Berlin • New York

About the Editors

Robert G. Evans is Professor of Economics and Faculty, Centre for Health Services and Policy Research, University of British Columbia. Dr. Evans is the author of *Strained Mercy: The Economics of Canadian Health Care,* and of many journal articles. He is a member of the editorial boards of a number of health services and health policy journals.

Morris L. Barer is Director, Centre for Health Services and Policy Research, and Professor, Department of Health Care and Epidemiology, University of British Columbia. He co-authored with Greg Stoddart the 1991 report *Toward Integrated Medical Resource Policies for Canada.* Dr. Barer is the author of numerous journal articles and research monographs. He served until recently as Senior Health Economics editor for *Social Science and Medicine.*

Theodore R. Marmor is Professor of Public Policy and Management at Yale University. Among his books are *The Politics of Medicare* (Aldine); *America's Misunderstood Welfare State: Persistent Myths and Enduring Realities,* co-authored with Jerry L. Mashaw and Philip Harvey; and *Social Security: Beyond the Rhetoric of Crisis,* co-edited with Jerry L. Mashaw.

Die Deutsche Bibliothek-CIP-Einheitsaufnahme

Why are some people healthy and others not? : The determinants of health of populations / ed. Robert G. Evans . . .
- Berlin ; New York : de Gruyter, 1994
(Social institutions and social change)
ISBN 3-11-014508-1 (Berlin . . .) brosch.
ISBN 3-11-014509-X (Berlin . . .) Geb.
ISBN 0-202-30490-6 (New York . . .) brosch.
ISBN 0-202-30489-2 (New York . . .) Geb.
NE: Evans, Robert G. [Hrsg.]

WG: 33 DBN 94.121715.9 94.05.25
0091 wi

Manufactured in the United States of America

10 9 8 7 6 5 4 3 2 1

To Fraser Mustard

Contents

PART III

PART IV

Preface

BACKGROUND

The question addressed in this book, Why are some people healthy and others not?, has generated a vast academic literature, spanning many disciplines and many decades. But few, if any, of the specialists who have written on different aspects of the topic—epidemiologists, biomedical scientists, psychologists, sociologists, economists, political scientists, historians, among others—confront the full range of available scholarship. Such a task is almost surely beyond the capability of a single scholar. And if one could assemble a large enough group of scholars, could they really communicate with each other?

Our aim is less ambitious than a complete synthesis of this literature. Instead we draw together a set of "anomalous findings" about the determinants of health, from a number of different disciplines. These findings challenge the conventional views of how health is gained and lost, recovered and maintained, which underlie most of the policies and activities through which members of modern societies try to improve their individual and collective health. They are extensive and secure enough, we believe, to support a "paradigm shift" in the scholarship of health.

One might expect such a shift to lead to a major alteration in the focus of policies and activities. In fact, changes in theory and practice seem as often to occur together, or to be led by the latter. But the two *are* connected: What we think has a significant influence on what we do.

Important changes in scholarly perspective do not occur, however, in response to simple exhortation. They occur when enough people find the old perspective unsatisfactory—because of a growing awareness of its inadequate explanatory power—and discover a new one that is both more enlightening and more interesting. We believe that this shift will only occur if the diversity of scholarship on this topic can be assembled and interpreted using a common framework, so that claims from different sources and perspectives can be related to one another in a coherent way.

Some of the "anomalous findings" discussed in this book are quite new; others have been known, within certain specialist communities at least, for years or decades. We offer no radically new interpretations of particular observations. But, to the best of our knowledge, no one has previously juxtaposed observations from as wide a range of disciplines, let alone attempted to integrate and interpret them within a single coherent framework. Yet they appear all to be pieces from the same large and complex jigsaw puzzle. This book is a start at assembling that puzzle. The resulting picture, while still very incomplete, has important implications for the evolution of public and private policies within and outside the conventional spheres of health and health care. A number of these are also explored in this book.

THE EVOLUTION OF THE BOOK

Even this modest beginning is the product of an unusual collective intellectual process, which in turn has occurred within a most unusual institution. The authors are drawn from a number of different disciplines, from genetics to economics, physiology to anthropology, but they share a common interest in population health. The ideas for the chapters were developed, and drafts subsequently polished, through a series of meetings over several years. In these meetings, the authors had to confront and attempt to understand the other disciplinary perspectives of their "pit bull" colleagues, while developing their own contributions to our collective understanding. They had then to defend their interpretations in a free and frank exchange of views, in which claims of disciplinary exclusiveness had no weight. The book is, as a result, a truly collective product, which no one of us could have written. While the group was producing the book, the book was also producing the group. The common effort has served to bind the authors together in a joint enterprise with a common intellectual understanding.

The unique institution that fostered this enterprise, among many others, is the Canadian Institute for Advanced Research (CIAR). The fundamental idea of the Institute is that complex scientific and social problems, demanding tools and ways of thinking spanning several scientific or social disciplines, will be most effectively addressed by networks of individuals unrestrained by institutional or disciplinary boundaries and brought together in an "institute without walls." The CIAR supports researchers in a number of fields, ranging from cosmology and evolutionary biology to economic growth and law.

The authors of this book are members of the Institute's Program in Population Health, initiated in 1987 through a generous grant of "venture capital" from Sydney Jackson of the Manufacturers Life Insurance Company on the occasion of the company's centennial. The program is assisted by an advisory committee, which in the case of the Program in Population Health is chaired by the president and founder of the Institute, J. Fraser Mustard. The structure and contents of this book were worked out during the ongoing series of formal meetings of that Program, three to four times a year.

The research interests and activities of the members of the Program in Population Health are as diverse as one might expect, but the linking thread is their common focus on trying to understand the determinants of the health of populations. The questions raised by this concern take one from the societywide to the subcellular level and back again, from economic and social policy to molecular biology. The individual person represents the point of contact between cellular and social aggregates. Determinants of health must ultimately show their effects on particular individuals, but their origins may be well "above" or "below" the individual level—mass unemployment, say, or genetic predisposition.

Arising out of this concern for better understanding of such determinants, from which presumably to develop more effective health policies, are two major corollary interests. One is the measurement of health at the population level, and the development of extended and improved data systems, to permit us to know with more precision how our health is evolving and what factors are affecting it. The second is improved understanding of the role of the formal health care system—both its strengths and its limits—as a vehicle for mobilizing our resources to improve our health.

AIMS

But why this particular book? It has played a central role within the broader activities of our group by organizing and making more coherent emerging ideas about the determinants and measurement of health and the appropriate role of health care. Equally important, it provides a vehicle for communicating the synthesis of those ideas to a wider audience in a common "voice," which we hope will be generally accessible. The book is then our collective attempt to explain what we believe we have learned.

Two sources provided evidence of the need in the wider community for such a vehicle. First, it is clear that the understanding of the determinants of health has been changing in recent decades. A variety of claims, from a variety of disciplines, communicated in a variety of settings to different audiences, have challenged earlier perspectives. To our knowledge there has been no serious attempt since the Lalonde report of the mid-1970s to bring this literature together and attempt to make sense of it within a unifying conceptual framework. Furthermore, there were significant problems both within and arising from the "Lalonde perspective."

Second, the effectiveness of traditional medical care as a determinant of the health and well-being of populations has been coming under increasing scrutiny. A burgeoning literature documents wide and unexplained variations in patterns of medical practice that do not seem traceable to differences in the needs of patients. These observations are complemented by a corresponding literature identifying specific forms of inappropriate care in a wide range of clinical settings. Moreover, similar questions are being asked about the activities of the medical research community. Pessimistic assessments of the results from a quarter century of intense international effort in the "war against cancer," and the more recent intense efforts in AIDS research, suggest that much is learned, many researchers are kept busy, much money is spent, but the health of the afflicted populations improves little, if at all.

These two bodies of work—the first focusing on changing perceptions of health and the second emphasizing the limits both of health care interventions and of the research underlying them—remain largely independent: two intellectual solitudes. Although their policy implications seem to us to be largely complementary, no literature explicitly addresses this interdependence. One purpose of this book, is an attempt to bridge that gap.

OUTLINE AND CONTENTS

The book has four parts. The first section begins with a paper describing and briefly synthesizing some of the leading "anomalous results," traditional and more recent, that have arisen from studies of the health of a number of different populations, human and nonhuman. It focuses attention on what we believe makes these observations fundamentally anomalous—why and how they challenge the conventional ways in which we think about health and health care. This then provides an empirical motivation for a change of perspective.

This first chapter also illustrates the methodological principle encapsulated in the title of the book, the identification and exploration of systematic differences—"heterogeneities"—in the health status not just of individuals but of groups of people. Systematic differences between the average health status of people in different regions, occupations, time periods, educational levels, and social classes, for example, contain important information about the determinants of health that is often not apparent, or ignored, when one looks only at individuals. The task is to extract that information, and find ways to use it.

Chapter 2 starts by asking how, on the basis of what we know today, one would seek to produce more "health" in populations. A distinction is drawn between any particular *definition* of health, and the range of factors that might *determine* its level, whatever the definition. The chapter then sets out a model for thinking about the determinants of health and disease, which casts the question of why some people get sick and others do not within a conceptual framework around which much of the rest of the book is organized.

This framework is, we believe, both sufficiently broad to encompass the many determinants of health, and consistent with current evidence on and understanding of the ways in which those determinants are linked. Within this model, medical care is but one of many socioeconomic "institutions" (e.g., income maintenance, social security, education) that affect health.

Few now contest the view that other factors—the air we breathe, the food we eat, how we work, what we earn and how we feel about its fairness, the housing in which we live, the nurturance we receive as youngsters, and the transportation we take as adults—are powerful influences on a population's health. These are the broad determinants of how we fare, how "healthy" we are as individuals and societies. The objective of Chapter 2 is to place this "common understanding" into a more rigorous conceptual framework, showing how a narrower "medical determinist" perspective is merely a component of the wider view.

More explicit frameworks, however, also permit—demand—more rigorous testing. The second section of the book opens with a chapter developing an "accounting framework" for assembling the now largely disparate bodies of evidence with which one could test the disarmingly simple question, What is the *evidence* on the factors that determine who gets ill and who does not? As Chapter 3 illustrates, the factors that determine the health status of a population are not only multiple and complicated, but they interact with each other in ways that are much more intricate than communicated by the popular media. They have their effects over long periods of time; the link between cause and effect is neither immediate nor direct. They show up in differential susceptibility to threats of illness; and the biological and social mechanisms underlying susceptibility are far from easy to understand, let alone to subject to clear and rigorous testing.

Chapter 4 addresses another source of complexity: the influence of culture on (the interpretation of) who is ill, and who is not, and with what consequences. The concept of culture is notoriously difficult to specify clearly, but also clearly impossible to ignore. This chapter makes plain the importance of cultural context for interpreting what represents ill-health, what are its causes, and what should be done about it. The relative clarity and universality of a broken bone or an acute infection, for example, are at one end of a continuum that shades into mental illness—"depression," for example, or "schizophrenia"—or for that matter the "menopause experience" or disability resulting from back injury. The cultural community surrounding the individual—from neighbourhood to nation—influences how threats to well-being are construed, or whether they are even perceived. But it also intervenes powerfully between the determinants of health and their effects; its mediating role may be buffering and protective, or may accentuate the effects of other risk factors.

The links between genetic factors and population health are explored in Chapter 5, which reviews the major presumptions and findings of modern genetics. Again the simplistic stories are confuted; in general, there is no simple connection between genetic inheritance and health effects. The exceptions to this generalization are well-known, and from a population perspective, not (quantitatively) very important. Much more significant is the way in which the *predispositions* in an individual's genetic endowment interact with other determinants of health in the physical and social environment. Whether or not such predispositions will be given expression depends upon this much broader range of factors.

Chapter 6 continues the effort to integrate the scientific understandings and the social accounts of the determinants of health—to bridge the evidence from aggregates of individuals, to that from aggregates of molecules or cells. How is it that apparently equivalent threats to health manifest so differently in different people? When one observes marked differences in health status among different socioeconomic groups, what actually happens (or does not happen) within the human mind and body to make those in lower strata more susceptible to disease? (Simplistic stories about deprivation or unhealthy life-style "choices" are not irrelevant, but woefully incomplete.) What, in short, are the biological processes underlying the heterogeneities we see in the health of populations?

The authors review a broad range of evidence, both experimental and population based, much of it from extended studies of nonhuman primates and other animals. This evidence includes the extraordinary collection of observations and interpretations referred to as *psychoneuroimmunology,* but it now appears that this label imposes too restrictive a view of the potential pathways. The immune system may play a powerful role in linking (perceptions of) the external environment to internal biological responses, but there are other pathways as well, particularly through the endocrine and cardiovascular systems.

The findings emerging from this rapidly advancing area of biological research can be expressed very simply as, How you fare depends upon how you feel, and how you cope. But that "folk maxim" level of understanding is being dramatically deepened by the insertion of scientific underpinnings that are unambiguously important even though they are far from fully understood.

Chapter 7 focuses on a particular set of diseases, those of the cardiovascular system, in order to offer a concrete example of the determinants, interactions, and pathways portrayed in the previous chapters. The authors lay out the complex links between disease causation and disease expression. In particular, they note that a proper understanding of cardiovascular disease requires that one distinguish between "hardening of the arteries," which is a natural part of the human aging process, and the modern epidemic (now receding somewhat) of "heart attacks," in which hardened arteries become occluded, or plugged.

The authors note that the history of heart disease in this century, and the complex evolution of its relationship with social class—first a disease of the affluent, more recently one striking more heavily at people of lower income and education—clearly implicate factors more complicated than individual habits and genetic inheritances. Earlier chapters had noted the inadequacy of measures of individual risk factors to explain observed differences across populations; in this chapter the authors go into more detail on both the physiology and the epidemiology of "heart disease" to illustrate basic themes of the book as a whole. In this specific context they trace out some of the biological pathways through which the social environment can influence the cellular and subcellular world, thus raising fundamental questions about the conventional conception of "risk factors."

The third section of the book shifts its focus from biological and epidemiological questions to the social and political realm. Chapter 8 sets the historical context for contemporary debates about medical care and health policy, in two parts. It begins by describing the movement for universal sickness insurance that arose in all industrial democracies in the early decades of the twentieth century, and culminated in the period after the Second World War with the establishment of various forms of national health insurance. This movement was driven by an enthusiasm for redistributing access to medical care—and an attendant faith in its health-improving consequences—that could be shared by patients, providers, and payers alike.

This earlier consensus is in marked contrast to the concern for containing medical costs that has become widespread in the developed world since the general decline in economic growth rates in the middle 1970s. Such efforts automatically and necessarily place payers in direct opposition to providers, with the general public in an ambiguous role in the middle.

It is in this latter context that there has emerged a greatly renewed interest in "health promotion," in the sense both of alternatives to conventional medical care, and of broader conceptions of health itself. But there is an obvious and direct conflict, though rarely acknowledged, between those who see health promotion as a means of containing the conventional health care system—saving money—and those who hope to expand opportunities for offering services and "doing good"—spending money.

The authors of Chapter 9 provide a review both of the various forms of evidence currently available on the effectiveness of medical care in different settings, and of the relationship, or lack of it, between this evidence and actual patterns of care provided. Some of the stories are old; the uncertain basis for much of medical intervention has been known for many years. But the research that demonstrates this uncertainty has been growing rapidly in quality and quantity, along with the growth of interest in "evidence-based medicine" (as opposed to the other kind) among clinicians themselves. The conclusions about the extent of unexplained variation in current medical practice, and of provision of ineffective or unevaluated care, or care of questionable quality, should be sobering.

But what to do about it? Chapter 10 addresses a number of problems that bedevil efforts to regulate the scope and quality of medical practice, from outside *or* inside. It outlines the difficulties faced in different societies in attempting to reduce or at least stabilize the growth of expenditures on medical services, whether in response to a more limited view of their relative contribution to health or simply because of "diminished expectations" for economic growth generally. But there are also significant barriers to efforts to increase the effectiveness with which resources are used within health care.

Changing the behaviour of medical practitioners and organizations can be extremely difficult, not only because of inherent inertia and conservatism, but because in many cases that behaviour represents a quite reasonable response to the circumstances in which they find themselves, even though from a broader perspective it may be inappropriate or counterproductive. The authors of this chapter offer some evidence on successful and unsuccessful efforts to increase the efficiency and effectiveness of medical care, and some suggestions for the way ahead.

They also consider ways to create a more balanced understanding of, and support for, social as well as medical investments in health, not only among those responsible for public policy but also among their masters—the general public.

Both improved management of the health care system itself—a recommendation made by virtually every "official" body of enquiry in the developed world over the last ten years—and understanding of and action upon the broader range of determinants of health outside that system, require more and better data. We need to know what we are doing now, what effect it is having, how to tell whether recommended changes are in fact occurring, and whether they are leading to improvements.

Chapter 11 describes in detail the contents and organization of the type of data system a society would need in order to mount and manage a really serious and broad-ranging *health* policy. It emphasizes the mismatch between the mountains of data now generated, usually for payment purposes, on the activities of medical practices and organizations, and the minimal information available as to the outcome from all such activity. Even such limited aggregate data as are available on the health of populations, are virtually impossible to relate to the extensive and expensive array of activity putatively addressing its improvement.

Concerned with the informational requirements for judging "value for money" in health, this chapter connects the conceptual framework of the book with the statistical requirements for informed policy formulation and evaluation. It sketches out a "template" or general system for defining and organizing health data that is not bound by the peculiarities of any one national environment but is intended for international application by those concerned with problems of measurement and evaluation.

Finally, the concluding chapter provides a far-reaching and speculative essay on the alternative futures, the paths through the twenty-first century, arising from alternative evolutions and uses of our emerging understanding of the determinants of health, and the role and effects of medicine. The picture is not in general an optimistic one, at least if the future is expected to be a simple extrapolation of present trends in health and health care policy. We would be very naive indeed to imagine that the steady expansion of biomedical knowledge and technological capability will lead to a general improvement in well-being, regardless of how our social and political structures may evolve.

Some of the futures look quite bleak: When H. G. Wells described the history of civilizations as a "race between education and disaster," he did not suggest that the race was fixed in our favour.

HOPES

We have in mind two primary audiences for this book. One is students of health and health care, broadly understood. But it may also be of interest to the generally informed citizen who is bombarded daily with nostrums for health improvement, apocalyptic visions of threats to personal and planetary health, and insistent calls for more expenditure, from whatever source, on medical care. Our hope is that this book demonstrates the importance (and the complexity) of the other factors that influence the health of populations, while offering a more balanced perspective on the potential, and limitations, of biomedical science and its clinical applications. A more balanced perspective, if widely shared, may support the development of a more balanced mix of social policy.

At the moment, we believe, there is a considerable degree of confusion about the importance of different determinants of health, and the relationship among them. Much of the confusion arises from the peddling of simple conceptualizations of complex phenomena. Improved diet, more exercise, less stress, better medical care, genetic engineering—each offers a simple remedy with a catchy label that may be easily understood. The problem is that when offered as explanations of why some people are healthy and others not, they are simplistic and incomplete.

ACKNOWLEDGMENTS

The members of the Program in Population Health have incurred a substantial number of debts in the course of producing this volume. Following the usual practice of authors, we acknowledge but are unlikely to repay them.

Sydney Jackson and Manufacturers Life played the critical catalytic role, investing in the risky venture of funding the collaboration among a group of intellectuals to work in a field—population health—that was not yet defined. We hope he will find this book a worthy part of the return on that investment. Fraser Mustard had a vision of the field long before our group was brought into existence; his role as president of the CIAR, chairman of our advisory committee, and intellectual collaborator, sounding board, and goad is reflected in virtually every stage of this project. Other members of the advisory committee have also taken a close interest in this project. They have been consistently supportive and encouraging, though that support and encouragement has from time to time taken the form of a free and frank exchange of views.

Our thinking has also been powerfully extended and enhanced by a number of scholars who have taken the time to come to our meetings, and discuss their work with us in a free-for-all setting quite unlike the usual academic seminar.

One of the principal benefits of membership in the CIAR programs is the opportunity to examine, at close quarters, really first-class work in disciplines other than one's own. The people who have generously shared their time and work with us will find their influence throughout the volume, usually but probably not always acknowledged, and we hope that they feel their efforts were worthwhile. While we hesitate to list them all, for fear that we will not, we wish to acknowledge the help of John Bienenstock, Max Cynader, Ellen Hall, James House, Naoki Ikegami, Jeffrey Johnson, Paul Lamarche, Ron Lévy, Margaret Lock, Dan Offord, Gérard de Pouvourville, Paul Sabatier, Robert Sapolsky, Steven Suomi, and Len Syme.

We have also received a great deal of support, intellectual as well as financial, from members of the various governments of Canada who are concerned with health and health care policy. Both at the political and at the civil service level, people have shown a lively interest in our activities and have been very open in discussing their perceptions and concerns with us. Members of the program have had particularly helpful continuing contacts with people in the governments of British Columbia, Manitoba, Ontario, and Quebec, and in the federal Department of Health.

But meetings, manuscripts, and money do not emerge out of thin air, or the good intentions of academics. A number of people have been involved in carrying out the actual organization of meetings, the handling the finances, and helping to keep track of the massive flow of paper that accompanies a project of this complexity. Staff at the central office in Toronto have carried a good part of the load, but we have been assisted by a number of people at each of our "nodes" and meeting sites—in Vancouver, Winnipeg, Hamilton, Toronto, Montreal, and New Haven.

Finally we are grateful to our editor and publisher, Richard Koffler. He helped to carry the project forward with his confidence and enthusiastic support, and resisted the impulse to alter our language substantially. For that, and for his cooperation throughout the production process, he deserves our thanks.

Being indebted to so many for so many things makes it tempting to share blame for errors or omissions widely and generously. But we will resist that temptation: those are ours.

The Editors

I

I

1

Introduction

R. G. EVANS

The prudent text-books give it
  In tables at the end—
The stress that shears a rivet
  Or makes a tie-bar bend—
What traffic wrecks macadam—
  What concrete should endure—
But we, poor Sons of Adam,
  Have no such literature,
    To warn us or make sure!

—Kipling, *Hymn of Breaking Strain*

Top people live longer. Moreover, they are generally healthier while doing so. This is not exactly news. Many studies, in many countries, over many years, have shown a correlation between life expectancy and various measures of social status—income, education, occupation, residence (Wilkinson, 1992). Studies of the living, while fewer because decent health information is so scarce (see Chapter 11), show that health status is also correlated with social status. And such studies confirm what most people knew anyway—poverty is bad for you. As Sophie Tucker said, "I've been poor, and I've been rich. Rich is better."

Yet this commonplace observation, when examined in detail, raises complex and important questions about the determinants of health, for individuals and populations.[1] Or in short, Why? Moreover, the correlation between social status and health is only one leading example of a much larger class of observations, of large differences in health status not just among individuals, but among well-defined groups: populations and subpopulations, both human and animal. Such aggregate observations, the "heterogeneities" discussed in Chapter 3, lead naturally to attempts to identify the group characteristics associated with good and bad health, in the hope of finding and then influencing the underlying causal factors.

At quite an early stage in any such analysis, it becomes apparent that many of the conventional explanations of the determinants of health—of why some people are healthy and others not—are at best seriously incomplete if not simply wrong. This is unfortunate, because modern societies devote a very large share of their wealth, effort, and attention to trying to maintain or improve the health of the individuals that make up their populations. These massive efforts are primarily channeled through health care systems, presumably reflecting a belief that the receipt of appropriate health care is the most important determinant of health.

But if this is not so, if the principal determinants of the health of populations lie elsewhere, then we may well have left undone those things that we ought to have done, and have done those things that we ought not to have done. And there will in consequence be less health in us than there could be. We may also, as a result, be less wealthy.

Nor is this situation likely to be improved by efforts to expand "preventive" activities, if these are also based on shaky assumptions about the determinants of health. The hypotheses about causality that underlie arguments for prevention are often no more able to explain differences in health status between different groups of people than are those which attribute all or most differences to the availability of "curative" services.

There is, of course, still a very real and important role for medical and other health care services in preserving life, relieving suffering, and maintaining or restoring function. It is difficult to understand the faintly sneering tone with which health care systems are sometimes dismissed as "illness care systems." Is caring for illness, usually effectively, something to be ashamed of? Health care services, and the people and institutions that provide them, have earned the high regard in which they are generally held, even though as shown in Chapter 9 the expectations of both providers and users are often greater than can be justified on the available evidence. But while they may be decisive in individual cases, the availability of such services—or their lack—cannot begin to explain observed differences among the health of populations. Nor is this any surprise to thoughtful clinicians, past or present.

In this chapter we introduce and link together a selection of studies that either report or bear upon various aspects of the relationship between status and health. This linkage permits us to extract and focus upon a series of propositions that, taken together, constitute at least the beginnings of a much more complex and comprehensive, yet coherent, understanding of the determinants of health. They are intended to provide a thread through what is now a vast labyrinth of particular findings. The subsequent chapters explore the underpinnings and implications of this synthesis. In the process we consider how a true *health* policy based on an understanding of the relative importance of the various determinants of health might differ from the *health care* policies that predominate today.

We start our story with the work of Marmot [1986; Marmot, Kogevinas, and Elston, 1987 (see especially pp. 126–28)]. His Whitehall Study has followed more than ten thousand British civil servants for nearly two decades, accumulating an extensive array of information on each of the individuals in the study. The data set is thus person specific and longitudinal, offering important advantages over the many studies of status and health based only on group average data, at a single point in time. Moreover, it is readily and unambiguously divisible into status groupings; the hierarchy of income and rank in the civil service is well defined.

Marmot found that the (age-standardized) mortality, over a ten-year period, among males aged forty to sixty-four was about *three and a half times* as high for those in the clerical and manual grades, as in the senior administrative grades (Marmot and Theorell, 1988). The correlation between status and health is alive and well in Whitehall. But that is only the beginning of the story.

There was an obvious *gradient* in mortality from top to bottom of the hierarchy. Mortality was significantly higher in the second rank, professional and executive personnel, than in the top, administrative, grades, and increased further as one went down the scale (see Figure 1.1). But in none of these groups are people impoverished or deprived (at least according to the common understanding of those concepts). All are employed, most in office jobs with low risk from the physical environment (or at least at no greater risk than those in the classes above them), and the professional and executive grades are relatively well paid compared with the general population.

Thus a common interpretation of the correlation between socioeconomic status and health—that "the poor" are deprived of some of the material conditions of good health, and suffer from poor diet, bad housing, exposure to violence, environmental pollutants, crowding, and infection—cannot explain these observations. Indeed a focus on poverty can block progress in understanding, because it can be dismissive of further questions.

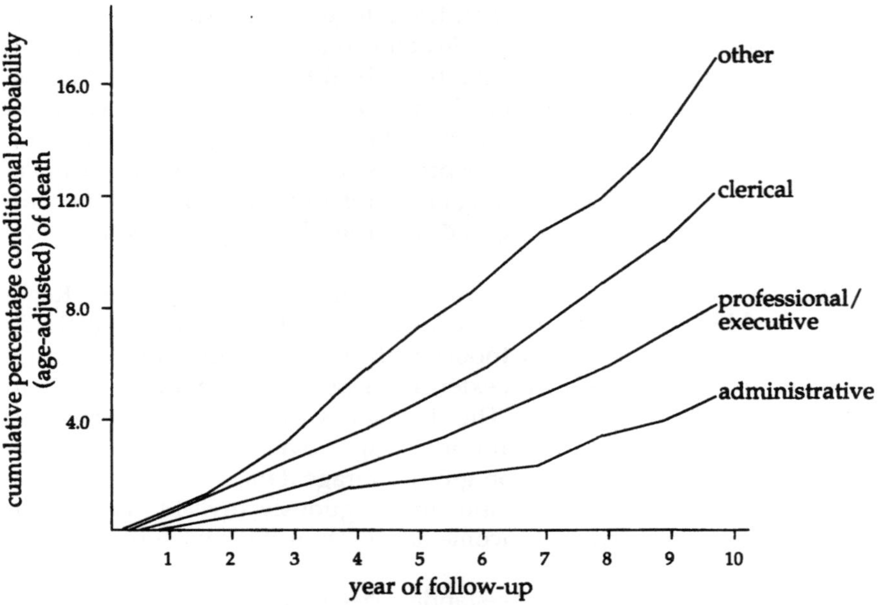

Figure 1.1. Whitehall study: all-cause mortality among total population by year of follow-up.
Source: Marmot (1986:23)

For some (on the right), "the poor ye have always with ye." One can never remove social differentiation; some people are just better than others, and some will always be at the bottom. Health differentials are thus inevitable (and probably deserved). "What can't be cured, must be endured." Fortunately most of us have the intestinal fortitude to bear with good grace the sufferings of someone else. For others (on the left), health differentials are markers for social inequality and injustice more generally, and are further evidence of the need to redistribute wealth and power, and restructure or overturn the existing social order.

Both preconceptions miss the main point of Marmot's findings, that there is *something* that powerfully influences health and that is correlated with hierarchy per se. It operates, not on some underprivileged minority of "them" over on the margin of society, to be spurned or cherished depending upon one's ideological affiliation, but on all of us. And its effects are *large*.

There is more. A gradient in mortality was found in each of a number of different diseases or causes of death (but not all).[2] Some were clearly correlated with smoking behaviour: Top people rarely smoke; bottom

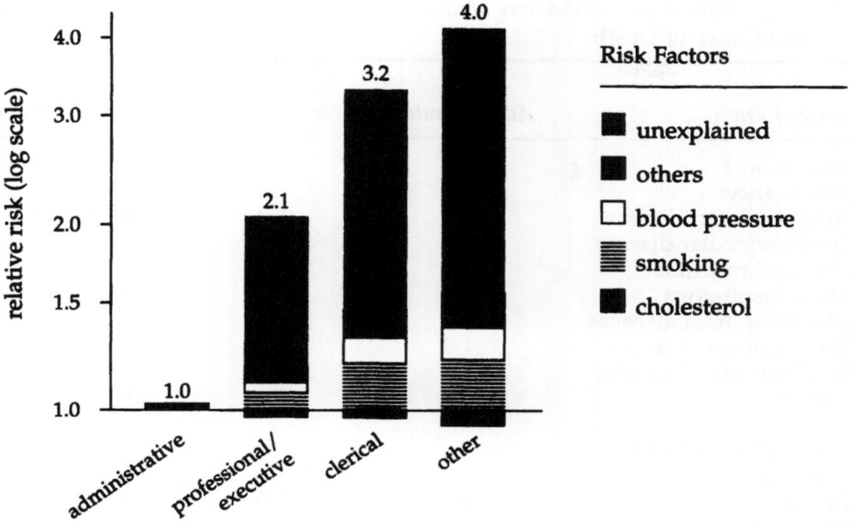

Figure 1.2. Relative risk of CHD death in different grades "explained" by risk factors (age-standardized).
Source: Marmot et al. (1978:248)

people often do. (That in itself is a very systematic pattern with major health implications. It cries out for explanation, rather than trivialization as "personal choice.") But a gradient was also observed in other causes of death that have no known relation to smoking (see Figure 1.2 and Tables 1.1 and 1.2). Moreover those few top people who *did* smoke were much less likely to die from smoking-related causes.

Nor is smoking behaviour the only "individual" risk factor that failed to explain the gradient.[3] On average, people in the lower grades were at greater risk for heart disease, because they had higher levels on the established triad of smoking, blood pressures, and cholesterol. But differences in mortality from heart disease persisted after adjustment for all these factors.

These observations suggest some underlying general causal process, correlated with hierarchy, which *expresses* itself through different diseases. But the particular diseases that carry people off may then simply be alternative pathways or mechanisms rather than "causes" of illness and death; the essential factor is something else.[4]

These two ideas—the gradient in mortality, and the disease as pathway rather than cause—are also suggested by a number of other studies of differential mortality by socioeconomic class (see Chapter 3). The British data (Table 1.3) on mortality rates by social class reviewed in the

Table 1.1. Age-Adjusted Relative Mortality[a] in Ten Years by Civil Service Grade and Cause of Death

Cause of death	*Administrators*	*Professional & executive*	*Clerk*	*Other*
Lung cancer	0.5	1.0	2.2	3.6
Other cancer	0.8	1.0	1.4	1.4
Coronary heart disease	0.5	1.0	1.4	1.7
Cerebrovascular disease	0.3	1.0	1.4	1.2
Chronic bronchitis	0.0	1.0	6.0	7.3
Other respiratory	1.1	1.0	2.6	3.1
Gastrointestinal diseases	0.0	1.0	1.6	2.8
Genitourinary diseases	1.3	1.0	0.7	3.1
Accidents and homicide	0.0	1.0	1.4	1.5
Suicide	0.7	1.0	1.0	1.9
Nonsmoking related causes				
Cancer	0.8	1.0	1.3	1.4
Noncancer	0.6	1.0	1.5	2.0
All causes	0.6	1.0	1.6	2.1

Source: Marmot (1986:25).
[a]Calculated from logistic equation adjusting for age.

Table 1.2. Age-Adjusted Mortality in Ten Years (and Number of Deaths from Coronary Heart Disease and Lung Cancer) by Grade and Smoking Status

Cause of death	*Administrators*	*Professional & executive*	*Clerk*	*Other*	*Total*
Nonsmokers					
CHD	1.40	2.36	2.08	6.89	2.59
Lung cancer	0.0	0.24	0.0	0.25	0.21
Ex-smokers					
CHD	1.29	3.06	3.32	3.98	3.09
Lung cancer	0.21	0.50	0.56	1.05	0.62
Current smokers					
CHD	2.16	3.58	4.92	6.62	4.00
Lung cancer	0.35	0.73	1.49	2.33	2.00

Source: Marmot (1986:26).

Table 1.3. Mortality by Social Class 1911–1981 (Men, 15–64 Years, England and Wales)[a]

Year	professional I	managerial II	skilled manual and non-manual III	semi-skilled IV	unskilled V
1911	88	94	96	93	142
1921	82	94	95	101	125
1931	90	94	97	102	111
1951	86	92	101	104	118
1961[b]	76 (75)	81	100	103	143 (127)
1971[b]	77 (75)	81	104	114	137 (121)
1981[c]	66	76	103	116	166

Source: Marmot (1986:2) and OPCS (1978:174).
[a]Figures are SMRs, which express age-adjusted mortality rates as a percentage of the national average at each date.
[b]To facilitate comparisons, figures shown in parentheses have been adjusted to the classification of occupations used in 1951.
[c]Men, 20–64 years, Great Britian.

Black report (Office of Population Censuses and Surveys, OPCS, 1972; Black, Morris, Smith, Townsend, and Whitehead, 1988; Wilkinson, 1986) are of particular interest, because they are available decade by decade over most of the twentieth century. They too show a gradient, but most interestingly they show it persisting, with not much change, over most of the period since the first data were collected in 1911, and apparently increasing in recent years.

Yet during that period the causes of death have changed radically. At the beginning of the century infectious diseases were the great killers, and (age-standardized) mortality rates were higher in the lower classes. At the end of the century heart disease and cancer are the killers; and they too hit harder the people lower in the social hierarchy. While death is ultimately quite democratic, deferral appears to be a privilege correlated with rank. The diseases change, the gradient persists, again suggesting (from a completely different data set) an underlying factor, correlated with hierarchy and expressing itself through particular diseases.

There has been another major change in the last fifty years. All developed societies have greatly expanded their health care systems, and (with the exception of the United States) have introduced systems of financing designed to make that care accessible to the whole population, regardless of ability to pay. And the use of health care has correspondingly increased dramatically, and become more equal across social classes. Yet the longitudinal data from the United Kingdom show no evidence that the introduction of the National Health Service has reduced the mortality gradient. There *is* some evidence in some countries of a reduction in the gradient in, as well as the rate of, infant mortality in response to more, and more generally accessible, health care, but it is far from conclusive (Wilkins, Adams, and Brancker, 1990). Whatever underlies the gradient does not seem to be very sensitive to the provision of health care.

This observation links the data on social class gradients with the well-known work of McKeown (1979) in historical epidemiology. He showed that the very large reductions in mortality from the principal infectious diseases, which have occurred over the last two centuries, took place prior to the development of any effective medical therapy. His data on tuberculosis are of particular importance (Figures 1.3A and 1.3B).

A common response is that public health measures, rather than medical therapy, were decisive. But the TB bacillus is not waterborne, so the decline cannot be attributed to clean water supplies—at least not directly. It may be that greater general cleanliness, made possible by clean water and sewage removal, played a role.

In particular, as Szreter (1988) points out, tuberculosis mortality could have fallen because people were less weakened by other infections whose incidence *was* reduced by public health measures, if not by medical care per se. He emphasizes that McKeown's own "explanation" for the TB decline—rising incomes and improved diet, with no significant

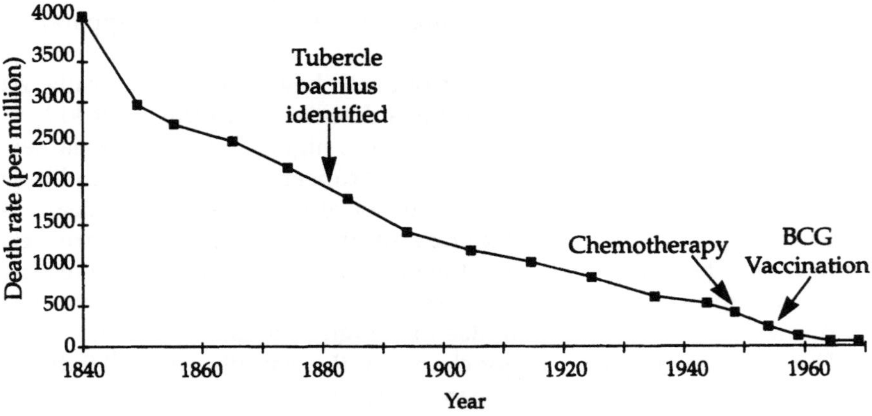

Figure 1.3A. Respiratory tuberculosis: mean annual death rates (standardized to 1901 population), England and Wales, 1840–1970.
Source: McKeown (1979)

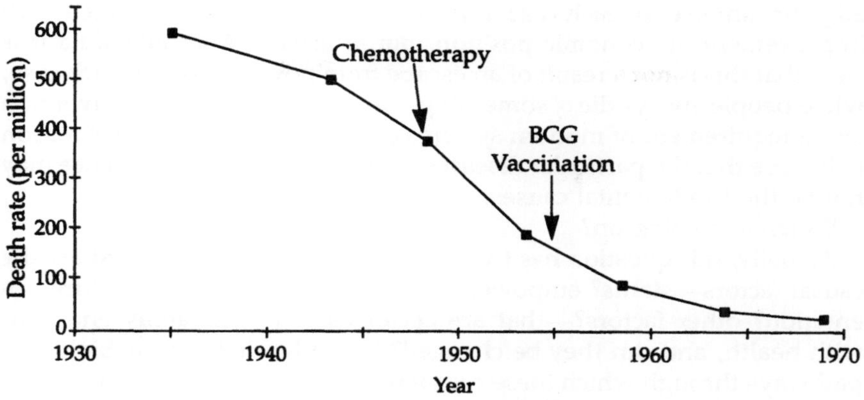

Figure 1.3B. Respiratory tuberculosis: mean annual death rates (standardized to 1901 population), England and Wales, 1935–1970.
Source: McKeown (1979)

influence from public health or other deliberate human agency—was at best a "diagnosis of exclusion," which appears to be unsustainable in the light of more recent evidence.

In any case, even as late as the 1940s most adults in the United Kingdom still showed evidence of having been exposed to the bacillus at some time. Unlike their ancestors, few of them developed the disease, and fewer died. One is still left with the interesting question of why people who were exposed to the "cause" of TB—the bacillus—in one century developed the disease, and in the next did not. And McKeown's central point—that the major decline in mortality from most infectious diseases predates effective therapy—remains unchallenged.

The tuberculosis data illustrate another important point, however, which is somewhat obscured in the long-term historical picture. The development of effective therapy in the 1940s *was*, in fact, a significant factor in the further reduction in mortality. The decline at that point was about 50 percent in a decade, a very large proportionate fall, so there is no argument here for therapeutic nihilism. But these gains are swamped, in the historical record, by the much larger impact of something else operating outside the health care system. The role of medicine was very real, but limited. While it accelerated the speed of decline, it was not the initiating force.

Thus McKeown observed very large changes in mortality in a society over time, and Marmot and the authors of the Black report found very large differences among social groups at particular points or over shorter periods in time, in each case apparently independent of medical knowledge or care use. In each case improvement in health is associated with improvement in economic position, but at least in Marmot's data it is clear that this is not a result of an escape from poverty. And in each case, while people always die *of* something—this is both a cultural convention and a requirement of modern systems of vital statistics—there is reason to believe that the particular diseases recognized by medical science may not be the fundamental causes.

So what is going on?

Actually, this question has two quite distinct parts. First, what are the causal factors—status? empowerment? stress? coping skills? future orientation? other factors?—that are correlated with hierarchy and thus with health, and can they be changed? Second, what are the biological pathways through which these causal factors operate? We do not believe in spooks and the supernatural; disease and death are biological phenomena. Whatever factors lie upstream in the sequence of causes, at some point in the chain there must be biological processes at work.[5]

Possible answers to these questions are only beginning to emerge, with pieces of the puzzle being supplied, in a relatively uncoordinated fashion, from the research of a number of different disciplines. The incomplete, tentative, and sometimes controversial nature of the answers to What is going on? must not, however, be permitted to obscure the fact that *something* is going on. While death rates are admittedly incomplete measures of health, they are unambiguous and "hard-edged" measures of difference. And a three-to-one difference, emerging from large numbers of individual observations, deserves attention. The lack of an adequate explanation for the phenomenon in no way negates the reality or the importance of the phenomenon itself.

Taking the second (biological) question first, some remarkable results are now coming from animal studies, both experimental and observational. Social hierarchies are not peculiar to humans. Other primates have them as well, both in their natural state and in experimental colonies.

Sapolsky (1990) has been observing the social relationships among free-ranging olive baboons in Kenya, taking physiological measurements in a way that would probably be unacceptably intrusive for most human subjects. He finds that a dominance hierarchy is readily identifiable among male baboons, and that there are, on average, significant differences between dominant and subordinate males in the functioning of their endocrine systems. In dominant males, the physiological responses to stress—the "fight or flight syndrome"—are turned off more rapidly after the stressful event has passed. In subordinate animals, there seems to be a break in the feedback loop, and the stress response continues. Top baboons thus cope with stress better than their subordinates, who seem to be in a continuous state of low-level readiness or anxiety. (Interestingly, there is a very similar break in the cortisol feedback loop for humans suffering from some forms of depression—see Chapter 6.)

Prolonged stress, or rather the responses it engenders, are known to have deleterious effects on a number of biological systems and to give rise to a number of illnesses. Could this be happening in other primate populations, such as free-ranging British civil servants? Interestingly, Marmot has found that, on average, all ranks in his study have similarly elevated blood pressure when at work (see Figure 1.4). But the blood pressure of senior administrators drops much more when they go home. They seem to be better able to turn off the stress response. There also appear to be systematic differences in the levels of fibrinogen circulating in the blood, which may be a marker for other differences in stress response.[6]

Another study of primate social hierarchies, among female macaques in an experimental setting, was primarily focused on the animals' responses to high-cholesterol diets. The intent was to induce heart disease, and this indeed occurred. But a striking finding was that the degree of stenosis of the coronary arteries was nearly *four times* as severe among the low-status as among the high-status monkeys. The possible physiological pathways to this outcome are discussed in Chapter 7; in

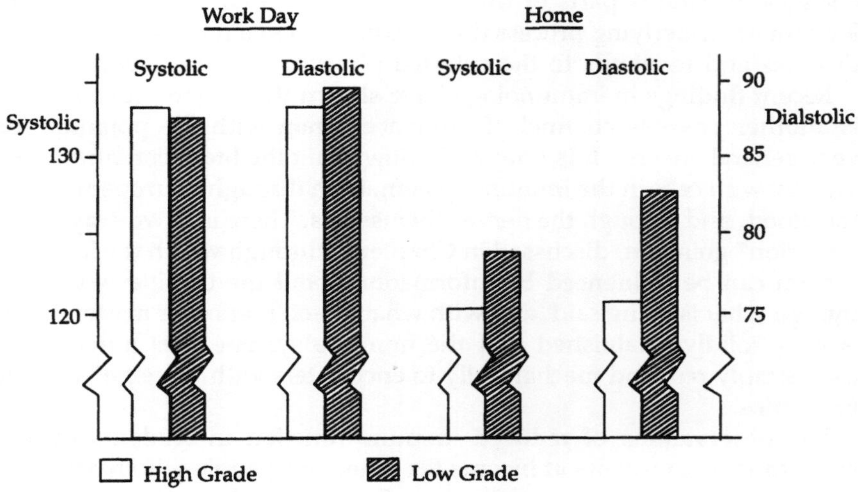

Figure 1.4. Blood pressure in British civil servants.
Source: Marmot and Theorell (1988:671)

general terms, prolonged stress can lead to injury to the arterial walls, and this in turn to clotting, atherosclerosis, and stenosis—coronary heart disease (CHD). CHD, of course, is the leading killer of human primates.

The external social environment, as interpreted by the various receptors of the nervous system, the senses, induces a generalized response by the endocrine system. This stress response, which we commonly experience as a burst of adrenalin, can if inappropriately prolonged result in a variety of forms of physiological damage, including heart disease. Still other animal experiments, with a variety of different subjects, have demonstrated that experimentally generated, prolonged, and unavoidable stress can lead to a variety of illnesses, and eventually death (Dantzer and Kelley, 1989).

But the stress response need not be inappropriate. The low-status baboons and macaques may have good reasons for continued anxiety—as may the low-ranking civil servants. You never know when some higher-ranking animal is going to turn up and drive you away from a meal or a female, or make some other threat to your sense of well-being. The "learned helplessness" that is experimentally induced in animals may also be a response by low-status humans or other free-ranging primates to a rather unsatisfactory social environment, and may be the behavioural counterpart to biological processes.

The endocrine system has the characteristics that it is strongly responsive to the nervous system, and induces a wide range of physiological changes in various parts of the organism. It is thus a natural place to look for an underlying process that is expressed in a number of different diseases and responds to the external physical or social environment.

Recent findings in immunology have shown that the immune system is another possible channel of influence, again with the potential for very general effects.[7] It is now well known that the brain communicates directly with cells in the immune system, both through neuropeptides in the blood, and through the nerves themselves. There is a two-way "conversation" going on, discussed in Chapter 6, through which the immune system can be influenced by information about the outside world, although what is being said, and with what effect, is another matter. But it is now solidly established that the immune system does much more than simply respond mechanically to encounters with "foreign" cells or molecules.

The observations of reduced immune function in students during exam time, accountants at income tax time, and people who have lost a spouse now begin to fit into the story. Studies of other primate populations once again provide support; they too have complex social structures, and respond to loss of a "social object" (a technical term for one's mate?) with a depression of immune function. (The response may include other generalized unhealthy "behaviours"—see Chapter 2.) If immune status is compromised by stressful events, then this may be an alternative pathway through which social status can have generalized health effects.[8]

So the biological pathways appear to be there, although there are still many careers to be made, and Nobel prizes to be won, in elucidating them in detail. But this brings us back to the prior question: What is it about hierarchies, or social structures more generally, that triggers the biological responses, and can anything be done about it? Our discussion has suggested that rank correlates inversely with stress, or with ability to cope with stress.

A common reaction, particularly among those who are themselves near the top of the social hierarchy, is that such a relationship is inevitable, inherent in either genetic endowment or human social structure. Fitter people rise to the top, and are also healthier—genetic selection. Alternatively human societies must have hierarchies—that's just how primates are—and the health effects follow. (The inevitability of both hierarchy and its rewards is usually more clearly visible from the top.) But is this reaction justified? As for most really interesting questions, the correct answer seems to be, yes and no.

On the "no" side, there is ample, indeed striking, evidence for the malleability of population health status, over time spans far too short for any change in genetic endowment. Studies of migrant populations demonstrate that as they take on the social patterns and customs of the host country, they take on its disease patterns as well. These changes can be very large indeed, over one or two generations (Doll and Peto, 1981). The classic study (Chapter 7) of Japanese in the home islands, in Hawaii, and in California shows very clearly the effects of successive migrations to social environments that pose greater risks of heart disease (Marmot, et al., 1975; Marmot and Syme, 1976).

Indeed the Japanese in Japan itself have in the last thirty years demonstrated that the health status of an entire population can change very rapidly, and that the current experience of Western countries does not represent an upper bound on the possible. Since 1960, Japanese mortality statistics (male and female life expectancy, infant mortality) have improved from markedly below most European countries to markedly above, and the trend may be continuing (see Figures 1.5A and 1.5B). The dramatic improvements of the 19th century, which were analysed in detail by McKeown, are not matters of historical interest only.

Also paralleling the tuberculosis story, the extraordinary increase in Japanese life expectancy does not appear to follow from better medical care (Marmor, 1992). All countries were greatly expanding their health

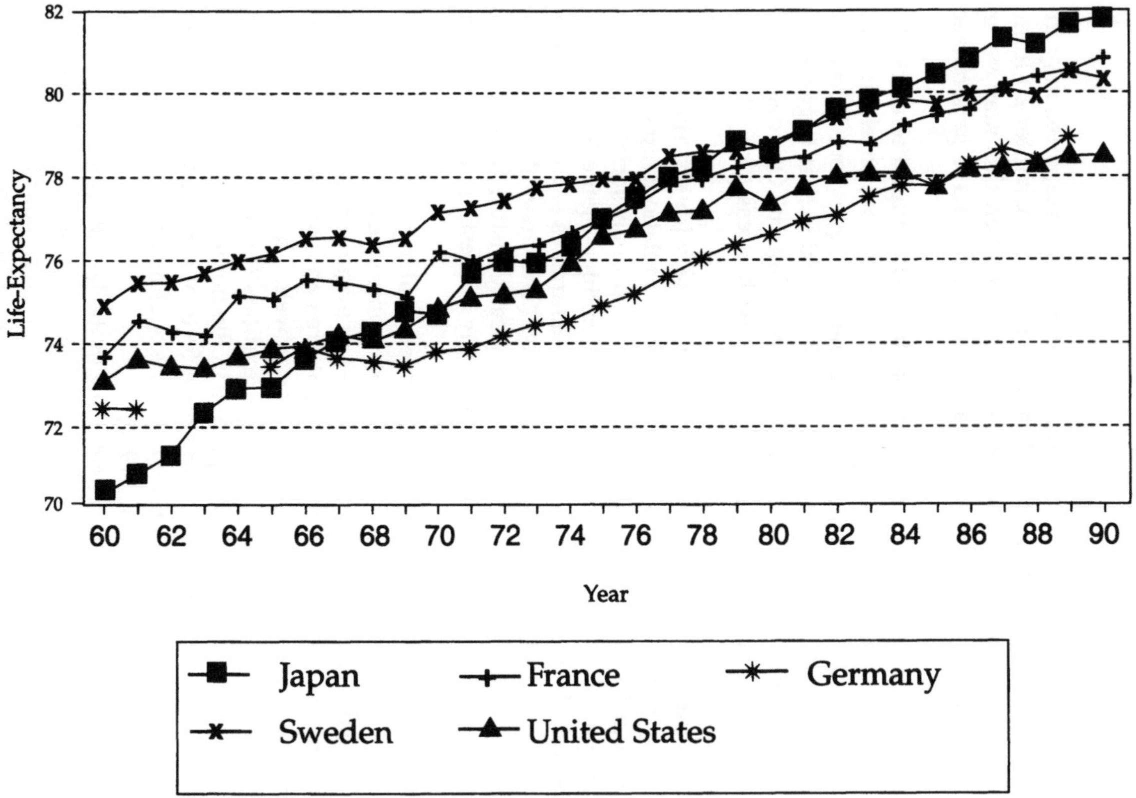

Figure 1.5A. Trends in female life expectancy. Selected OECD countries, 1960–1990.
Source: Schieber et al. (1992)

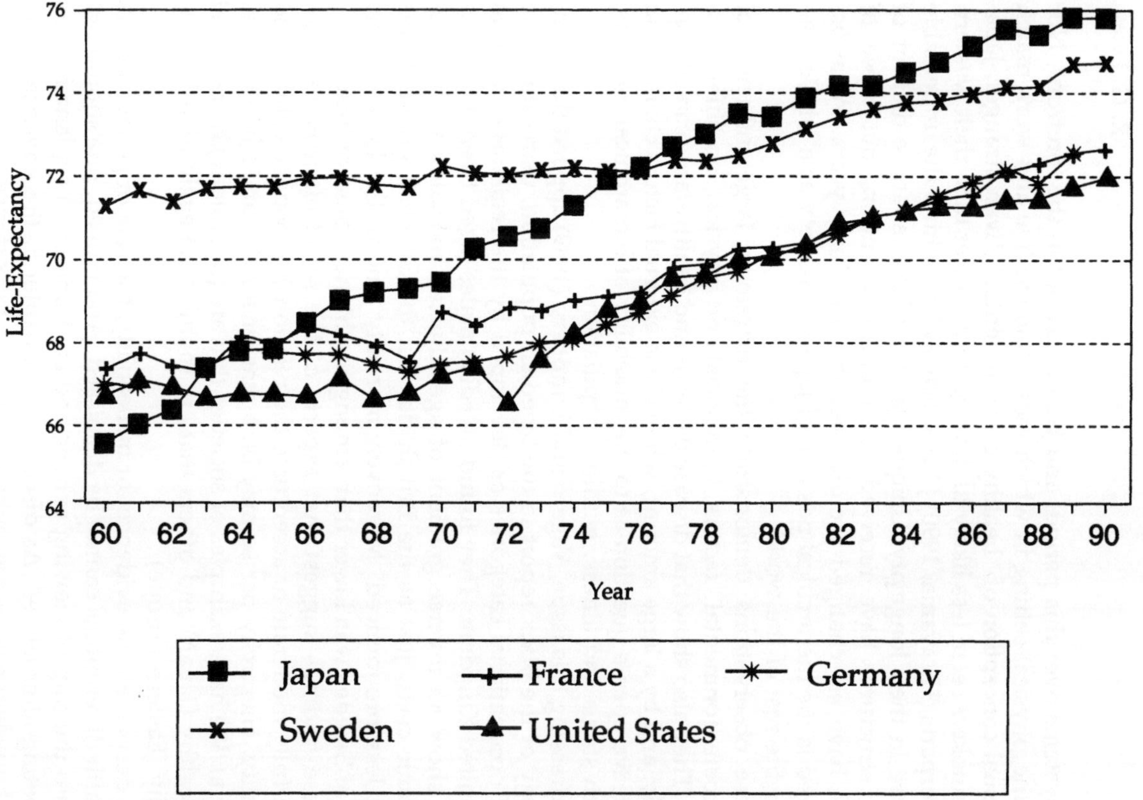

Figure 1.5B. Trends in male life expectancy. Selected OECD countries, 1960–1990.
Source: Schieber et al. (1992)

care systems over this period, and Japan was not in the forefront. Nor does the physical setting in which most Japanese live and work match our usual conception of "healthy environments." [Even stranger, Japanese smokers seem less likely to develop lung cancer than their western counterparts (Hirayama, 1990).] Yet *something* lies behind the undeniable increase in their longevity. Unique features of the Japanese diet, or of social structure, have received considerable attention, but these of course have *not* changed rapidly over the last thirty years. What *has* changed is the hierarchical position of Japanese society as a whole relative to the rest of the world.

These observations demonstrate the extremely large influence of "macroenvironmental" factors, both social and physical, on illness patterns. They also show that disease patterns and health status can change rapidly, and by a large amount, when these external factors change. But they leave open a question as to the mutability of hierarchical patterns, of both status and illness, within a population.

Addressing this issue, Vagero and Lundberg (1989) applied the methodology of the Black report to the Swedish population, using the same set of occupational categories as developed by the registrar-general in the United Kingdom. They found Swedish males (aged twenty to sixty-four) show an inverse gradient of age-adjusted mortality with socioeconomic class, just as the British do. But the Swedish gradient was much less pronounced. Moreover, mortality among the lowest social class of Swedes was lower than among the highest class of Britons.

These findings suggest that aspects of the social environment can powerfully moderate or accentuate the relationship between status and mortality. Hierarchy per se may be a marker for the underlying causal factor(s): We have examples of societies that are (nominally) hierarchical but healthy (Japan) and others that are (nominally) egalitarian but unhealthy (Eastern Europe).

Yet despite all the evidence for malleability, the role of genetic factors in health differentials cannot be dismissed. And indeed, one should not fall into the trap of viewing genetic and environmental explanations as competing alternatives. As discussed in Chapter 5, the advance of genetic knowledge is increasingly revealing the importance of genetic predispositions, based on clusters or networks of interacting genes, whose expression depends in a complex way on the environment experienced by the individual. The genetic endowment may be fixed at birth, but its effects generally are not.

Moreover the expression of genetic predispositions depends on environmental influences over the *history* of the individual. As discussed in Chapter 3, previous environments and particularly those in early childhood (and before birth) can play a very important role in determining the subsequent status of the individual, both health and socioeconomic. But their influences will depend in part on their interaction with the genetic endowment.

Looking again at the animal studies, Sapolsky found that the superior physiological functioning of the dominant males in his study population —their ability to turn off the fight-or-flight syndrome more quickly and completely—was impaired when the dominance hierarchy was disrupted. When status was uncertain, all the animals began to show the continuing anxiety and low-level stress response characteristic of subordinates. This indicates the importance of contemporaneous circumstances, rather than that some are "born to rule." It is supported by other animal studies showing that deliberate manipulations of a hierarchy—removing and inserting dominant animals—have measurable and reversible physiological effects. Physiological function follows status, not the other way around.

On the other hand, Sapolsky also found that only a subset of the observably dominant animals showed the more effective endocrine response. Others were physiologically more similar to subordinates. The "true" dominants shared a cluster of personality traits that did appear to be inherited.

The relationship between personality and reaction to stress has been explored in considerable depth by Suomi (1991) working with rhesus monkeys in both experimental and free-ranging environments. He has identified about 20 percent of his primate population as having "highly reactive" personalities, and has shown that this behaviour pattern is inherited. These animals show extreme reactions, both behavioural and physiological, to stress. Interestingly, while their behavioural reactions differ at different stages in the life cycle, the underlying physiological reactions are the same.[9]

Suomi's findings clearly establish a genetic basis for differential responses to stress, with extreme reactions being associated with symptoms similar to clinical depression in humans. On the other hand, he also found that the adverse health and social consequences of the reactive personality could be mitigated or avoided if the animals were reared by a particularly nurturing mother (not necessarily biological). An exceptionally supportive early environment could offset the effects of a genetic predisposition.

These findings recall those of the cohort study, still underway, of all of the children born on the island of Kauai in 1955. The Kauai Longitudinal Study (Werner and Smith, 1982; Werner, 1989) has focused on the long-term consequences of prenatal and perinatal stress, and the effects of adverse early rearing conditions, on various aspects of child development. One of the findings has been that children who suffer moderate or severe perinatal stress, but are subsequently reared in "good" environments (as measured by family stability or high socioeconomic status), suffer little or no disadvantage in development at twenty months.[10] Children with no perinatal stress likewise showed little disadvantage despite poor, unstable households. But two negative factors together had quite severe consequences for child development.

Other recent studies have shown that very early intervention programs can compensate for a deprived rearing environment. Educational day care (starting between six and twelve weeks of age) has been found to be protective for children at high risk for intellectual impairment, especially those with mentally retarded mothers (Martin, Ramey, and Ramey, 1990; see also Chapter 3). And both nutritional supplementation and psychological stimulation were found by Grantham-McGregor, Powell, Walker, and Himes (1991) to have significant and independent beneficial effects on the mental development of growth-retarded children.

Thus an initial disadvantage, whether reactive personality (Suomi) or perinatal stress (Werner), can be buffered by a sufficiently supportive early environment. At the same time, an inadequate early environment can be remedied by specific interventions. Genetic and congenital factors are not unimportant, but the expression or nonexpression of their effects depends on the social environment. This offers a possible reconciliation of the old "nature/nurture" debate. Even if genetic or congenital problems were equally distributed across the population, their expression would still depend to some extent upon buffering factors whose availability and strength in turn is correlated with socioeconomic position.

In reality, of course, such "initial" problems or predispositions are not equally distributed across social groups. Birth outcomes depend on the condition and behaviour of the mother, and possibly the father as well, and these are affected by social factors. Most obvious is the social class gradient in maternal smoking; still more extreme and tragic are the children of crack addicts. What is "nature" for the individual is influenced by the social environment of the parent—again no [one] is an island.

How such buffering factors might work, and have their long-term effects, is unclear. One thinks naturally in terms of "learned" responses, of people consciously or unconsciously adopting styles of behaviour and ways of responding to their environments. But one must be careful not to allow the use of words like learning to lead us to confuse this process with learning the multiplication table. Who (or what) learns and what does he, she, or it learn?

For example, it has been shown that *immune systems* can "learn," and not just in the obvious sense of learning to recognize and attack foreign material. The immune systems of mice can be classically conditioned, by feeding them saccharin and cyclophosphamide (an immunosuppressive drug), such that when they are later fed saccharin-flavoured water *alone*, their immune systems do not respond to challenge. Some part of the nervous system of the mouse receives the taste sensation . . . and something happens. Is this true of men as well as mice? Can various forms of experience condition the human immune system (or the endocrine system)—perhaps quite independently of consciousness? If so, then this might provide a pathway for very long term effects of experience on health, through a wide array of different diseases.

An analogy from engineering may be helpful in pulling these threads together. Suppose we think of people becoming ill, or injured, or dying, as similar to the failure, in whole or in part, of a material or structure. That failure is in response to some external force—some stress—acting either all at once, or over a long period of time, or both. The individual, like the material or the structure, responds to an external force by becoming strained, deformed to some degree. But how much it is strained, and with what consequences, will depend both upon the amount of stress and the characteristics of the material itself.

Neither stress, the external force, nor strain, the response of the person or material, is necessarily harmful. For both persons and materials there is a range of "working strain" that is normal and healthy. Over this range, deformations are reversible and the material is resilient. Some have introduced the terms *eustress* and *distress* to distinguish "good" and "bad" stress. These terms reflect the important point that stress is not per se bad. But what is eustress for one person may be distress for another, so we prefer to focus on the extent of the strain response, which depends on what one is made of.

Trouble arises when the strain is too great, and one is (irreversibly) "bent out of shape," or broken. This unfortunate outcome can be prevented either by avoiding overloading—do not let the stress level get too high—or by using stronger materials or construction. The strength of the materials themselves depends on their inherent characteristics, and on how they have been worked and processed. These may be analogous to genetic endowment and early rearing environment, which interact to influence the resilience of the individual just as they do for steel, wood, or plastic. (Heat treatment and tempering can toughen steel; it is not recommended for wood.)

But one can also make a structure more resistant to stress—reduce the degree of strain—by the way in which it is supported. A horizontal beam can carry much larger loads if it is part of a structure, supported at several points along its length, than if it is simply fastened at one end and otherwise projecting into empty space. The same is true of people—a supportive environment helps one to bear heavier loads without breaking.

From this perspective, Marmot's data indicate a social gradient in the degree of breakage. Is it because people in the lower ranks are under greater stress, or because they are in themselves less able to bear the strain that follows from stress, or because their environments, at work or at home, do not provide the supports that would permit them to transfer some of the strain? These possibilities are, of course, interactive, not mutually exclusive.

There is now a very large literature on the third point, the supportiveness of the social environment in assisting the individual in coping with stress. House, Landis, and Umberson (1988), for example, report widespread and strong correlations between mortality and social support networks—friends and family keep you alive. They interpret the evidence as suggesting that the sheer number of contact persons is protective, regardless of the nature of the interaction. Others, however, emphasize the "quality" of the social interaction, its cultural context and interpretation (see Chapter 4). More is not always better; social contacts can generate as well as mitigate stresses.[11]

Syme, Karasek, Theorell, and others focus in particular on the nature of the work environment and the characteristics of the job (Karasek and Theorell, 1990; Johnson and Johansson, 1991). They find a connection between job demand and job latitude, and morbidity and mortality. Looking at heart disease among male workers, they show that people in jobs that impose unpredictable and uncontrollable demands, yet that leave very little room for individual discretion in responding, and that in addition underutilize the individual's skills and abilities—no opportunity for personal growth—tend to have higher rates of heart disease, and death.

In Marmot's Whitehall study, lower-ranked workers are more likely to report that their work is dull and underutilizes their abilities—perhaps not surprising. And experimental animal studies confirm that exposure to stress (e.g., electric shock) that is unpredictable and uncontrollable imposes much greater strain—and health damage—than stress that the animal can learn to predict and control.

Such findings suggest, plausibly, that it may be the quality of the "microenvironment," both social and physical, that is critical to health, rather than some mechanical connection between "health and wealth." Prosperity and health are certainly highly correlated, whether one looks at different income groups within a society or trends over time, or compares different societies. Increasing prosperity is both an indicator of past success in coping with one's environment and a basis for future possibilities—a source of both self-esteem and empowerment. And it may be difficult to maintain high-quality microenvironments in a society where overall income levels are static or declining. But as discussed in Chapter 3, one can find examples of both "health without wealth," and "wealth without health," not only among individuals, but across societies.

Caldwell (1986) shows that within the strong cross-national correlation between health and wealth, certain societies achieve aggregate health status measures that are much higher than their income levels would "predict," while others are much lower. He also notes that there are particular social characteristics (in particular, high levels of maternal education) that seem consistently to be associated with good population health even at low levels of average income. Wilkinson (1992) presents evidence that the health of a population depends upon the *equality* of income distribution, rather than the *average* income, so that rising average incomes can be associated with declining health, if the resulting wealth becomes concentrated in fewer pockets. Or, as Sir Francis Bacon observed: "Money is like muck—not good unless it be well spread."

And so on. Our purpose here is not to try, in an introductory chapter, to summarize this vast literature, or collection of potentially related literatures. Rather we have tried, through a selection of leading studies and findings, to sketch out the basis for an argument that factors in the social environment, external to the health care system, exert a major and potentially modifiable influence on the health of populations, through biological channels that are just now beginning to be understood.

The interpretation of these observations and their translation into health policy represent a massive challenge, to which the subsequent chapters of this book attempt to offer a first response. But the observations themselves are facts, which cannot be dismissed simply because they are incompletely understood. They do not fit comfortably, or at all, into the simplistic "repair shop" model of health and health care on which most current health policy is based.

Relative to that simplistic view, the observations outlined above are "anomalous findings" on the determinants of health. They emerge from a number of different disciplines whose members rarely, if ever, read each other's work. They do not follow the same journals, or use the same jargons or metaphors. Yet we believe that enough such anomalous results have now been observed that, if they could be assembled and interpreted in a common framework and related to one another in a coherent way, they would be seen, in Kuhn's terms, to justify a paradigm shift.

Such shifts of perspective, however, do not occur in response to exhortation. They only occur when enough people find the old perspective unsatisfactory—because of a growing awareness of its lack of explanatory power—*and* find a new one more interesting as well as more enlightening.

Many of the "anomalous findings" described above have long histories, though new observations are accumulating rapidly. But, to the best of our knowledge, this diverse set of observations has never been brought together and examined within a single coherent framework. Yet they appear all to be pieces from the same large and complex jigsaw puzzle. This book is a start at assembling that puzzle, and at drawing out some of the implications for social policy of the resulting (still sketchy) picture.

It must be admitted that at present these implications are far from clear. We cannot offer a detailed prescription of "What is to be done," and much remains to be learned about the development of effective *health* interventions. But the evidence does suggest that the potential for improvement, in directions not addressed by conventional health care systems, is great. And relevant new knowledge is emerging rapidly, from both the biological and the social disciplines.

ACKNOWLEDGMENTS

This introductory chapter, written by R. G. Evans, is to be understood as a collaborative effort, growing out of the continuing research and seminars of the Population Health Programme of the Canadian Institute for Advanced Research.

NOTES

1. Our work proceeds from a particular notion of "health" about which it is important to be clear at the outset. For the most part we simply assume that health is the absence of disability or disease. That is, when free of illness as experienced by patients (e.g., aching muscles or sinus congestion associated with cold or flu), of disease as understood by clinicians (e.g., arthritis, diabetes, or cancer), or of injury (e.g., broken leg or hip fracture), one is "healthier." For any given state of disease or illness, capacity to function may vary dramatically among individuals, and it is this functional capability, in combination with the absence of clinically defined disease, that is implicit throughout.

There are, of course, other conceptions of health. It is by now pretty well accepted that the WHO's broader definition—a state of complete well-being—is rather unhelpful operationally. Health, on that conception, is everything and hence nothing in particular. But there is in some contemporary intellectual circles productive ferment about different understandings of health.

2. Sooner or later, the reader should question the rather morbid focus on death rates, as (inverse) measures of health. There is, after all, much more to good health than simply being alive. But for research purposes, deaths have the advantage of being quite unambiguously countable, and partly for that reason have been widely collected for a long time. Measurements of illness rates are much less complete, and more subject to differences in concept and definition over time and across regions. Measurements of health status are still more debatable conceptually, and are only sporadically collected.

But patterns of illness are also hierarchical. Marmot's later studies have found a gradient in morbidity, as measured by rates of sickness absence, which is at least as steep as the mortality gradient (North et al., 1993). It would have been rather surprising if the people who died earlier died in better health.

3. Are *any* risk factors truly "individual"? Donne is a better guide than Defoe. "No man is an island," and Robinson Crusoe is fiction.

4. The relation of this "something else" to one's position in a hierarchy may recall Maslow's concept of a "hierarchy of needs." All those in Marmot's study may have enough to eat, clothing and shelter, and personal safety. But the levels of "self-actualization" and self-esteem are probably quite different, on average, from top to bottom. So high status may correlate with satisfaction of high-level needs. But what exactly is low self-esteem (if that *is* the something else), and how does it kill you? It is somewhat easier to measure starvation or exposure and to understand their mechanisms of action.

5. In the subsequent discussion, we focus primarily on the possible relationships between hierarchy, stress, and health. But the reader should keep in mind that hierarchy is simply one example of the more general concept of heterogeneities. As discussed in Chapter 3, one also observes systematic differences in health status among cultures, geographic areas, and the sexes. And even in the explanation of differences within hierarchies, we have no basis for assuming a priori that stress is the only biological pathway.

6. Fibrinogen, in conjunction with thrombin, produces fibrin, which promotes normal clotting of blood. This may be very helpful, if one has sustained or is about to sustain a physical injury. It is much less so if the "clots" are on the interior walls of the arteries. In Marmot's studies, lower-ranking civil servants had on average higher levels of circulating fibrinogen, although the differences are not, in themselves, large enough to explain the differences in heart disease rates.

7. These are not alternatives; hormones released by the endocrine system may enhance or depress the functioning of the immune system.

8. Norman Cousins has done much to disseminate to clinicians and the general population the significance of brain-body links. But his emphasis seems to be on "self-improvement" and small-group support in a clinical context, rather than on the influence of broader social structures and networks, on predispositions as well as outcomes. Like many of the "health promoters" of the 1980s (Chapter 8), he focuses on the attitudes and behaviour of the individual rather than the physical and social environment from which that behaviour arises. Similarly Friedman (1991) describes "jobs that are disturbing and uncontrollable" as giving rise to "psychological impotence," but then without pausing for breath attributes this latter to the "disease-prone personality" (p. 43)! Both thus fit their work comfortably into the "medical model," in which the individual patient has (is) a problem, and one-on-one or small group therapy is the solution. No challenges are raised to the existing social and economic order.

9. Perhaps coincidentally, Offord, Boyle, Fleming, Blun, and Grant (1989) found in the Ontario Child Health Study that 18.1 percent of the child population met the study criteria for presence of some degree of psychological problem.

10. One of the most well-known findings of the Kauai Study has been the identification of a small group of "vulnerable but invincible" or "indomitable" children who, despite "high-risk" perinatal experiences and home environments, grew into successful adults. The common characteristics seemed to be close bonding with and high level of attention from *some* adult—not necessarily a parent or even a family member—very early in life. But these children also had personalities that "elicit positive responses"—presumably enabling them to "recruit" emotional support.

11. Again there is a mechanical analogy. In the case of the simple beam above, more supports lead to greater strength. But in complex structures, with each part transferring stresses to others in an overall pattern that is difficult to deduce a priori, reinforcing one part may in fact weaken the whole structure. Hence Seppings's maxim: "Partial strength produces general weakness" (quoted in Gordon, 1978:69).

2

Producing Health, Consuming Health Care

R. G. EVANS and G. L. STODDART

People care about their health, for good reasons; and they try in a number of ways to maintain it, to improve it, or to adapt to its decline. Individually and in groups at various levels—families, associations, work groups, communities, and nations—they engage in a wide range of activities that they believe will contribute to their health. People also attempt to avoid activities or circumstances that they see as potentially harmful. Implicit in such behaviour are theories, or more accurately loosely associated and often inconsistent collections of causal hypotheses, as to the determinants of health.

In particular, but only as a subset of these health-oriented activities, modern societies devote a very large proportion of their economic resources to the production and distribution of *health care,* a particular collection of goods and services that are perceived as bearing a special relationship to health. The *health care industry,* which assembles these resources and converts them into various health-related goods and services, is one of the largest clusters of economic activity in all modern states (Schieber and Poullier, 1989; OECD Secretariat, 1989).[1] Such massive efforts reflect a widespread belief that the availability and use of health care is central to the health of both individuals and populations.

This concentration of economic effort has meant that public or collective health policies have been dominated by health *care* policy. The provision of care not only absorbs the lion's share of the physical and

Reprinted with permission from *Social Science and Medicine,* vol. 31, no. 12, pp. 1347–63.
 Reprinted with slight authorial and editorial revision.

intellectual resources that are specifically identified as health related, it also occupies the centre of the stage when the rest of the community considers what to do about its health.

Health care, in turn, is overwhelmingly *reactive* in nature, responding to perceived departures from health, and identifying those departures in terms of clinical concepts and categories: diseases, professionally defined. The definition of health implicit in (most of) the behaviour of the health care system, the collection of people and institutions involved in the provision of care, is a negative concept: the absence of disease or injury. The system is in consequence often labeled as a "sickness care system."[2] The label is usually applied by critics, but there is no justification for devaluing the contribution of sickness care.

Yet this definition of health was specifically rejected by the World Health Organization (WHO) more than forty years ago. Its classic statement, "Health is a state of complete physical, mental, and social well-being, and not merely the absence of disease or injury," expressed a general perception that there is much more to health than simply a collection of negatives—a state of *not* suffering from any designated undesirable condition.

Such a comprehensive concept of health, however, risks becoming the proper objective for, and is certainly affected by, *all* human activity. There is no room for a separately identifiable realm of specifically health-oriented activity. The WHO definition is thus difficult to use as the basis for health policy, because implicitly it includes *all* policy as health policy. It has accordingly been honoured in repetition, but rarely in application.

Moreover, the WHO statement appears to offer only polar alternatives for the definition of health. Common usage, however, suggests a continuum of meanings. At one end of that continuum is well-being in the broadest sense, the all-encompassing definition of the WHO, almost a Platonic ideal of the Good. At the other end is the simple absence of negative biological circumstances—disease, pain, disability, or death.[3]

But the biological circumstances identified and classified by the health care disciplines as diseases are then experienced by individuals and their families or social groups as illnesses—distressing symptoms. The correspondence between medical disease and personal illness is by no means exact. Thus the patient's concept of health as absence of illness need not match the clinician's absence of disease. Further, the functional capacity of the individual will be influenced but not wholly determined by the perception of illness, and that capacity too will be an aspect, but not the totality, of well-being.

There are no sharply drawn boundaries between the various concepts of health in such a continuum; but that does not prevent us from recognizing their differences. Different concepts are neither right nor wrong, they simply have different purposes and fields of application. Whatever the level of *definition* of health being employed, however, it is important to distinguish this from the question of the *determinants* of (that definition of) health (Marmor, 1989).

Here, too, there exists a broad range of candidates, from particular targeted health care services, through genetic endowments of individuals, environmental sanitation, adequacy and quality of nutrition and shelter, stress and the supportiveness of the social environment, to self-esteem and sense of personal adequacy or control. It appears, on the basis of both long-established wisdom and considerable more recent research, that the factors affecting health at all levels of definition include but go well beyond health care per se (Dutton, 1986; Levine and Lilienfield, 1987; Marmot, 1986; McKeown, 1979; McKinlay, McKinlay, and Beaglehole, 1989; Black, Morris, Smith, and Townsend 1982).

Attempts to advance our understanding of this broad range of determinants through research have, like the health care system itself, tended to focus their attention on the narrower concept of health: absence of disease or injury. This concept has the significant advantage that it can be represented through quantifiable and measurable phenomena: death or survival, the incidence or prevalence of particular morbid conditions. The influence of a wide range of determinants, in and beyond the health care system, has in fact been observed in these most basic—negative—measures.

Precision is gained at a cost. Narrow definitions leave out less specific dimensions of health that many people would judge to be important to their evaluation of their own circumstances, or those of their associates. On the other hand, it seems at least plausible that the broad range of determinants of health whose effects are reflected in the "mere absence of disease or injury," or simple survival, is also relevant to more comprehensive definitions of health.

The current resurgence of interest in the determinants of health, as well as in its broader conceptualization, represents a return to a very old historical tradition, as old as medicine itself. The dialogue between Asclepios, the god of medicine, and Hygieia, the goddess of health—the external intervention and the well-lived life—goes back to the beginning. Only in the twentieth century did the triumph of "scientific" modes of inquiry in medicine (as in most walks of life) result in the eclipse of Hygieia. Knowledge has increasingly become defined in terms of that (and only that) which emerges from the application of reductionist methods of investigation, applied to the fullest extent possible in a "Newtonian" frame of reference (Reiser, 1978).

The health care system has then become the conventional vehicle for the translation of such knowledge into the improvement of health:

more, and more powerful, interventions, guided by better and better science. Nor have its achievements been negligible. Medical science *has* enhanced our ability to prevent some diseases, cure others, and alleviate the symptoms or slow the progress of many more. Thus by midcentury the providers of health care had gained an extraordinary institutional and even more an intellectual dominance, defining both what counted as health and how it was to be pursued. The WHO was a voice in the wilderness.

But the intellectual currents have now begun to flow in the other direction. There has been a growing unease about the exclusive authority of classically "scientific," positivist methods, both to define the knowable and to determine how it may come to be known (McCloskey, 1989; Dreyfus and Dreyfus, 1988), an unease that has drawn new strength from developments in subatomic physics and more recently in artificial intelligence and mathematics.[4] In addition, the application of those methods themselves to the exploration of the determinants of health is generating increasing evidence—in the most restricted scientific sense—of the powerful role of contributing factors outside the health care system (House, Landis, and Umberson, 1988; Dantzer and Kelley, 1989; Bunker, Gomby, and Kehrer, 1989; Renaud, 1987; Sapolsky, 1990).

Simultaneously, the more rigorous evaluation of the health care system itself has demonstrated that its practices are much more loosely connected with scientific or any other form of knowledge than the official rhetoric would suggest (Banta, Behney, and Willems, 1981; Eisenberg, 1986; Feeny, Guyatt, and Tugwell, 1986; Lomas, 1990a). And finally, the very success of that system in occupying the centre of the intellectual and policy stage, and in drawing in resources, has been built upon an extraordinarily heightened set of social expectations as to its potential contributions. Some degree of disappointment and disillusion is an inevitable consequence, with corresponding concern about the justification for the scale of effort involved.

There is thus a growing gap between our understanding of the determinants of health, and the primary focus of health policy on health care. This increasing disjunction may be partly a consequence of the persistence, in the policy arena, of incomplete and obsolete models, or intellectual frames of reference, for conceptualizing the determinants of health. How a problem is framed will determine which kinds of evidence are given weight, and which are disregarded. Perfectly valid data—hard observations bearing directly on important questions—simply drop out of consideration, as if they did not exist, when the implicit model of entities and interrelationships in people's minds provides no set of categories in which to put them.

There is, for example, considerable evidence linking mortality to the (non)availability of social support mechanisms, evidence of a strength that House et al. (1988) describe as now equivalent to that in the mid-1950s on the effects of tobacco smoking. Retirement and the death of a spouse are documented as important risk factors. Similarly, some correlate or combination of social class, level of income or education, and position in a social hierarchy is clearly associated with mortality (Dutton, 1986; Marmot, 1986). None of this is denied, yet no account is taken of such relationships in the formulation of health (care) policy.

Such policy is, by contrast, acutely sensitive to even the possibility that some new drug, piece of equipment, or diagnostic or therapeutic manoeuvre may contribute to health. That someone's health may perhaps be at risk for lack of such intervention is prima facie grounds for close policy attention, and at least a strong argument for provision. Meanwhile the egregious fact that people are suffering, and in some cases dying, as a consequence of processes not directly connected to health care, elicits neither rebuttal nor response.

The explanation cannot be that there is superior evidence for the effectiveness, still less the cost-effectiveness, of health care interventions. It is notorious that new interventions are introduced, and particularly disseminated, in the absence of such evidence (Banta et al., 1981; Eisenberg, 1986; Feeny et al., 1986). If (some) clinicians find it plausible that a manoeuvre might be beneficial in particular circumstances, it is likely to be used. The growing concern for "technological assessment" or careful evaluation *before* dissemination is a response to this well-established pattern. But those who might wish to restrain application, fearing lack of effect or even harm, find themselves bearing the burden of rigorous proof. If the evidence is incomplete or ambiguous, the bias is toward intervention, subject to the limits imposed by financial constraints.

This bias is encouraged when the causal relationships from sickness, to care, to cure are expressed by a simple mechanical model. The machine (us) is damaged or breaks, and the broken part is repaired (or perhaps replaced) by the doctor-mechanic. Although this mental picture may be a gross oversimplification of reality, it is easy to hold in mind.

By contrast, it is not at all obvious how one should even think about the causal connections between "stress" or "low self-esteem," and illness or death—much less what would be appropriate policy responses. Where there are multiple causal pathways (see Chapter 3), the picture is even more difficult to envision. The whole subject has a somewhat mysterious air, with overtones of the occult, in contrast to the (apparently) transparent and scientific process of health care.[5] There being no set of intellectual categories in which to assemble such data, they are ignored.

In this chapter, we propose a somewhat more complex framework, which we believe is sufficiently comprehensive and flexible to represent a wider range of relationships among the determinants of health. The test of such a framework is its ability to provide meaningful categories in which to insert the various sorts of evidence that are now emerging as to the diverse determinants of health, as well as to permit a definition of health broad enough to encompass the dimensions that people—providers of care, policymakers, and particularly ordinary individuals—feel to be important.

Our purpose is *not* to try to present a comprehensive, or even a sketchy, survey of the current evidence on the determinants of health, some of which is discussed in subsequent chapters. Even a taxonomy for that evidence, a suggested classification and enumeration of the main heads, would now be a major research task, on which Chapter 3 offers a beginning. Rather, we propose an analytic framework within which such evidence can be fitted, and which will highlight the ways in which different types of factors and forces can interact to bear on different conceptualizations of health. A precedent is the Canadian government's white paper, *A New Perspective on the Health of Canadians* (Canada, 1974), which likewise presented very little of the actual evidence on the determinants of health, but offered a very powerful and compelling framework for assembling it.

The white paper offered no more than the most cursory indication of what the implications of such evidence might be for health policies, public or private. These issues are, however, addressed explicitly in this book. Policy implications will arise from the actual evidence on the determinants of health, not from the framework per se. If the framework is useful it should facilitate the presentation of evidence in such a way as to make its implications more apparent. But there is of course much more to policy than evidence; "the art of the possible" includes most importantly one's perceptions of who the key actors are and what their objectives might be (see Chapter 10).

Finally we must emphasize that the components of our framework are themselves categories, with a rich internal structure. Each box and label could be expanded to show its complex contents (Chapters 4 and 11). One must therefore be very careful about, and usually avoid, treating such categories as if they could be adequately represented by some single homogeneous variable, much less subjected to mathematical or statistical manipulations like a variable. Single variables may capture some aspect of a particular category, but they are not the same as that category. Moreover, in specific contexts it may be the interactions between factors from different categories of determinants, and their timing, that are critical to the health of individuals and populations. These are discussed in more detail in the following chapter.

DISEASE AND HEALTH CARE: A (TOO) SIMPLE FOUNDATION

We build up our framework component by component, progressively adding complexity both in response to the demonstrable inadequacies of the preceding stage, and in rough correspondence to (our interpretation of) the historical evolution of the conceptual basis of health policy over the last half-century. The first and simplest stage defines health as absence of disease or injury and takes as central the relation between health and health care. The former is represented in terms of the categories and capacities of the latter. The relationship can be represented in a simple feedback model, as presented in Figure 2.1, exactly analogous to a heating system governed by a thermostat.

In this framework, people "get sick" or "get hurt" for a variety of unspecified reasons represented by the unlabeled arrows entering on the left-hand side. They may then respond by presenting themselves to the health care system, where the resulting diseases and injuries are defined and interpreted as giving rise to "needs" for particular forms of health care. This interpretive role is critical, because the definition of need depends on the state of medical technology. Conditions for which (it is believed that) nothing useful can be done may be regrettable and

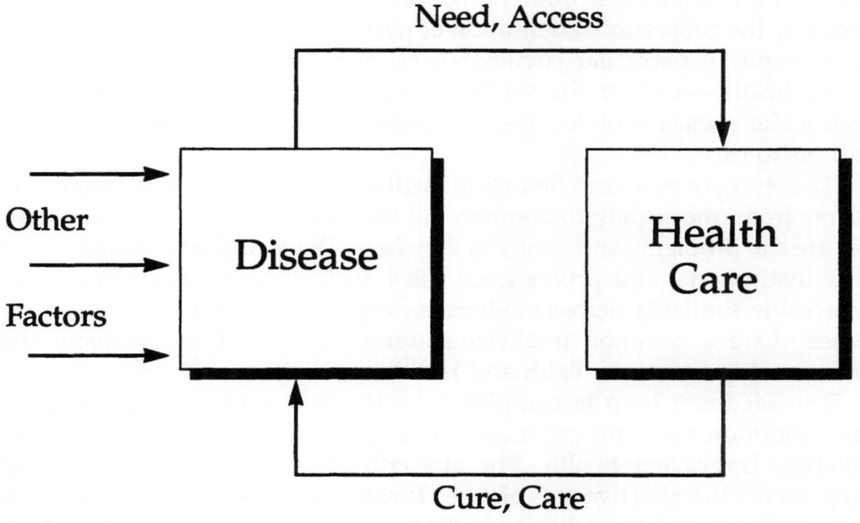

Figure 2.1. Simple feedback model of relationship between health and health care.

very distressing, but do not represent needs for care. The patient feels the distress, but the health care system defines the need.

Potential needs for health care are, however, prefiltered before they reach the care system, an important process that is reflected explicitly neither in Figure 2.1 nor in most of health policy.[6] Whether or not people respond to adverse circumstances by contacting the health care system, seeking "patient" status, will depend on their perceptions of the severity of the problem and their expectations of the formal system, relative to their own coping capacities and their informal support systems. These expectations and reactions are thus included among the "other factors" that determine the set of presenting conditions to which the health care system responds.

The health care system then combines the functions of thermostat and furnace, interpreting its environment, determining the appropriate response, and responding. The level of response is determined by the "access" to care that a particular society has provided for its members. This access depends both on the combination of human and physical resources available—doctors, nurses, hospitals, diagnostic equipment, drugs, etc.—and also on the administrative and financial systems in place that determine whether particular individuals will receive the services of these resources, and under what conditions.[7]

The top arrow in Figure 2.1 thus reflects the positive response of the health care system to disease: the provision of care. But the form and scale of the response is influenced, through a sort of "two-key" system, both by the professional definition of needs—what should be done to or for people in particular circumstances, suffering particular departures from health—and by the whole collection of institutions that in any particular society mobilize the resources to meet the needs and ensure access to care.

Those organizing and financing institutions have very different structures from one society to another, but their tasks are essentially similar, as are the problems and conflicts they face. The actual technologies, and the institutional and professional roles, in health care also show a remarkable similarity across modern societies, suggesting that those societies share a common intellectual framework for thinking about the relationship between health and health care.

The feedback loop is completed by the lower arrow, reflecting the presumption that the provision of care reduces the level of disease, thereby improving health. The strength of this negative relationship represents the effectiveness of care. These effects include the restoration and maintenance of health (providing "cures"); preventing further deterioration; relieving symptoms, particularly pain; offering assistance in coping with the inevitable; and providing reassurance through authoritative interpretation.

The important role of health care in providing comfort to the afflicted fits somewhat ambiguously in this framework, since services that can clearly be identified as making people feel good, but having no present or future influence on their health status however defined, can readily be seen to include a very wide range of activities, most of which are not usually included as health care (Evans, 1984, Chapter 1).

The provision of services that *are* generally recognized as health care should obviously take place in a context of consideration for the comfort of those served. There is no excuse for the gratuitous infliction of discomfort, and patients should not be made any more miserable than they have to be. But for those services that represent *only* comfort, it is important to ask both: (1) Why should they be professionalized, by assigning "official" providers of health care a privileged right to serve? and (2) Why should the clients of the health care system be awarded privileged access to such services? There are many people, not by any sensible definition ill, who might nevertheless have their lives considerably brightened by comforting services at collective expense.[8]

In this conceptual framework, the level of health of a population is the negative or inverse of the burden of disease. This burden of disease in Figure 2.1 is analogous to the temperature of the air in a house in a model of a heating system. The health care system diagnoses that disease and responds with treatment; the thermostat detects a fall in air temperature and turns on the furnace. The result is a reduction in disease/increase in room temperature. The external factors—pathogens, accidents—that "cause" disease are analogous to the temperature outside the house; a very cold night is equivalent to an epidemic. But the consequences of such external events are moderated by the response of the heating/health care systems.

The thermostat can, of course, be set at different target temperatures, and the control system of the furnace can be more or less sophisticated depending on the extent and duration of permissible departures from the target temperature. Similarly access to care can be provided at different levels, to meet different degrees of "need" and with tighter or looser tolerances for over- or underservicing.

The systems do differ, insofar as the house temperature can be increased more or less indefinitely by putting more fuel through the furnace (or adding more furnaces). In principle, the expansion of the health care system is bounded by the burden of remediable disease. When each individual has received all the health care that might conceivably be of benefit, then all needs have been met, and health in the narrow sense of absence of (remediable) disease or injury has been attained. Health is bounded from above; air temperature is not. The occupants of the house do not of course *want* an ever-increasing temperature, whether or not it is possible. Too much is as bad as too little. Yet no obvious meaning attaches to the words "too healthy." More is always better, a closer approximation to the ideal of perfect, or at least best attainable, health.[9]

The differences are more apparent than real, however, since in practice the professionally defined needs for care are themselves adjusted according to the capacity of the health care system, and the pressures on it. The objective of health, René Dubos' (1959) mirage, ever recedes as more resources are devoted to health care. As old forms of disease or injury threaten to disappear, new ones are defined. There are always "unmet needs."[10]

Furthermore, though one cannot be too healthy, obvious meanings *do* attach to the words "too much health care," on at least three levels. First, too much care may result in harm to health in the narrow sense—iatrogenic disease—because potent interventions are always potentially harmful. But even if care contributes to health in the narrow sense—keeping the patient alive, for example—it may still be "too much." Painful interventions that prolong not life but dying are generally recognized as harmful to those who are forced to undergo them. More generally, the side effects of "successful" therapy may in some cases be, for the patient, worse than the disease.

Second, even if the care *is* beneficial in terms of both health and well-being of the recipient, it may still represent "too much" if the benefits are very small relative to the costs, the other opportunities forgone by the patient or others. If health is an important, but not the only, goal in life, it follows that there can be "too much" even of effective health care (Woodward and Stoddart, 1990).

And finally, an important component of health is the individual's *perception* of his or her own state. An exaggerated sense of fragility is not health, but hypochondria. Too much emphasis on the number of things that can go wrong, even presented under the banner of "health promotion," can lead to excessive anxiety and a sense of dependence on health care—from annual checkup to continuous monitoring. This is very advantageous economically for the "health care industry,"[11] and *perhaps* may contribute in some degree to a reduction in disease, but does not correspond to any more general concept of health (Illich, 1975; Haynes, Sackett, Taylor, Gibson, and Johnson, 1979; Toronto Working Group on Cholesterol Policy, 1989).

Unlike a heating system, however, health care systems do not settle down to a stable equilibrium of temperature maintenance and fuel use. The combination of the "ethical" claim that all needs must be met and the empirical regularity that, as one need is met, another is discovered, apparently ad infinitum, leads to a progressive pressure for expansion in the health care systems of all developed societies. It is as if no temperature level were ever high enough; more and more fuel must always be added to the furnace(s).[12]

CONCERNS ABOUT COST, EFFECTIVENESS, AND THE MARGINAL CONTRIBUTION OF HEALTH CARE

The result is shown in Figure 2.2, in which the top arrow, access to health care, has been dramatically expanded to reflect a "health care cost crisis."[13] A comparison of international experience demonstrates that the *perception* of such a crisis is virtually universal, at least in Western Europe and North America. It is interesting to note, however, that the countries that perceive such a crisis actually spend widely differing amounts on health care, either absolutely or as a proportion of their national incomes (Schieber and Poullier, 1989; OECD Secretariat, 1989).

Nevertheless, whether they spend a little or a lot, in all such countries there is an expressed tension between ever-increasing needs and increasingly restrained resources. Even in the United States, one finds providers of care claiming that they face more and more serious restrictions on the resources available to them (Reinhardt, 1987), despite the

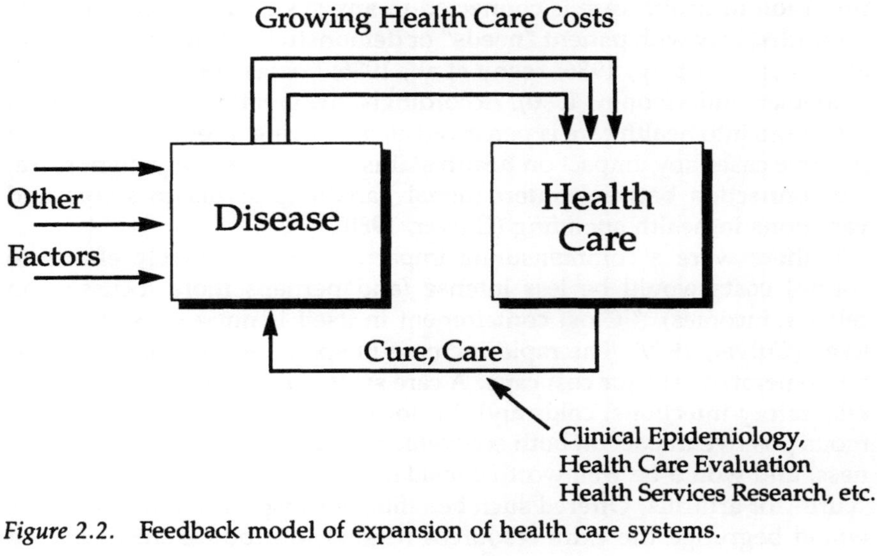

Figure 2.2. Feedback model of expansion of health care systems.

egregious observation that the resources devoted to health care in that country are greater, and growing faster, than anywhere else in the world.

We interpret this observation as implying that perceptions of "crises" in health care finance arise from conflicts over the level of expenditure on health care (and thus by definition also over the levels of incomes earned from its provision). Such conflicts develop whenever paying agencies attempt to limit the rate of increase of resources flowing to the health care system. They are independent of the actual level of provision of health care to a population, or of its expense, let alone of the level of health, however defined, of that population. They also appear to develop independently of the particular payment system in a country.

Nor, as the American example shows, does it matter whether the attempts to limit cost escalation are successful. Perceptions of crisis emerge from the attempt, not the result. Accordingly one should not expect to find any connection between the health of a population and allegations of crisis in the funding of its health care—or at least not among the countries of Western Europe and North America.

On the lower arrow, and intimately connected with the perceptions of cost crisis, we find increasing concern for the effectiveness with which health care services respond to needs. The development and rapid expansion of clinical epidemiology, for example, reflects a concern that the scientific basis underlying much of health care is weak to nonexistent. More generally, the growing field of health services research has accumulated extensive evidence inconsistent with the assumption that the provision of health care is connected in any systematic or scientifically grounded way with patient "needs" or demonstrable outcomes (Banta et al., 1981; Eisenberg, 1986; Feeny et al., 1986; Lomas, 1990a; Ham, 1988; Andersen and Mooney, 1990). Accordingly, the greatly increased flow of resources into health care is perceived as not having a commensurate, or in some cases any, impact on health status. Nor is there any demonstrable connection between international variations in health status and variations in health spending (Culyer, 1988).

If there were a commensurate impact, then presumably efforts to control costs would be less intense (and perhaps more focussed on relative incomes). "[C]ost containment in itself is not a sensible objective" (Culyer, 1989). The rapid increase in spending on computers has not generated calls for cost caps. A care system that could "cure" upper respiratory infections, colds and flu, for example, would have an enormous positive impact on both economic productivity and human happiness, and would be well worth considerable extra expense. So would a "cure" for arthritis. Offered such benefits, we suspect that few societies would begrudge the extra resources needed to produce them; indeed these resources would to a considerable extent pay for themselves in higher productivity.[14]

The combination of virtually universal concern over cost escalation, among payers for care, with steadily increasing evidence from the international research community that a significant proportion of health care activity is ineffective, inefficient, inexplicable, or simply unevaluated, constitutes an implicit judgment that the "expanding needs" to which expanding health care systems respond are either not of high enough priority to justify the expense, or simply not being met at all.

It is not that no needs remain, that the populations of modern societies have reached a state of optimum health. This is obviously not the case. Nor is it claimed that medicine has had no effect on health. This too is clearly false. The concern is rather that the remaining shortfalls, the continuing burden of illness, disability, distress, and premature death, are less and less sensitive to further extensions in health care. We are reaching the limits of medicine. At the same time the evidence is growing in both quantity and quality that this burden may be quite sensitive to interventions and structural changes outside the health care system.

These concerns and this evidence are by no means new—they go back at least two decades. Yet most of the public and political debate over health policy continues to be carried on in the rhetoric of "unmet needs" for *health care*. There is a curious disjunction in both the popular and the professional conventional wisdom, in that widespread concerns about the effectiveness of the health care system, and acceptance of the significance of factors outside that system, coexist quite comfortably with continuing worries about shortages and underfunding.

The periodic "shortage" of hospital nurses in Canada and indeed in much of the industrialized world, provides a good example. Nursing "shortages" have been cause for concern in Canada for more than a quarter century. Yet throughout that time, there has been virtually uniform agreement among informed observers that utilization of inpatient beds in Canada is substantially higher than needed, and efforts have been ongoing to reduce such use. Taking both positions together, this suggests that there is a "shortage" of nurses to provide "unnecessary" care.

The significant point is not the validity or otherwise of either perception, but the fact that they do not confront one another. In terms of the thermostatic model, public discussion still consists almost entirely of claims by providers (with considerable public support) that the room temperature is not high enough, or is in danger of falling, or that a severe cold spell is on the way . . . but in any case it is imperative that we install more and bigger furnaces immediately, and buy more fuel.

Meanwhile payers—in Canada, provincial governments—wring their hands over the size of the fuel bill and seek, with very little external support, ways of making the existing heating system more efficient.

A more efficient heating system is indeed a laudable objective, although it is understandable that the providers of health care, as the owners of the fuel supply companies, may give it a lower priority than do those who are responsible for paying the bills. But there is a much more fundamental question. The people who live in the building are primarily concerned about the level and stability of the room temperature, not the heating system per se. They become drawn into an exclusive focus on the heating system, if they perceive that this is the only way to control the room temperature. But as was (re)learned in North America after the oil shock of 1974, this is not so.

Similarly the health care system is not, for the general population, an end in itself. It is a means to an end, maintenance and improvement of health (Evans, 1984). And while few have followed Ivan Illich (1975) in arguing that the health care system has no positive—and indeed net negative—effects on the health of those it serves, nevertheless as noted above, the evidence for the importance of health-enhancing factors outside the health care system is growing rapidly in both quantity and quality.

But the intellectual framework reflected in Figures 2.1 and 2.2 pushes these other, and perhaps more powerful, determinants of health off the stage and into the amorphous cluster of arrows entering from the left-hand side of the diagram. By implication they are unpredictable, or at least uncontrollable, so there is no point in spending a great deal of intellectual energy or policy attention on identifying or trying to influence them. For most of the twentieth century, rapid advances in the scientific, organizational, and financial bases of health care have encouraged, and been encouraged by, this dismissal. We have given almost all our attention to the heating contractor and the fuel salesman, and have had no time or interest to consider how the house is insulated.

By the early 1970s, however, all developed nations had in place extensive and expensive systems of health care, underpinned by collective funding mechanisms, which provided access for all (or in the United States, most) of their citizens. Yet the resulting health gains seemed more modest than some had anticipated, while the "unmet needs," or at least the pressures for system expansion, refused to diminish. Simple trend projections indicated that, within a relatively short span of decades, the health care systems of modern societies would take over their entire economies. As public concerns shifted from expansion to evaluation and control, the alternative tradition began to reassert itself. In such an environment, a growing interest in alternative, perhaps more effective, hopefully less expensive, ways of promoting health was a natural response.

The resurgence of interest in ways of enhancing the health of populations, other than by further expansion of health care systems, was thus rooted both in the concern over growing costs and in the observation of the stubborn persistence of ill-health. As detailed in Chapters 8 and 10, the former development has been particularly important in "recruiting new constituencies" for the broader view of the determinants of health. Financial bureaucrats, both public and private, have become (often rather suspect) allies of more traditional advocates (Evans, 1982; McKinlay, 1979).

THE HEALTH FIELD CONCEPT: A NEW PERSPECTIVE

The broader view was given particularly compact and articulate expression in the famous Canadian white paper referred to above, which came out, presumably by complete coincidence, in the same year as the first "energy crisis." Its "four-field" framework for categorizing the determinants of health was broad enough to express a number of the concerns of those trying to shift the focus of health policy from an exclusive concern with health care. In Figure 2.3 this framework is superimposed upon the earlier "thermostat/furnace" model of health care and health.

The New Perspective proposed that the determinants of health status could be categorized under the headings of "life-styles," "environment," "human biology," and "health care organization." As can be seen in Figure 2.3, the first three of these categories provided specific identification for some of the "other and unspecified" factors entering on the left hand side of Figures 2.1 and 2.2. By labeling and categorizing these factors, the white paper drew attention to them and suggested the possibility that their control might contribute more to the improvement of human health than further expansions in the health care system. At the very least, the "health field" framework emphasized the centrality of the objective of *health*, and the fact that health care was only one among several forms of public policy that might lead towards this objective.

The white paper was received very positively in Canada and abroad; no one seriously challenged its basic message that who we are, how we live, and where we live are powerful influences on our health status. But the appropriate policy response was less clear, because the document could be read in several different ways. At one end of the ideological spectrum, it was seen as a call for a much more interventionist set of

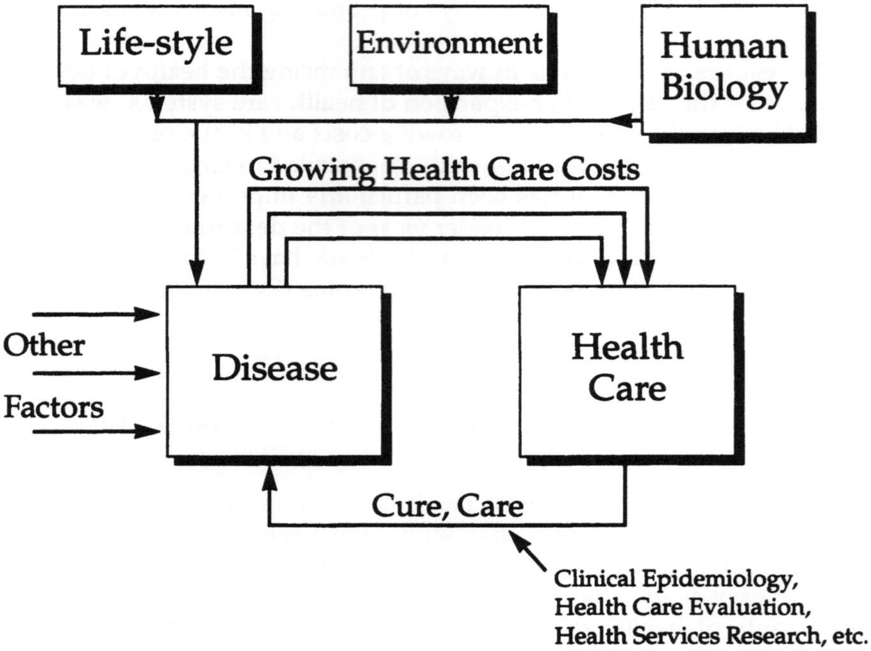

Figure 2.3. Four-field framework for health care determinants added to the model.

social policies, going well beyond the public provision of health care per se in the effort to improve the health of the Canadian population and relieve the burden of morbidity and mortality.

At the other end, however, the assumption that life-styles and to a lesser extent living environments are *chosen* by the persons concerned could be combined with the white paper framework to argue that people are largely responsible for their own health status—have in fact chosen it. If so, then the justification for collective intervention, even in the provision of health care, becomes less clear.[15] This appears to have been far from the intention of the authors of the paper, but the framework in Figure 2.3 lends itself to "victim-blaming" as well as to arguments for more comprehensive social reform (Evans, 1982).

Whatever the original intent, however, the white paper led into a period of detailed analysis of *individual* risk factors, i.e., both individual hazards and individual persons, as contributors to "disease" in the traditional sense.[16] The potential significance of processes operating on health at the level of groups and populations was obscured, if not lost (Buck, 1985). Smoking, for example, was viewed as an individual act predisposing to specific diseases. Specific atmospheric pollution contributes to lung disease. Genetic defects result in well-defined genetic diseases. The central thermostatic relationship is preserved, with health as absence of disease, and health care as response to disease in order to provide "cures" or relieve symptoms, individual by individual.

To illustrate the distinction, one can formulate health policy to address cancer across a spectrum from the individual to the collective. One can increase facilities for the treatment of cancer patients, a wholly individualized, reactive response. One can increase research on cancer treatment, an activity with a collective focus only insofar as the specific recipients of new treatments may not be known in advance. One can launch antismoking campaigns, trying to induce certain individuals whose *characteristics* are known—they smoke—to change their behaviour voluntarily. These campaigns may in turn be wholly individualized —paying or otherwise encouraging physicians to provide counselling, for example—or advertising campaigns aimed at the general population. Or one can try to limit involuntary exposures by regulating the presence of carcinogens in the environment, establishing mandatory smoke-free zones (hospitals, restaurants, aircraft, workplaces, . . .) or regulating industrial processes.

The focus on individual risk factors and specific diseases has tended to lead not away from but back to the health care system itself. Interventions, particularly those addressing personal life-styles, are offered in the form of "provider counselling" for smoking cessation, seatbelt use, or dietary modification (American Council of Life Insurance and Health Insurance Association of America, 1988; Lewis, 1988). These in turn are subsumed under a more general and rapidly growing set of interventions attempting to modify risk factors through transactions between clinicians and individual patients.

The "product line" of the health care system is thus extended to deal with a more broadly defined set of "diseases": unhealthy behaviours. The boundary becomes blurred between, e.g., heart disease as manifest in symptoms, or in elevated serum cholesterol measurements, or in excessive consumption of fats. All are "diseases" and represent a "need" for health care intervention. Through this process of disease redefinition, the conventional health care system has been able to justify extending outreach and screening programs, and placing increased numbers of people on continuing regimens of drug therapy and regular monitoring.

The emphasis on individual risk factors and particular diseases has thus served to maintain and protect existing institutions and ways of thinking about health. The "broader determinants of health" were matters for the attention of individuals, perhaps in consultation with their personal physicians, supported by poster campaigns from the local public health unit. The behaviour of large and powerful organizations, or the effects of economic and social policies, public and private, were not brought under scrutiny. This interpretation of the white paper thus not only fitted in with the increasingly conservative *zeitgeist* of the late 1970s and early 1980s, but protected and even enhanced the economic position of providers of care, while restricting sharply the range of determinants, and associated policies, considered. Established economic interests were not threatened—with the limited exception of the tobacco industry.

This tendency was reinforced by attempts to estimate the relative contribution of the four different fields or sets of factors to ill-health. Such a simple partitioning of sources of mortality, morbidity, or care utilization into four discrete "boxes" is, as Gunning-Schepers and Hagen (1987) have pointed out, fundamentally misguided. The following chapter provides a more sophisticated and flexible framework for partitioning effects. Nevertheless, "expert opinion" suggested that, of the three fields external to the health care system, "life-styles" had the largest and most unambiguously measurable effect on health. Life-styles—diet, exercise, substance use— were also the factors most readily portrayed as under the control of the individual. They thus lent themselves to the politically innocuous, inexpensive, highly visible, and relatively ineffective intervention of health education campaigns—carried on through the public health arm of the health care system.

Smoking cessation provides a partial counterexample, which illustrates the difficulty of breaking out of the disease–health care intellectual framework. Tobacco is not only toxic, but addictive, and addiction most commonly commences in childhood. Consequently the presumption that users rationally and voluntarily "choose" smoking as a "life-style" is particularly inappropriate. Furthermore, the observation that smoking behaviour is very sharply graded by socioeconomic class undercuts the argument that it represents an individual choice, and indicates instead a powerful form of social conditioning.[17]

Partly for these reasons, Canadian health policy has gone beyond educational campaigns to spread information about the ill effects of smoking, and includes limitations on the advertising and marketing of tobacco products. The political resistance to these limitations has been much more intense, suggesting prima facie that the marketers of such products fear that they might be effective. But the broader question, of the social determinants of tobacco use, is still left open.[18]

The intellectual framework of the white paper, at least as it has been applied and as represented in Figure 2.3, has thus supplemented the thermostatic model of health as absence of disease and health care as response, but has failed to move beyond the core relationship. Since as noted above, "disease" is defined through the interpretation of individual experience by the providers of health care, it is perhaps not surprising that the "health care organization" field tended to take over large parts of the other three, when they were presented as determinants of disease.

EXTENDING THE FRAMEWORK: HEALTH AND ITS BIOLOGICAL AND BEHAVIOURAL DETERMINANTS

Yet in the years since the publication of the white paper, a great deal of evidence has accumulated, from many different sources, which is difficult or impossible to represent within this framework. The very broad set of relationships encompassed under the label of "stress," for example, and factors protective against "stress" (Dantzer and Kelley, 1989; Sapolsky, 1990), have directed attention to the importance of social relationships, or their absence, as correlates of disease and mortality. Feelings of self-esteem and self-worth, or hierarchical position and control, or conversely powerlessness, similarly appear to have health implications quite independent of the conventional risk factors (Dutton, 1986; Marmot, 1986; House et al., 1988; Sapolsky, 1990).

These sorts of factors suggest explanations for the universal finding, across all nations, that mortality and (when measurable) morbidity follow a gradient across socioeconomic classes. Lower income and/or lower social status are associated with poorer health.[19]

This relationship is not, however, an indication of deprivation at the lower end of the scale, although it is frequently misinterpreted in that way. In the first place, the socioeconomic gradient in health status has been relatively stable over time (Townshend and Davidson, 1982), although average income levels have risen markedly in all developed societies. The proportion of persons who are deprived of the necessities of life in a biological sense has clearly declined. But even more important, the relationship holds across the whole socioeconomic spectrum. Top people appear to be healthier than those on the second rung, even though the latter are above the population averages for income, status, or whatever the critical factors are (Marmot, 1986).

It follows that the variously interpreted determinants of health that lie outside the health care system are not just a problem of some poor, deprived minority whose situation can be deplored and ignored by the rest of us. *De te fabula narratur,* we are all (or most of us) affected. And that in turn implies that the effects of such factors may be quantitatively very significant for the overall health status of modern populations. The issues involved are not trivial, second- or third-order effects.

Moreover, the gradients in mortality and morbidity across socioeconomic classes appear to be relatively stable over long periods of time, even though the principal causes of death have changed considerably. *This implies that there are underlying factors that influence susceptibility to a whole range of diseases.* They are general rather than specific risk factors. Whatever is going around, people in lower social positions tend to get more of it, and to die earlier—even after adjustment for the effects of specific individual or environmental hazards (Marmot, Shipley and Rose, 1984).

This suggests that an understanding of the relationship between social position, or "stress," and health will require investigation at a more general level than the etiology of specific diseases. It also raises the possibility that disease-specific policy responses—through health care or otherwise—may not reach deeply enough to have much effect. Even if one "disease" is "cured," another will take its place.

An attempt to provide a further extension to our intellectual framework, to encompass these new forms of evidence, is laid out in Figure 2.4. Two major structural changes are introduced. First, a distinction is drawn between disease, as recognized and responded to by the health care system, and health and function as experienced by the individual person. Such a distinction permits us to consider, within this framework, the common observation that illness experienced by individuals

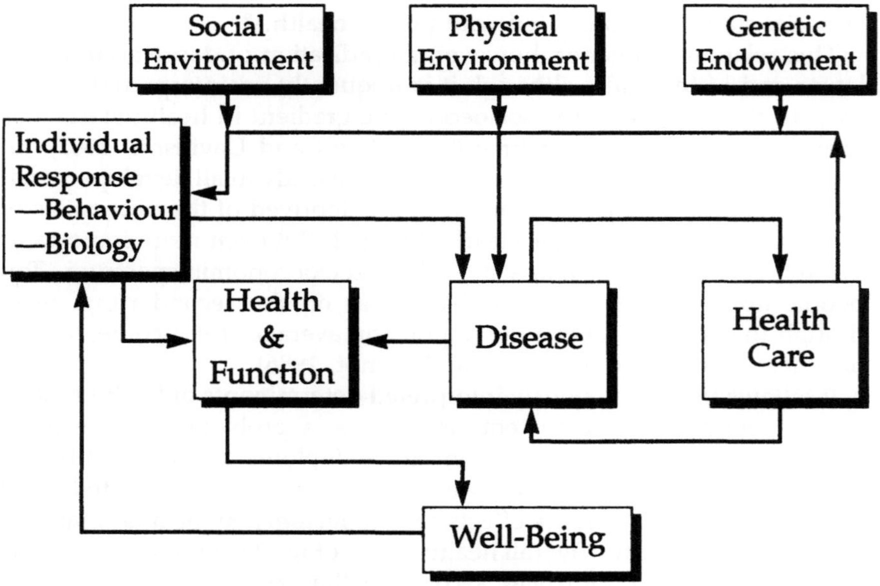

Figure 2.4. Relationship between social and individual factors and health.

(and their families or other relevant social groups) does not necessarily correspond to disease as understood by the providers of care. Persons with "the same" disease, from the point of view of the health care system—similar biological parameters, prognoses, and implications for treatment—may experience very different levels of symptoms and distress, and effects on their ability to function in their various social roles. These individual differences arise in turn from the very different cultural settings that govern their interpretation of and accommodation to the disease, as elaborated in Chapter 4. Arthritis, and musculoskeletal problems more generally, are leading examples of conditions for which the patient's sense of "illness" bears no very close relationship to the clinician's interpretation of "disease."

This is not to say that one perspective is right and the other wrong; the two modes of interpretation simply have different purposes. The clinician's concept of disease is intended to guide the appropriate application of available medical knowledge and technology, and so is formulated in terms of that knowledge and technology. Patients, on the other hand, are ultimately concerned with the impact of illness on their own lives. The clinician's interpretation may be an important part of that impact but is by no means the only relevant factor.

Moreover, from the point of view of the individual's well-being and social performance—including economic productivity—it is the individual's sense of health and functional capacity that is determinative—as shown in Figure 2.4. The "diseases" diagnosed and treated by the health care system are important only insofar as they affect that sense of health and capacity—which of course they do. But health, even as interpreted by the individual, is not the only thing in life that matters. Figure 2.4 introduces the category of "well-being," the sense of life satisfaction of the individual, which is or should be (we postulate) the ultimate objective of health policy. The ultimate test of such policy is whether or not it adds to the well-being of the population served.

Going back to the original WHO definition of health, we are relabeling that broad definition as well-being. Our concept of health is defined, in narrow terms but from the patient's perspective, as the absence of *illness* or injury, of distressing symptoms or impaired capacity. Disease, as a medical construct or concept, will usually have a significant bearing on illness, and thus on health, but is not the same thing. Illness, in turn, is a very important (negative) influence on well-being—but not the only one. The WHO broad definition of health is, as noted above, so broad as to become the objective, not only of health policy, but of all human activity.

Hypertension screening and treatment gives a clear and concrete example of this distinction, as well as bringing out the limitations of the static framework expressed in all the accompanying figures. It is sometimes said that hypertension does not hurt you, it only kills you. Target organ damage proceeds silently and without symptoms; a sudden and possibly fatal stroke announces both the presence of the long-term condition, and its consequences. Until that point the individual concerned may have no illness, although a clinician who took his/her blood pressure might identify a disease.

Studies of the impact of hypertension screening and treatment programs, however, have made it clear that the fact of *diagnosis*, "labeling," makes the patient ill, in ways that are unambiguous and objectively measurable (Haynes et al., 1979). Treatment exacerbates the illness, through drug side effects, although those who comply with treatment may suffer less severe labeling effects. Screening and treatment of hypertension thus spread illness among the beneficiaries and reduce their functional capacity, in a real and literal sense, even as their disease is alleviated.

Of course, such screening is not carried out from clinical malice! The long-term consequences of hypertension as a disease may be expressed in very definite forms of illness, including death. The immediate consequences of discovery and treatment of disease may be increased illness; the longer term consequences are reduction in illness, and very severe illness at that, for some of those under care. There is substantial evidence that screening and treatment of moderate to severe hypertension have very significantly reduced both morbidity and mortality from stroke; this is widely regarded as one of the leading "success stories" in clinical prevention (Hypertension Detection and Follow-Up Program Cooperative Group, 1979). But regardless of their relative strength, the static framework of Figure 2.4 does not reflect this pattern of off-setting movements in different time periods.

Indeed there is an implicit time structure to all of the figures. "Cures" are rarely instantaneous, so health care has its negative effect on disease only with a time lag of variable length. The life-style and environmental factors displayed in Figures 2.3 and 2.4 have long-term and cumulative effects on health/disease. But the extra problem in Figure 2.4 arises because the relationship being displayed may reverse itself over time. Health care can have a negative effect on health in the short term, and a positive one in the longer term.[20]

The possibility of "long-term gain" may, but does not necessarily, justify the "short-term pain," and analysts and evaluators of preventive programs are acutely aware of the necessity of weighing the health benefits and health costs against each other. Overzealous intervention can do significant harm to the health of those treated, even if at some later date it can be shown to have "saved lives," or more accurately postponed some deaths.

The debate over cholesterol screening, and the contradictory recommendations arising from "experts" in different jurisdictions, is a current case in point (Toronto Working Group on Cholesterol Policy, 1989; Moore, 1989; Anderson, Brinkworth, and Ng, 1989). At issue are not merely differing interpretations of the epidemiological evidence, or different weightings of "lives and dollars"—program resource costs versus mortality outcomes. The prospect of converting a quarter of the adult population of North America into "patients" with chronic illness requiring continuous drug therapy gives at least some clinicians (and others!) pause.

The framework of Figure 2.4 enables, indeed encourages, one to consider this distinction. Large-scale cholesterol screening and drug therapy, in this framework, would represent an epidemic of new illness, a deterioration in "health and function" from both labeling effects and drug side effects. As the hypertension studies remind us, these negative effects are real and concrete, measurable in people's lives. Against this, there would be a reduction in disease, as measured first in serum cholesterol, and subsequently in heart disease. The latter would then contribute positively to health, but the conflicting health effects of disease reduction, i.e., deterioration in health now, improvement later, must be weighed against each other in assessing their net impact on well-being.

In addition to distinguishing explicitly disease from illness, Figure 2.4 extends the categorization of the determinants of health provided in the white paper framework. This permits us to incorporate within the framework the diverse and rapidly growing body of research literature on the determinants of health that does not fit at all comfortably within the white paper categories.

The key addition is the concept of the *individual (host) response*, which includes but goes beyond the usual epidemiological sense of the term. The range of circumstances to which the organism/individual may respond is also wider than is usually encompassed within epidemiology (Cassel, 1976). This host response now includes some factors or processes that were previously assembled under the labels of life-style and human biology.

The implications of this change can be seen when one considers (yet again) smoking behaviour. In the white paper framework, tobacco use is labeled as a "life-style," from which one can draw the implication that its use is an "individual choice." That in turn leads not only to victim-blaming, but also to an emphasis on informational and educational strategies for control, which are notoriously ineffective. The powerful ethical overtones of "choice," with its connections to "freedom" and "individual self-expression," introduce not only political but also intellectual confusions into the process of control of an addictive and toxic substance.

Yet it is widely observed that tobacco use is strongly socially conditioned. Income, status, and prestige rankings in modern societies have become strongly negatively correlated with smoking, such that differential smoking behaviour is now a significant factor in the social gradient in mortality. This was not always so; prior to the widespread dissemination of information about its health effects, smoking was positively correlated with status. It seems clear that, far from being simply an individual choice, smoking is an activity engaged in—or not—by groups of people in particular circumstances. Understanding why some people smoke, and others do not, and a fortiori developing successful strategies to discourage this self-destructive behaviour, requires that one explore these group processes and their conditioning circumstances. To smoke or not to smoke is obviously an individual *action*, but it may not be an individual *choice*. To treat it as such is simply to throw away the information contained in the clustering of behaviour.

This is not to reduce the individual to an automaton, or deny any role for individual choice. Nor is smoking the only activity that is socially conditioned—far from it. But the well-defined clustering of smoking and nonsmoking behaviour within the population suggests that such behaviour is also a form of "host" (the smoker) response to a social environment that does or does not promote smoking. Heavy tobacco advertising promotes, for example, while legislated smoke-free environments discourage, quite separately from the "individual choice."

The psychological dynamics of status and class may have even more powerful, if subtler, effects. The sense of personal efficacy associated with higher social position encourages beliefs both in one's ability to break addictions and in the positive consequences of doing so. Beliefs in the effectiveness (or lack of it) of one's own actions are both learned and reinforced by one's social position.

The distinction between social environment and host response also permits us to incorporate conceptually factors that influence health in much less direct and obvious ways than smoking. It has been observed that the death of a spouse places an individual at increased risk of illness, or even death. This may be due to a reduction in the competence of the immune system, although the causal pathways are by no means wholly clear. Evidence is accumulating rapidly, however, that the nervous and immune systems communicate with each other, each synthesizing hormones that are "read" by the other, so that the social environment can, in principle, influence biological responses through its input to the nervous system. Data from animal experiments have shown the power of these effects (Dantzer and Kelley, 1989).

Biological responses by the organism to its social environment are not restricted to the immune system. Forms of stress that one feels powerless to control—associated with hierarchical position, for example—may be correlated with differences in the plasma levels of reactive proteins such as fibrinogen (Markowe, et al., 1985), or with the efficiency of the hormonal responses to stress (Sapolsky, 1990). The adequacy or inadequacy of nutrition in early infancy may "program" the processing of dietary fats in ways that have consequences much later in life (Barker, Winter, Osmond, Margetts, and Simmonds, 1989; Birch, 1972). The range of possible biological pathways is only beginning to emerge, and is at present still quite contentious, but it seems clear that the sharp separation between human biology and "other things" is crumbling.

Accordingly we have in Figure 2.4 unbundled that field, and restricted it to the genetic endowment. This endowment then interacts, as described in more detail in Chapter 5, with the influences of the social, cultural, and physical environments, to determine both the biological and the behavioural responses of the individual (Baird and Scriver, 1990). Some of these responses will be predominantly unconscious—few of us are aware of how our immune system is performing (unless it is overwhelmed), much less can deliberately affect it. Other responses will be behavioural—smoking, for example, or buckling seatbelts. Both forms of response, or rather the continuum of such responses, will influence the ability of the individual to deal with external challenges, either to resist illness or to maintain function in spite of it. They will also affect the burden of disease, separately from illness. The decision to seek care, compliance with therapy, and response to therapy (or to self-care) are also part of the host response.

An example of the significance of changes in such host responses may be given by the decline in tuberculosis in the United Kingdom over the last century. This dramatic change in mortality patterns occurred prior to the development of any effective responses from either public health measures or medical therapy (McKeown, 1979). The decline was apparently *not* due to a reduced rate of exposure to the bacillus, as the majority of the population continued to test positive for the TB antibody as late as 1940 (Sagan, 1987). The resistance of the population simply increased. McKeown offers improved nutrition as an explanation, but the issue still seems to be open (McKeown, 1979; Sagan, 1987).[21] The point for our purposes is that the *biological* response of the organism is malleable.

Indeed, progress in genetics is also extending the older picture of a fixed genetic endowment, in which well-defined genetic diseases follow from single-gene defects. It now appears that particular combinations of genes may lead to predispositions, or resistances, to a wide variety of diseases, not themselves normally thought of as "genetic" (see Chapter 5). Whether these predispositions actually become expressed as disease, will depend inter alia on various environmental factors, physical and social.

The insertion of the host response between environmental factors, and both the expression of disease and the level of health and function, provides a set of categories sufficiently flexible to encompass the growing but rather complex evidence on the connections between social environment and illness. Unemployment, for example, may lead to illness (quite apart from its correlation with economic deprivation) if the unemployed individual becomes socially isolated and stigmatized. On the other hand, if support networks are in place to maintain social contacts, and if self-esteem is not undermined, then the health consequences may be minimal.

The correlation of longevity with status in a hierarchy may be an example of reverse causality: The physically fitter rise to the top. But it is also possible that the self-esteem and sense of coping ability induced by success and the respect of others results in a "host response" of enhanced immune function or other physiological strengthening. The biological vulnerability or resilience of the individual, in response to external shocks, is dependent on the social and physical environment in interaction with the genetic endowment. While as noted the biological pathways for this process are only beginning to be traced out, the observed correlations continue to accumulate. Figure 2.4 provides a conceptual framework within which to express such a pattern of relationships, while Chapter 3 takes up in more detail alternative explanations such as reverse causality.

In this extended framework, the relationship between health care and the health of a population becomes even more complex. The sense of self-esteem, coping ability, powerfulness, may conceivably be either reinforced or undermined by health care interventions. Labeling effects may create a greater sense of vulnerability in the labeled, which itself influences physiological function. Such a process was an important part of Illich's (1975) message. Yet the initiation of preventive behaviour, or of therapy, may also result in positive "placebo" effects, perhaps reflecting an increased sense of coping or control, independently of any "objective" assessment of the effectiveness of such changes.

That medical interventions may have unintended effects is inevitable. Our framework includes both placebo and iatrogenic effects in the causal arrow from care to disease. But one could presumably also show an effect, of ambiguous sign, from care to host response.

The protective sense of self-esteem or coping ability may well be a collective as well as an individual possession. Being a "winner," being on a "winning team," or simply being associated with a winning team—a resident of a town whose team has won a championship—all seem to provide considerable satisfaction, and may have more objectively measurable influences on health.

A FURTHER EXTENSION: ECONOMIC TRADE-OFFS AND WELL-BEING

But there is still another feedback loop to be considered. Health care, and health policies generally, have economic costs that also affect well-being. Once we extend the framework, as in Figure 2.4, to reflect the fact that the ultimate objective of health-related activity is not the reduction of disease, as defined by the health care system, or even the promotion of human health and function, but the enhancement of human well-being, then we face a further set of trade-offs, which are introduced in Figure 2.5.

Health care is not "free"; as noted above, the provision of such services is now the largest single industry or cluster of economic activities in all modern societies. This represents a major commitment of re-

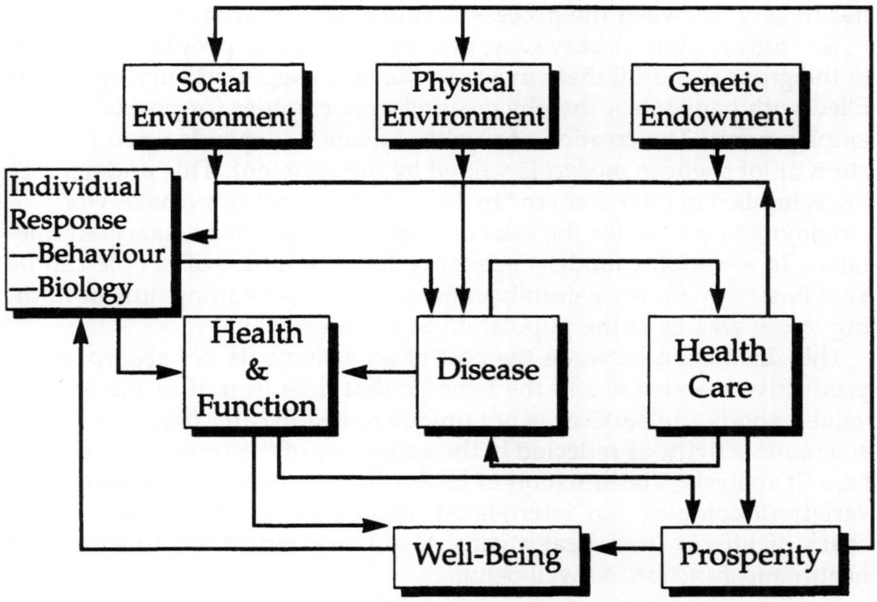

Figure 2.5. Feedback loop for human well-being and economic costs.

sources—human time, energy, and skills, raw materials, and capital services—which are therefore unavailable for other forms of production. To the extent that health care makes a positive contribution to health, it thereby contributes to human happiness both directly and through the economic benefits of improved productivity and functioning.

The latter effect is frequently referred to as an "investment in health"; spending on health care may even pay for itself through increased capacity of the population to work and to produce wealth. The increasing concentration of health care on those outside the labour force, the very elderly or chronically ill, has, however, severely weakened this particular linkage. For most health care now provided, the benefits must be found in the value of the resulting improvements in health and function, not in productivity gains.

Whatever the form of the payoff to health care, the resources used in its provision are a net claim on the wealth of the community. The well-being and economic progress of the larger society are thus affected *negatively* by the extension of the health care system per se. The fallacious argument frequently put forward by the economically naive, that health care, or any other industry, yields economic benefits through the creation of jobs, rests on a confusion between the job itself—a resource-using activity or cost—and the product of the job, the output. It is in fact an extension into the general economic realm of a common confusion in health care, between the process of care and its outcome.[22]

Yet "job creation" is very easy; one can always hire people to dig holes in the ground and fill them in again. (Keynes suggested burying bottles filled with banknotes, thereby creating opportunities for profitable self-employment.) The creation of wealth, however, depends upon the creation of jobs whose *product* is valued by the recipient. This understanding is implicit in references to "real jobs," as distinct from make-work, or employment purely for the sake of keeping people busy—and remunerated. In a complex modern economy, large numbers of people can be kept busy, apparently gainfully employed, and yet adding little or nothing to the wealth of the population as a whole.[23]

This distinction between the cost of an activity, its net absorption of productive resources, and the benefits that flow from it in the form of valued goods and services is not unique to health care. It applies to any economic activity, as reflected in the generality of the techniques of cost-benefit analysis. The situation of health care is different, however, for a variety of complex and interrelated reasons, which are implicit in the chain of effects from health care, to disease reduction, to improved health and function, to well-being.

Health care has characteristics that make it intrinsically different from "normal" goods and services traded through private markets, and this is reflected in the peculiar and complex collection of institutional arrangements that surround its provision. As a consequence both of these intrinsic peculiarities and of the institutional responses to them, the mechanisms that for most commodities maintain some linkage between the resource costs of a commodity and its value to users are lacking.

These problems are discussed in detail in the literature on the economics of health care (e.g., Evans, 1984, Chapters 1–5). For our purposes, however, the important point is that overexpansion of the health *care* system can in principle have negative effects not only on the well-being of the population, but even on its *health*. These dual effects are shown in Figure 2.5.

The possible negative impact of overprovision on well-being is straightforward. As emphasized, the provision of health care uses up economic resources that could be used for other valued purposes. In 1990 Canadians spent about 9 percent of their national income on health care, and these resources were thus unavailable for producing consumer goods like clothing or furniture, building rapid transit systems, improving the educational system, etc. In the United States, over 12 percent of national income was spent on health care; in Japan, about 6 percent. The Japanese correspondingly have a larger share of their income available for other purposes, the Americans a smaller proportion.

Less obviously, but implicit in Figure 2.5, the expansion of health care draws resources away from other uses that may also have health effects. In public budgets, for example, rising health care costs for the elderly draw funds that are then unavailable for increased pensions or other forms of social support; rising deficits may even lead to pension reductions. Increased taxes or private health insurance premiums lower the disposable income of the working population. Environmental clean-up programs also compete for scarce resources with the provision of health care.

Once we recognize the importance and potential controllability of factors other than health care in both the limitation of disease and the promotion of health, we simultaneously open for explicit consideration the possibility that the direct positive effects of health care on health may be outweighed by its negative effects through its competition for resources with other health-enhancing activities. *A society that spends so much on health care that it cannot or will not spend adequately on other health-enhancing activities may actually be reducing the health of its population.*

Two points of clarification may be helpful here, along with one of qualification.

First, we are *not* referring to iatrogenesis, the direct negative effects of health care on health. Powerful interventions have powerful side effects; the growing reach of medical technology often brings with it increased potential for harm.[24] Clinical judgment includes the balancing of probabilities for benefit and harm—the best care will sometimes work out badly. Moreover, all human systems involve some degree of error—inappropriate and incompetent care, or simply bad luck. Expansion of the health care system thus carries with it a greater potential for harm as well as good, as a direct result of care, but that is not the point here.

Second, the potential effects we are postulating are the economist's *marginal* effects. The global impact of health care, on either health or the resources available for other activities, is not addressed. Perhaps Ivan Illich is right, and the health care system as a whole has a net negative impact on the health of the population it serves. But we do not know that, and we do not know how one could come to know it.

The point we are making is a much more limited one, and one that within the framework of Figure 2.5 may be self-evident. The health of individuals and populations is affected by their health care, but also by other factors as well. Expansion of the health care system uses up resources that would otherwise be available to address those other factors. (Whether they would be so used or not, is another matter, which is taken up in Chapter 8.) It follows that an expansion of the health care system may have negative effects on health. A *health* policy, as opposed to policies for *health care,* would have to take account of this balance.

The qualification, however, arises from the fact that when we speak of the health of a population, we are aggregating across all the individuals in it. Different policies benefit different individuals. A decision to reallocate resources from health care to other health-enhancing or productivity-enhancing activities might indeed result in a population that was in aggregate both healthier and wealthier, but particular individuals in it would be worse off. Most clearly, of course, these will include persons who either make or intended to make their living from the provision of health care. But in addition, health care services respond to the circumstances of identified individuals, in the present. A more limited commitment of resources to health care might leave such persons worse off, even though in future there would be fewer of such persons.

Such trade-offs, between the interests of those who are now ill and those who may become so, may be inevitable. In any case it is important to note their possibility, because they are hidden from view in the aggregate framework. But conversely, it should also be noted that there is no obvious ethical, much less prudential, basis for resolving this trade-off in favour of more health care. We need to be clear as to whether we have, as a community, undertaken a collective obligation of concern, and support, for each other's *health,* or only for those aspects of health that can be enhanced through *health care*. If the latter, we may find that we are as a society both poorer, and less healthy, than we could otherwise be, and we may want to rethink the details of our (self-imposed) ethical obligation. The need for such rethinking, and the capacity to act upon it, varies markedly from one society to another.

In this context, as in so many others, the Japanese experience is startling, and may provide an illustration of the feedback loop from prosperity to health included in Figure 2.5. The extraordinary economic performance of Japanese society is not a new observation; the phenomenon goes back forty years, and indeed a similar period of extraordinary modernization and growth began after the Meiji restoration in 1868. What is new is that within the last decade Japan has begun to shift from the very successful copying of innovations elsewhere in the world, to being increasingly on the leading edge of both economic growth and technological change.

Over the same period there has been a remarkable growth in Japanese life expectancy, which in the 1980s has caught up with and then surpassed that of the rest of the developed world (Marmot and Smith, 1989). Like the Japanese economy and per capita wealth, average life expectancy is continuing to rise on a significantly faster trend than in other industrialized countries. This experience is now setting new standards for the possible in human populations.

On the other hand, Japanese health care absorbs one of the lowest shares of national income in the industrialized world, and has been described by a recent American observer as "an anachronism" in the context of modern Japanese society (Iglehart, 1988). And the popular external image is that life in Japan is very crowded, highly stressful, and quite polluted. How then does one explain the extraordinary trends in life expectancy?

One causal pattern suggested in Figure 2.5 would lead from extraordinary economic performance, to rapid growth in personal incomes and in the scope and variety of life, to the greatly enhanced sense of individual and collective self-esteem and hope for the future. A number of observers, concerned not with comparative health status but with international economic competitiveness, have noted the extraordinary Japanese sense of self-confidence and pride arising from their rapid progress toward world economic leadership. Individually and as a nation the Japanese are seeing themselves as harder-working, brighter, richer, and just plain better than the rest of the world. Could this attitude be yielding health benefits as well?

Conversely, the formerly centrally planned economies of Eastern Europe and the Soviet Union had on most measures of economic success performed dismally for many years, to the extent that their rulers as well as their populations were willing to undertake a massive and indeed revolutionary political restructuring. Corresponding to this extended period of economic decline, measures of life expectancy in those nations were stagnant or even falling, in marked contrast to the universal improvements in Western Europe (Hertzman, 1990).

Uncontrolled environmental pollution and unhealthy life-styles are commonly cited explanations, and are certainly part of the explanation. But the observation is at least consistent with the hypothesis of a relationship between collective self-esteem and health—a relationship that could be expressed through unhealthy life-styles.

The factors underlying the shift in world economic leadership are no doubt complex and diverse. One of several recurring explanatory themes, however, is the Japanese advantage in access to low-cost long-term capital, which is channeled into both research and development, and plant and equipment investment embodying the latest technology. This low-cost capital is generated by the very high savings rates of the Japanese people. The U.S., by contrast, has an exceedingly low savings rate, and now relies heavily on savings borrowed from the rest of the world—particularly Japan.

To maintain a high savings rate, one must limit the growth of other claims on public and private resources—such as health care.[25] The difference between Japanese and United States rates of spending on health care amounts to over 5 percent of national income and could account for a significant proportion of the large difference between Japanese and American aggregate savings rates. (The difference in military spending accounts for another large share.)

One can then speculate that by limiting the growth of their health care sector, the Japanese have freed up resources that were devoted to capital investment, both physical and intellectual. The consequent rapid growth in prosperity, particularly relative to their leading competitors, has greatly enhanced (already well developed) national and individual self-esteem, which has in turn contributed to a remarkable improvement in health.

It must be emphasized that this is a rough sketch of a possible argument, not a well-developed case, much less a "proof." There are other candidate explanations for Japanese longevity—diet, for example, or prenatal care, or the peculiar characteristics of Japanese society that may be protective against the ill effects of stress. (On the other hand, there are different forms of stress, and the stress of success is much less threatening to health than the stress of frustration and failure.)

Equally problematic, there is good evidence that environmental effects on morbidity and mortality may operate with very long lags, so that present Japanese life expectancies may reflect factors at work over the past fifty years. And in any case, what has been observed is that the Japanese live a long time. Whether they are relatively healthy in any more comprehensive sense is another matter. But the Japanese gains in life expectancy are occurring across the whole age spectrum, with both the world's lowest infant mortality, and extended lives among the elderly.

Whatever the explanation, it is clear that something very significant is happening (or has happened) in Japan—something reflected in trends in life expectancy that are remarkable relative to any other world experience. These observations are at least consistent with the rough sketch above. A good deal of closer investigation would seem warranted.

It is not our intent in this paper to lay "the Decline of the West" at the feet of the health care system of the United States, or even those of North America and Western Europe combined. Rather our point is to show that the framework laid out in Figure 2.5 is capable of permitting such a relationship to be raised for consideration. Its network of linkages between health, health care, the production of wealth, and the well-being of the population are sufficiently developed to encompass the question, without overwhelming and paralyzing one in the "dependence of everything upon everything."

FRAMEWORKS IN PRINCIPLE AND IN PRACTICE

The test of this framework will be the extent to which others find it useful as a set of categories for portraying complex causal patterns. The understanding of the determinants of a population's health, and the discussion, formulation, and evaluation of health policies, have been seriously impeded by the perpetuation of the incomplete, obsolete, and misleading framework of Figure 2.1. There is a bigger picture, but clearer understanding, and particularly a more sensible and constructive public discussion, of it requires the development of a more adequate intellectual framework. The progression to Figure 2.5 is offered as a possible step along the way.

In this chapter we have suggested several important features of such a framework. It should accommodate distinctions among disease, as defined and treated by the health care system, health and functioning, as perceived and experienced by individuals, and well-being, a still broader concept to which health is an important, but not the only, contributor. It should build on the Lalonde health field framework to permit and encourage a more subtle and more complex consideration of both behavioural and biological responses to social and physical environments.

Finally, it should recognize and foster explicit identification of the economic trade-offs involved in the allocation of scarce resources to health care instead of other activities of value to individuals and societies, activities that may themselves contribute to health and well-being.

To date, health care policy has in most societies dominated health policy-making, because of its greater immediacy and apparently more secure scientific base. One may concede in principle the picture in Figure 2.5, then convert all the lines of causality into "disease" and "health and function" into thin dotted ones, except for a fat black one from "health care." That is the picture implicit in the current emphasis in health policy, despite the increasing concern among health researchers as to the reliability and primacy of the connection from health care to health.

One lesson from international experience in the post-Lalonde era is that appropriate conceptualization of the determinants of health is a necessary but not a sufficient condition for serious reform of health policy. Intellectual frameworks, including the one offered here, are only a beginning. Simply put, to be useful, they must be used. The chapters of this book represent an attempt to do so.

ACKNOWLEDGMENTS

We wish to thank colleagues in the CIAR Population Health Program, the Health Polinomics Research Workshop at McMaster University, and the Health Policy Research Unit at the University of British Columbia for stimulating comments on earlier versions of this paper. We take responsibility for remaining errors or omissions.

NOTES

1. The language varies from one country to another. In Canada, *medical care* usually refers to the services of physicians, while *health care* includes hospitals, dentists, drugs, etc. In the United States, *medical care* and *health care* are used interchangeably to refer to this latter, broader range of activities, which in Sweden are termed *sickness care* (*sjukvard*).

2. The rhetoric of "prevention" has penetrated the health care system to a significant degree; reactive responses to identified departures from health may be labelled secondary or tertiary prevention insofar as they prevent further deterioration of an adverse condition. But even when components of the health care system move from a reactive to a promotive strategy—screening for cholesterol, for example, or hypertension—the interventions still consist of identifying departures from clinically determined norms for particular biological measure-

ments, and initiating therapeutic interventions. Elevated blood pressure or serum cholesterol measurements become themselves identified as "diseases," to be "cured."

3. The representation of mental illness is always troublesome: Where is the borderline between clinical depression and the "normal" human portion of unhappiness? The difficulty of definition persists, however, across the whole continuum; the WHO definition of health does not imply perpetual bliss.

4. This does not represent a rejection of rational modes of enquiry; the universe is still seen as, on some levels, a comprehensible and orderly place. But there appear to be fundamental limits on its comprehensibility—not just on our ability to comprehend it—and the relevant concepts of order may also be less complete than was once hoped. Whether or not Nietzsche turns out to be right about the death of God (Hawking, 1988), Laplace's Demon appears definitely defunct (Dreyfus and Dreyfus, 1988; Gleick, 1987; Holton, 1988).

5. The actual interventions themselves may be very far from transparent; "medical miracles" are an everyday occurrence, and the processes are presented as beyond the capacity or ken of ordinary mortals. But the application of a high degree of science and skill is still within the conceptually simple framework of a mechanical model: fixing the damaged part.

6. To the extent that overt policy does recognize this process, it tends to respond with marketing activities encouraging people to seek care. A surprising proportion of so-called health promotion includes various forms of "see your doctor" messages, and might more accurately be called "disease promotion." Measures to encourage "informal" coping should inter alia include recommendations *not* to contact the health care system in particular circumstances; the latter are virtually unheard of.

7. The experience of the United States is a clear demonstration of the distinction between the resource and administrative/financial dimensions of access. The United States devotes a much larger share of its national resources to producing health care than does any other nation, and spends much more per capita (Schieber and Poullier, 1989; OECD Secretariat, 1989). Yet the peculiarities of its financing system result in severely restricted (or no) access for a substantial minority of its citizens. On the other hand, nominally universal "access" to a system with grossly inadequate resources would be equally misleading.

8. Providers of care, particularly nurses, often emphasize their caring functions. The point here is not at all that caring is without importance or value, but rather that it is by no means the exclusive preserve of providers of health care. Furthermore, the "social contract" by which members of a particular community undertake collective (financial) responsibility for each other's health narrowly defined does not necessarily extend to responsibility for their happiness. "Caring" independently of any contemplated "curing," or at least prevention of deterioration, represents an extension of the "product line"—and sales revenue—of the health care system. If collective buyers of these services, public or private, have never in fact agreed to this extension, its ethical basis is rather shaky.

9. Best attainable health begs the question of by what *means* health may be attained. A hypothetical situation in that the members of a population had each received all the health *care* that might benefit them might nevertheless be one in which the population fell well short of attainable health because other measures outside the health care system were neglected.

10. A classic example has been provided by the response of paediatrics to the

collapse of the baby boom in the mid-1960s. The "new paediatrics"—social and emotional problems of adolescents—was discovered just in time to prevent underemployment. At the other end of the paediatric age range, progress in neonatology will ensure a growing supply of very low birth weight babies surviving into childhood, with a complex array of medical problems requiring intervention. An equally dramatic example is provided by dentistry. The declining incidence of dental caries has led, not to unemployment among general dentists, but to the emergence of new forms of caring for the mouth. We do not suggest that these system responses are the result of conscious and deliberate self-seeking by providers; such is almost certainly not the case. But the outcome is what it is.

11. The quotes are needed because the health care system, and the people in it, are not simply an "industry" in the sense of a set of activities and actors motivated solely by economic considerations. But to the extent that they are—and it is undeniable that economic considerations *do* matter, even if they are not the exclusive motivations—then this observation holds.

12. If building environmental standards were set by fuel supply companies, would we have similar problems with the regulation of thermostats?

13. The rhetoric of "cost crises" rarely if ever recognizes an extremely important distinction between expenditures or outlays and the economist's concept of resource or opportunity costs. Expenditures on health care may rise (fall) either because more (fewer) resources of human time, effort, and skills, capital equipment, and raw materials are being used in its production, or because the owners of such resources are receiving larger (smaller) payments for them—higher (lower) salaries, fees, or prices. The arrow from health care to disease represents a response in the form of actual goods and services provided—real resources. But much of the public debate over underfunding and cost crises is really about the relative incomes of providers of care, not about the amount and type of care provided. For obvious political reasons, income claims are frequently presented as if they were assertions about levels of care (Evans, 1984, Chapter 1; Reinhardt, 1987).

14. There might still, however, be quite justifiable interest in the patterns of prices and incomes generated by such care (see note 13). A competitive marketplace can generate intense pressures that automatically control prices and incomes, as the computer example has demonstrated. Health care, however, is nowhere provided through such a market (not even in the United States), and has not been for at least a hundred years. There are excellent reasons for this (e.g., Evans, 1984; Culyer, 1982), and the situation is not in fact going to change in the foreseeable future. It follows that other mechanisms, with associated controversy, will remain necessary to address issues of income distribution.

15. *Not* nonexistent. There is no basis in ethical theory or institutional practice for the proposition that creeps into so much of normative economics, that individual choice is the ultimate and even the only ground of obligation (Etzioni, 1988).

16. We do not mean to imply that the authors of the white paper had the relatively limited view that we present below, still less that all of their subsequent interpreters have been so intellectually constrained. But it is our perception that the principal impact of the white paper framework on debates about, and the development of, health policy *has* been limited in the way we describe.

17. None of which is news to tobacco marketers.

18. One should note, however, that the very limited experience in the early

1970s with *antismoking* advertising on television appeared to be sufficiently successful that tobacco companies were willing voluntarily to abandon this medium in order to get the "opposition" off the air.

19. Wilkins, Adams, and Brancker (1989) and Wolfson, Rose, Gentleman, and Tomiak (1990) provide recent Canadian data.

20. One might point out that this is true of much therapy. Surgery, for example, typically has a very powerful negative effect on health and function in the immediate intervention and recovery phase, while (when successful) yielding later improvements. In the hypertension case, however, healthy individuals are introduced to prolonged low-level illness, in order to receive large but uncertain benefits in the farther future. Such a difference of degree becomes one of kind.

For people with short time horizons, painful or disabling interventions with longer term payoffs may not be justified. Elderly people, in particular, will quite rationally discount future benefits more heavily. The finding that elderly cancer patients are more likely to choose radiation treatment over surgery, even if the latter has a greater five-year survival rate (McNeil, Weichselbaum, and Pauker, 1978), illustrates the point. The enthusiasm among dentists to provide "optimum" oral health to residents of nursing homes raises similar concerns. Would you want to spend a day in a dentist's chair if you expected to die tomorrow? Next week? Next month? . . .

21. "Improved" nutrition is ambiguous. For impoverished and deprived populations better is simply more, and more nutritious. But for a high proportion of modern populations better is probably less, and particularly less fats. It is not clear when in the historical record "better" shifted from more to less, for the majority of industrialized populations, such that (from a health perspective) nutrition may have begun to deteriorate.

22. The operation was a success, but the patient died.

23. The common identification between private sector jobs as by definition "real" and public sector ones as "unreal" is, however, simply ideological nonsense—"real" and "unreal" exist in both sectors, wherever activity is being carried on with no output, or none of any value. It includes, but is not restricted to, the caricature of the lazy or obstructionist bureaucrat.

A strong argument can be made, for example, that most of the jobs in the private health insurance sector in the United States—complex, demanding, and highly paid—are not "real" jobs, because they actually yield nothing of value and in all other health care funding systems are dispensed with. That is, of course, another story, but one that emphasizes the invalidity of an equation between "unreal jobs" and "lazy public servants." One can have valuable skills, apply them hard and conscientiously, both individually and as a group, and yet be completely useless or even get in the way. Parallels with public bureaucracies in centrally planned economies are not inapt.

To the individual concerned, the symbolism of "real jobs" is extremely important. The hard-working farmer producing grain or butter, to be stockpiled at public expense, is in no doubt about the difficulty and worth of an effort. Yet the product cannot be sold—has no value.

24. Often, but not always. Improvements in the techniques of diagnostic imaging, for example, have reduced the degree of risk and distress associated with earlier forms of diagnostic imaging; and the substitution of lithotripsy for kidney surgery has yielded similar benefits. On the other hand, less risky or uncomfortable procedures tend to be offered to many more patients.

25. It would, of course, be quite possible for a nation to maintain both high savings rates and high spending on health care—or the military—simply by cutting back on consumption. But there is strong resistance at both bargaining table and ballot box to a reduction in current consumption through higher taxes or lower wages. Citizens do not want to accept a reduction in present living standards to pay for more health care.

A neoclassical economist might argue that the living standard is *not* reduced; what is given up in smaller houses, poorer roads, or fewer electronic gadgets is gained in more cardiac bypass grafts, laboratory tests, MRI procedures, and months in nursing homes. But the average individual is, quite rightly, unconvinced. Health care, like military spending, is not valued for its own sake. What, after all, are the direct satisfactions from a tonsillectomy or a tank? Each is simply a regrettable use of resources, a service for which in a better world one would have no need. Hence the tendency for health spending increases to be drawn from savings, whether through government budget deficits or reduced corporate retained earnings.

II

3

Heterogeneities in Health Status and the Determinants of Population Health

C. HERTZMAN, J. FRANK and R. G. EVANS

As noted in Chapter 1, human populations display marked diversity in their patterns of health and disease. This diversity is not simply a consequence of the trivial observation that "every individual is different." Individual variations can be canceled out by aggregation; but there are also significant differences between entire populations, or among subgroups of "the same" population. And these differences in health status—life expectancy, for example, or functional capacity, injury rates, or the incidence or prevalence of particular illnesses—can be correlated with other distinguishing characteristics of those populations or subgroups.

Of particular interest is that there are ways of partitioning populations that consistently define subgroups differing greatly and systematically in their average health status. For instance, large gradients in life expectancy by income level, educational attainment, and social class have been repeatedly discovered in various parts of the developed world during the twentieth century. Higher status is consistently associated with longer life. Moreover this association holds across most major disease processes; as noted in Chapter 1, it appears to reflect some more general effect that expresses itself through particular diseases. But there are obviously many other characteristics that when used as a basis for partitioning a population, also yield groups differing markedly in their aggregate health status.

We use the term *heterogeneities* to refer to differences in aggregate measures of health status between or among population groups, which appear to be consistently associated with some defining characteristics of those groups. Such differences, particularly when associated with differences in income or social class, are commonly referred to as *inequalities* or *inequities* in health—which of course they are. But the term *heterogeneity* is somewhat less value-laden. It encompasses variations in health status that do not necessarily have a normative dimension—those between males and females, for example. In a world of genetic diversity, there is no presumption that under ideal conditions, heterogeneity as we have defined it would disappear.[1]

These heterogeneities represent more than an academic curiosity. Their study can provide insights into the fundamental determinants of health status. And these in turn should contribute to formulating public policies to enhance health.

We have already identified in Chapter 1 some of the more intriguing observations indicating the great diversity of factors influencing the health of human populations. In Chapter 2 we developed a conceptual framework that enabled us to trace the different classes of factors at work. The framework highlights features of the social and physical environment, the genetic endowment and the learned biological and behavioural responses of the individual, and access to and responses of the health care system, and suggests how they might interact. But that framework was presented at quite a high level of generality; each of its conceptual categories or "boxes" contained many different specific factors on which one might assemble evidence and test hypotheses. The progress from such a framework to understanding of causal relationships securely based in empirical evidence—what one would like to know when making policy—requires a great deal of additional work.

Much of this work consists of the assembly and evaluation of evidence, which comes in many forms, from many sources. Some of that evidence, but only a small part of it, is dealt with elsewhere in this volume. But as Wolfson points out in Chapter 11, much of it does not yet exist. Generating more information relevant to the health of populations is a major research enterprise for the future. As Wolfson quotes the WHO, "The road leading to Health For All by the Year 2000 passes through information."

But how to handle this mammoth "assembly and evaluation" task? In this chapter we offer another type of conceptual scheme for classifying the range of different factors influencing health status, and assessing their relative importance. It is not an alternative to the framework in the previous chapter. Rather it is a type of intellectual tool—which is all any conceptual scheme can be—with which to organize the process of filling the boxes of Chapter 2 and measuring the signs and strengths of their interconnections. Considering the massive amount of potentially relevant information, we believe that the use of some such tool is likely to be a good deal more effective than trying to work with one's "bare hands."

We demonstrate the use of our "assembly and evaluation" scheme with emphasis on differences in health status across socioeconomic classes. But we are also able to represent explicitly the various ways in which the effects of different influences on human health unfold over the life cycle. This is of particular importance for those determinants of health status that long precede their effects.

Finally, we review the implications of this framework for the direction and conduct of health research intended to inform public policy. The ultimate objectives of this chapter and of this book are both understanding and effective action, to assist social and health policymakers to address the fundamental determinants of health status in formulating public policies designed to enhance health.

In Chapter 1 we identified several common themes that emerged from consideration of a diverse array of intriguing observations of heterogeneities in health. A number of these observations link health and socioeconomic status.

Marmot's studies of U.K. civil servants, for example (Marmot, 1986; Marmot, Kogevinas, and Elston, 1987), found health differentials that were *unambiguous and large* (three-to-one differences in standardized mortality rates) and that showed a *gradient* across groups—linked to hierarchy per se, *not* to deprivation. Nor could these differentials be explained as simply the consequences of differences in life-style "choices" or other conventional risk factors, although life-styles do indeed vary with one's position in the hierarchy. And finally the gradient was found for many different diseases as causes of death, indicating a *common underlying factor or factors*.

Marmot's findings support those of the most widely known study of class and health, the Black report, which presented data from the U.K. Office of Population Censuses and Surveys (OPCS) showing large and persistent differences in mortality by socioeconomic class over the whole U.K. population. But Marmot's data have the important strength of being *population based and person specific* (Chapter 11), thus escaping some of the methodological criticisms leveled at the Black report.

The OPCS data, however, span much of the twentieth century. They thus demonstrate the stability of the gradient despite massive changes in the extent, effectiveness, and accessibility of health care. The observation that the mortality gradient did not respond to changes in medical care is the obverse of McKeown's findings, that the dramatic declines in deaths from particular infectious diseases over the nineteenth and early twentieth centuries occurred in the *absence* of any effective medical therapy.

While the relative contributions to this decline of nutrition, child spacing/family size, housing, and public sanitation are much debated (McKeown, 1979; Reeves, 1985), the (non-) role of medical care remains clear-cut. Life expectancy at birth increased in many now "developed" countries, roughly from forty to sixty years, with little assistance from individual patient treatment or medically delivered prevention aimed at specific diseases. Socioeconomic factors, broadly defined, have a major effect not only on the relative health of groups within a population, but on the health of "the same" population at different points in time.

This is not to say that medical care is ineffective: McKeown's work in historical epidemiology quite clearly *does* show the effects of improvements in medical therapy and in public health on certain diseases. But it demonstrates the limits to the effects of medical intervention on populations—a theme taken up by Roos and Roos in Chapter 9—and the extraordinarily powerful effects, from a long-term perspective, of factors external to the health care system.

For populations over time, as for population groups at a point in time, these "other factors" are associated with income and wealth. But they do not reflect simply the presence or absence of poverty and deprivation. Recall the dramatic improvements that have taken place in Japanese life expectancy in recent decades; precisely the opposite has occurred in the stagnant societies of Eastern Europe. There, life expectancy has actually fallen (Jozan, 1990). But in neither setting has there been a major shift out of or into poverty in an absolute sense.

The way in which income is distributed and used in a society may be more important than its average level. Marmot and Davey Smith (1989) note that Japan has not only the fastest rate of GNP growth of any OECD country, but also the smallest relative difference between the average incomes of the richest and the poorest 20 percent of the population. Cross-national comparisons of income distributions are difficult, but developed countries show rather strong correlations between the degree to which national income is equitably distributed and average health status (Wilkinson, 1992).

Certainly populations of some less developed countries are much healthier than those in others with similar per capita incomes (Caldwell, 1986). Costa Rica, Sri Lanka, and Kerala state in India, for example, have about the same average level of income as Pakistan, Afghanistan, and Morocco. Yet the infant mortality rates for the former group average 64 per 1,000 live births, compared with 173 in the latter. Average life expectancy is 61 years in the first group, 45 in the second.

The difference seems to be that the countries with better health status have placed a greater emphasis on the importance of women and children in their culture and social environment, and in their social policies.

Several observers have suggested that it is only when women are sufficiently educated to experience some sense of control over their lives and those of their children (e.g., by being able to achieve child spacing) that infant and child mortality rates really begin to fall (Caldwell, 1986; Caldwell and Caldwell, 1991).

These examples show that major shifts in the health status of whole populations over time do not necessarily depend upon the implementation of public health or medical control measures against specific diseases. They point instead to a profound linkage between health and the social environment, including the levels and distribution of prosperity in a society.

Other studies focus our attention on early life experiences. A longitudinal study of all children born on the Hawaiian island of Kauai during 1955 found that the early childhood developmental problems associated with severe perinatal stress were counteracted over time in families of high socioeconomic status or stability, but not in unstable families or those of low socioeconomic status (Werner and Smith 1982).

A long-term follow-up of an early childhood enrichment program in an inner-city ghetto in the United States demonstrated that at age nineteen the intervention group were much better off than the controls. More graduated from high school and went on to college; less than half as many were ever classified as mentally retarded; 40 percent fewer were ever arrested or detained; 50 percent more were employed; 45 percent fewer were on welfare; and they had only half as many teenage pregnancies (Schweinhart, Berrueta-Clement, Barnett, Epstein, and Weikart, 1985).

Martin, Ramey, and Ramey (1990) recently found that very early educational day care (starting between six and twelve weeks of age) protected children at high risk for intellectual impairment, especially those with mentally retarded mothers. At six months, all study children with retarded mothers had "normal" IQ scores; by age four and one-half, all of those children in the educational day care program were still evaluated as normal, while 86 percent of the "controls" had slipped below the normal ranges. Overall, only 7 percent of the study children were below normal at four and one-half, compared with 31 percent of those not provided with educational day-care.

Such studies highlight the critical role of early experience in influencing health and well-being over the course of the life cycle. They show that the impact of such experience goes well beyond the very narrowly defined "outcome"—mortality—compared in the larger population studies. Psychological and social performance measures also show heterogeneity. And, optimistically, they suggest the possibility of effective interventions in these domains—interventions by changing and enriching the social environment rather than through more traditional medical or public health measures.

THE NEED FOR A BROAD CONCEPTUAL FRAMEWORK

Taken together, these observations argue strongly against the view that the health of a population can be explained entirely in terms of the characteristics of individuals—biological, psychological, or otherwise. The whole is clearly different from the simple sum of the parts. The advantage of a broad analytic framework for understanding the determinants of health is that it allows impartial "lateral" consideration of a full range of causal hypotheses.

As an example, years of schooling is associated with a reduced risk of developing dementia in old age. At least one investigator has been troubled by the observation that the variable "years of schooling" seems to "confound" the measured performance of elderly individuals on mental status examinations (Berkman, 1986). The conventional view is that these examinations are less reliable for well-educated subjects, who are better able to "mask" the less severe forms of dementia by clever exam-writing tricks.

A compelling alternative hypothesis, however, is that education somehow conditions the brain to resist the physiological processes that lead to dementia, producing biochemical changes or altered neuro-anatomic networks in the brain, which might be directly protective against later dysfunction. The former view treats education as a "nuisance variable," which interferes with the ascertainment of a "hard" pathological outcome. The latter challenges the medical construct of dementia as a purely biological disease process and of education as a purely "social" exposure. It suggests that serious dysfunction in some of today's elderly may reflect social and educational policy failures decades ago.

Both views may hold some truth. But the prospect of linking health status to such policies is not readily accommodated within the prevailing medical framework for conceptualizing the determinants of health. Thus important policy implications of research into the causes of dementia, and many other illnesses, may be ignored if the emphasis in such research is entirely on narrowly disease-based models of causation.

Our framework for representing heterogeneities in population health status is presented as a cube (Figure 3.1), with the three axes representing three key dimensions for analysis. These are labeled:

- stages of the life cycle
- subpopulation partitions
- sources of heterogeneity.

Each of these dimensions is in turn divided into discrete levels. Any combination of individual levels forms a box or cell within the overall cube. The cells in the front face of the cube record the variation in average health status, by stage in the life cycle, across the subpopulations defined by partitioning a given population according to a particular characteristic. The successive vertical slices behind the front face then attribute this variation according to its possible sources.

As an illustration, socioeconomic status would be represented by a layer of the cube, or a row of the front face. A single cell from this row would then contain data on the relationship between various measures of health status and of socioeconomic status, for a particular stage of the

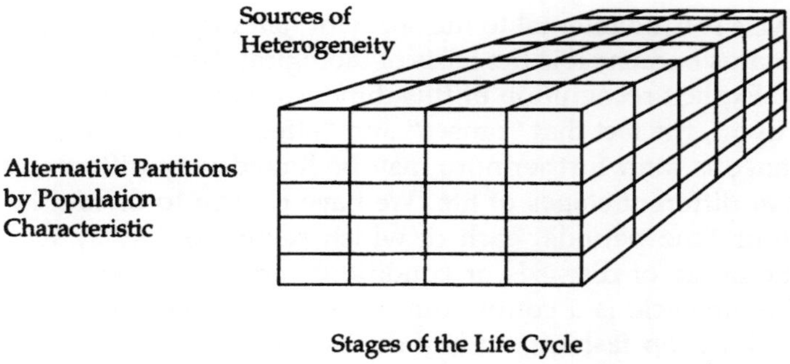

Stages of the Life Cycle	*Characteristics*	*Sources of Heterogeneity*
1. Perinatal: preterm to 1 year	1. Socioeconomic status	1. Reverse causality
2. Misadventure: 1–44 years	2. Ethnicity/migration	2. Differential susceptibility
3. Chronic disease: 45–74 years	3. Geographic	3. Individual life-style
4. Senescence: 75+ years	4. Male/female	4. Physical environment
	5. Special populations	5. Social environment
		6. Differential access to/ response to health care services

Figure 3.1. Model for investigation of heterogeneities in population health status.

life cycle, e.g., perinatal death rate or standardized mortality between the ages of fifteen and forty-five, by income quintile.

The dimensions of the cube were chosen to organize data on heterogeneities in population health, in order to use them more effectively as clues to the determinants of health status at the individual level. They do not purport to constitute a general model of health and disease. In particular, they presuppose a measure or measures of health status that can be established for any subpopulation at each stage of the life cycle. For example, perinatal mortality rates can be seen to refer, for any given subpopulation, to a well-defined life cycle stage. An observation of differential perinatal mortality rates across subpopulations in any society ("partitions"—which might be geographic, ethnic, socioeconomic, etc.) can then arise from a number of alternative sources.

Stages of the Life Cycle

The life cycle is fundamental to the study of heterogeneities in *population* health status because it is the basis of biological change in *individuals* as they age. Explicit recognition of this dimension enables us to reflect, and reflect upon, the fact that "causes" and "effects" are not necessarily contemporaneous, and furthermore may be linked very differently for individuals at different stages of life. We have chosen to divide the life cycle into four time periods, each of which seems to display its own characteristic range of diseases or conditions, and vulnerabilities. Admittedly, the life cycle is a continuum, and human development does not occur in lockstep fashion, so any division into discrete stages will create distortions. There is always room for argument about the precise age cutoffs and the number of divisions that should be used; and different diseases—and populations—will display different patterns. But we believe that our four stages are broadly representative of human populations and their ills.

The *perinatal* period is a subdivision of the life cycle so important, and with such steep mortality gradients globally and historically, that its statistics have often been used as major indicators of the overall health of entire populations (e.g., perinatal mortality rates and birth weight distributions).

If one survives unscathed this period of relatively high vulnerability, one enters the period of *misadventure*, which extends from less than one year of age to middle-age—roughly the midforties. During this time, the principal threats to health in industrialized countries are not disease based but rather accidents, violence, and suicide. The external threat of infectious disease in early life (with the important exception of AIDS) has been largely eliminated, due in part to the past success of public health measures. But the historical disappearance of these sources of mortality has thrown into more prominent relief the residuum in young persons of congenitally acquired disease, or predisposition-to-disease, which may result from either *in utero* or perinatal exposures, or genetic mechanisms. The prevalence of these conditions has also been increased by improvements in their treatment, which have lengthened the lives of their victims. Examples include cystic fibrosis, spina bifida, cerebral palsy, and asthma.

From forty-five to seventy-four years is termed the period of "premature" *chronic degenerative disease*. During this period, specific diagnostic entities like heart disease, stroke, cancer, and arthritis are the principal threats to health, function, and life. We use the term *degenerative* not to indicate predestination or inevitability, but to highlight the fact that previous decades of "wear and tear" (as well as a "rich" diet, lack of exercise, smoking, etc.) are significant causal influences here. In developed countries, these chronic conditions are so prevalent in the final years of life, usually in the next age range, that one may rightly term "premature" their occurrence by midlife. This premature occurrence reflects an accelerated natural history in some individuals, often due to adverse life-style exposures over preceding decades, acting in concert with particular genetic susceptibilities.

We have identified the age of seventy-five as the onset of more generalized senescence. Here health status is often determined by the late and usually less specific effects of more than one chronic degenerative disease process, leading to multiple organ system dysfunction. It may often, therefore, be difficult or impossible to assign an unambiguous single cause of disability or death.

Population Partitions

A population can be partitioned according to any number of different characteristics. But the interesting partitions are those which consistently demonstrate clear heterogeneity of health status across their subgroups in many diverse settings. Socioeconomic status, for example, has been represented by dividing a population into quintiles based on income, occupation, or education (or combinations thereof). A number of studies have found significant gradients in life and health expectancy across such quintiles (Hertzman, 1986). These gradients have persisted over decades despite major public policy initiatives, in both health and social services, aimed at reducing them (Davey Smith et al., 1990). Each basis for partition would be represented by a row or layer in the cube;

other partitions defining additional layers might include gender, ethnicity/migration, geographic location, and isolation of various "special populations."

Special populations are those which are not defined by particular values of some general characteristic—location, say, or gender or class—displayed in different ways by each member of the population. Rather members of such a subpopulation share some special characteristics peculiar to their group, which are expressed through, or at least correlated with, especially marked health status differentials. Aboriginal peoples, for example, in Canada and elsewhere, display markedly unfavourable patterns of health status (Schaefer, 1981; Millar, 1981). On the other hand, certain groups with "unusual life-styles"—Mormons, Seventh-Day Adventists, vegetarians—are known to have unusually good health, on average.

Sources of Heterogeneity

Observed heterogeneities in health status can arise through several different causal pathways or mechanisms operating across different population partitions and stages of the life cycle. The Black report (Black, Morris, Smith, and Townsend, 1982) identified four possible "explanations" for the large social class differentials in mortality observed in Britain: artifact, selection, material factors, and cultural factors. The effect of that classification was to stimulate debate about the relative importance of each explanation, because each has radically different implications for how one might think about the determinants of health and disease, and about policies to address them (West, 1991).

The six "explanations" in our model begin from those in the Black report, and are motivated by the same desire to understand the determinants of health in a way that will be relevant to policy formulation. But they are meant to apply more generally, to all possible population partitions and not just social class. We seek also to represent a broader range of potential determinants of health than those suggested in the Black report.

1. *Reverse causality*. The classic example of this is the "selective drift" hypothesis, the claim that mortality differentials by income level can be explained by the fact that the sick become poor, not that the poor become sick (Carr-Hill, 1987). The form of explanation, "If population characteristic X is correlated with sickness, that is because sick people develop characteristic X, not because X causes sickness," can be offered for a number of observed heterogeneities, but not all. Geographic varia-

tions might arise because the sick stay home while the healthy emigrate, for example, but differentials associated with gender, special populations, or ethnicity are not readily explained in this way.

To the extent that reverse causality "explains" observed health differentials across a particular partition, it reduces the plausibility of the associated characteristic as a *determinant* of health, and thus undermines support for policies to address it. But while reverse causality is easy to allege, it has been difficult to find in the longitudinal population studies, which are the best study design for establishing its occurrence (West, 1991). (Chronic mental illness is an exception to this generalization.)

2. *Differential susceptibility.* In the Black report, the explanatory category "selection" actually combined two different processes: selective drift (described above) and another described by West (1991) as "a process of sorting or allocation of individuals with different health potentials via the educational/training/occupational complex into an achieved (occupational) social class" (pp. 375–76). In general, one's potential for being discriminated against (e.g., on the basis of appearance or height) influences both health status and the subgroup a person reaches within a population partition.[2] For instance, height is known to be a predictor of intergenerational social class mobility in Britain, and perhaps of health status as well.

Several explanations have been offered for this phenomenon. Height might be a marker for genetic fitness, which is in turn a predictor of upward social mobility. Alternatively, height differences within a social class (as identified at birth) might reflect the level of well-being in the early childhood environment, which again predicts social mobility. Finally, taller people may be perceived as being more attractive than shorter people and therefore throughout life gain progressive educational and occupational advantages that are key ingredients of upward mobility. There is, in fact, substantial evidence that, unlike reverse causality, differential susceptibility may be important in explaining heterogeneities in population health status by social class (West, 1991).

3. *Individual life-style.* This category represents the effects of differences in specific health habits and behaviours on the average health status of persons in different subgroups of a population. The observation that heterogeneities in health status are associated with differences in the relative frequency of known risky or unhealthy behaviours (smoking, obesity, drunken driving, etc.) can, like the assertion of reverse causality, be used to close off discussion or divert policy attention from the heterogeneities themselves. After all, "It's a free country," and "They chose their life-styles."

But there are a number of different pathways that may lead to differences in health habits. "Free" (informed, deliberate, unconstrained) choice is not the only or even the most plausible explanation for marked differences in average life-style patterns *between large groups*. Health habits may be conditioned by the social environment of the individual, whose behaviour then constitutes a "host response" to environmental stimuli (see Chapter 2). Such social environmental risk factors can then operate to produce a pattern of negative health habits in a particular subgroup, greatly influencing their average health status.

Indeed, the correlation between unhealthy environments and unhealthy individual "behaviours" can lead to (upward) biases in measures of the importance of such behaviours. It has recently been shown, for instance, that failing to consider confounding by socioeconomic factors can lead to overestimating the strength of the relationship between smoking and mortality (Davey Smith and Shipley, 1991). Smoking is inversely associated with status, education, and income. But these factors have an independent negative correlation with mortality even in the absence of smoking. If they are not separately controlled for, their effects will be inappropriately attributed to smoking.

The cube framework permits us to take this point a stage further, by transforming the concept of life-style from an *individual* characteristic into an *average* characteristic of subgroups within the population. This allows us to consider what might otherwise be described as "socioeconomic confounding" as the central relationship, the "main effect" in some situations. The habit itself (smoking, or its absence) is then a "host response" to the socioeconomic environment, one of the pathways through which that environment exerts its influence.

4. *Physical environment.* This includes the potentially harmful effects of exposure to physical, chemical, and biological agents at home, at work, and anywhere else. For instance, if one partitions a population of workers according to their level of exposure to toxicants such as asbestos, some obvious heterogeneities in occupational disease rates emerge. But the "physical environment" can be interpreted more broadly. There is increasing evidence that the social structure of workplaces and the level of job demand and job discretion strongly influence workers' risks of heart disease and overall mortality rates (Marmot and Theorell, 1988). These job characteristics will be only partly reflected in the physical features of the workplace, so these influences might also be classified under the social environment.

5. *Social environment (and psychological response).* Here we include a diverse range of findings on the health effects of social support and isolation, emotional deprivation, stress and its relation to the learned coping capacity of the individual, and so on. Such notions encompass, broadly speaking, all aspects of social organization that might affect

health status. As an example, spousal bereavement and widowhood carries a clearly elevated mortality risk for some time after its occurrence. However, it is still unclear exactly what the protective factors are that mitigate such effects in some persons (House et al., 1988).

6. *Differential access to/response to health care services.* Heterogeneities in health status may result from systematic differences in care-seeking behaviour, in access to health services, or in availability of other resources or characteristics that influence the effectiveness of care. Also included here would be differential survival rates for a given disease when effective therapy has been provided. It is well known, for example, that disadvantaged blacks in the United States have a worse prognosis for hypertension, which may only partially be attributed to less adequate medical care (McCord and Freeman, 1990). Environmental factors, both social and physical, may be important, but one cannot completely rule out genetic differences in response to care.

ACCOUNTING FOR THE CORRELATES OF HEALTH: THE CASE OF SOCIOECONOMIC GRADIENTS

As noted above, higher socioeconomic status (SES), however measured, seems to be associated with better health, however measured. Certain diseases are important exceptions, correlating *positively* with higher status: breast cancer in developed countries, coronary heart disease in some newly industrialized societies. But these can be explained by marked differences in particular causal factors (such as lactation history, parity, or diet) across social groups. There are virtually no examples of societies in which the overall health status is (or was) inversely related to wealth, income, or social status.

The possible explanations for this association are precisely the six sources of heterogeneity arrayed along one axis of our cube (Figure 3.1). Quantifying the relative contribution of each would be an interesting study. Here, however, we wish to use the SES-health association to explore the connection between measures of health status, and the incidence or prevalence of particular diseases. If we accept that at least some part of the relationship between SES and health *is* causal, there remains the important question of the role played by particular diseases in linking more general characteristics of environments and life-styles with measures of health.

There appear to be two quite distinct perspectives on this question. One we may call the classical epidemiological view; the second does not (to our knowledge) have a satisfactory name as yet, but is essentially one in which specific diseases are not the centre of attention. We might call it the *generalized vulnerability* view.

From the classical epidemiological perspective, differences in SES are associated with differences in behaviour or environment that increase one's risk of particular diseases. People in lower SES groups are more likely to be exposed to pathogens. They are more likely to smoke, so have more heart and lung disease. They have lower incomes, and/or worse eating habits, so are less well fed, and suffer nutritional deficiencies. And so on. Differences in morbidity and mortality are thus seen as arising largely from specific disease processes.

It follows that if one could block the specific pathogenic mechanism, by immunization against infectious disease, for example, or taxation high enough to discourage smoking, then the SES differentials would be narrowed or eliminated. The phenomenon of heterogeneity could be successfully attacked in a reductionist way, by isolating particular diseases whose incidence and/or prevalence differs across SES groups, and then initiating curative or preventive measures against each of those diseases, or their specific risk factors—such as smoking.

This approach to improving the public's health—which accords with common sense—has gained classical epidemiology some tremendous victories. Improvements in basic sanitation toward the end of the last century, and arguably the more recent gains in the fight against stroke, coronary heart disease, and smoking-related illness, have their origins in this focus on disease-specific pathways. However, the historical data on health differentials by SES have some implications that are inconsistent with this point of view, and that suggest that it has inherent limitations.

The British data on mortality differences by social class, for example, indicate that these have been remarkably stable over decades—going back to the turn of the century (OPCS, 1972; Davey Smith et al., 1990). Yet the causes of death have clearly changed greatly over this time. People now die of very different things. But whatever people die of, poor people continue to die sooner.[3] Furthermore, in well-designed cohort studies with information at baseline about all suspected risk factors, adjusting for smoking, drinking, diet/serum-lipids, and other specific life-style differences across social class does not eliminate the overall SES health status gradient (Marmot et al., 1987; Davey Smith and Shipley, 1991).

These observations suggest that the factors responsible for SES and other differentials have more subtle and complex effects than can be represented by a direct connection between particular "causal" variables and particular diseases—smoking and lung cancer, for example. They suggest a more fundamental difference in "health" or "vitality," which expresses itself through risk gradients for most of whatever the currently predominant diseases might be. From this perspective, we would not necessarily expect that a successful campaign to eliminate smoking would reduce SES differentials for all-cause mortality (i.e., longevity per se). It might reduce or even eliminate the SES differentials in lung cancer or heart disease rates. However, if nothing else changed, the overall SES mortality differential would simply express itself through death due to some other disease entities.

Disease-based epidemiology borrows from the biomedical model, in two distinct and important ways. That model implicitly treats diagnostic labels as tightly attached to a well-defined underlying pathological state: either people do, or do not, have disease X. But in addition, this state is understood as resulting from an equally well-defined set of equally well-defined agents or events. The task of epidemiology is to identify these precursors.

For certain pathological states, such as fractured hip, this view is hard to challenge. Both the condition and the "agent" can be unambiguously labeled: The patient was hit by a truck, or fell on a patch of ice.[4] In other cases, such as advanced lung cancer or acute myocardial infarct, the diagnostic label is clear even if the underlying pathological determinants are not.

But it gets worse. A number of "patients" are not so easily or unambiguously labeled, and these appear to represent an increasing proportion of the workload of the health care system. From the generalized vulnerability perspective, they may simply have "something" wrong with them. The health care system and the rest of the society assign a label in accordance with current convention (or fashion) and formulate a corresponding therapeutic or palliative response.

SES differences might then underlie differences in the prevalence of "something wrong"; the particular label attached (e.g., "losing one's memory" versus "having early Alzheimer's disease") would depend on the current knowledge, perceptions, practices, and conventions in the health care system and surrounding society at the time. Alternatively, as in the case of heart disease, the labeling would not be context dependent, but this unambiguous end state might still have its origins in the generalized vulnerability associated with low status.

But the real problem, and it *is* real, is that underlying state of vulnerability that is expressed in various diseases. Its sources and remedies might be a more ultimately fruitful focus of study.

Indeed, the gradual demise of disease-based epidemiology, as a clue to the real determinants of population health status, may be forced upon us by the passage of time itself. Ironically, as developed societies "age," the vast majority of deaths and serious illness events become concentrated in the very elderly. Yet, as already noted, it is often impossible in such circumstances to assign a clear diagnostic label to the final illness process. Several interrelated failures of multiple organ systems are a better representation of what kills such patients. These persons have gone on for decades with subclinical damage to many anatomic sites by chronic diseases such as arteriosclerosis, when suddenly a modest event, such as the "flu," precipitates an overall "physiological crisis." The attribution of major illnesses and death at advanced age to specific diseases is often a futile academic exercise; the epidemiological statistics so generated are frequently unworthy of analysis.

Moreover, it can be argued that the study of serious physical illness and premature death, as health outcomes, becomes increasingly irrelevant in the extremely healthy populations of industrially advanced nations. This is because such events have become so rare, at least within the bulk of the population under seventy-five years of age, that they have limited social importance compared to the vastly more frequent and burdensome causes of human misery that are fundamentally nonmedical: underemployment, poverty, family stress, deviant behaviour, or failure of a loved one to succeed in one of life's main arenas (school, work, marriage, parenting, etc.). It is these conditions that affect at least 25–50 percent of the members of a modern industrialized population in any given year (S. M. Taylor, personal communication, 1990).

To spend a great deal of energy studying the causes of medically diagnosable disease and death—extremely rare events for all but the very elderly, in whom they are more or less inevitable and nonspecific—may not represent a very sensible definition of health-related research activity. Yet we find that the steadily growing effort and expense devoted to health care systems in industrialized societies is being increasingly concentrated on this smaller and smaller share of the population. This may not be unrelated to the growing sense of public dissatisfaction and unease with health care systems, in all developed societies—as reflected in almost universal calls for some degree of "reform," all across the political spectrum. Systems that increasingly focus on problems that most people do not have or that are not remediable, and in the process draw resources from relieving those problems they *do* have, may find their constituencies eroding (and with good reason).

TIME AND LATENCY

Time lays another serious trap in the way of understanding the determinants of health. The cube framework, as represented in Figure 3.1, explicitly includes time as one of its dimensions of classification. But it does not capture fully the complexity of the influence of time, and thus does not highlight the methodological problems it raises for studying the health of populations. As drawn, the cube appears to confine the effects of time to the stage of the life cycle at which heterogeneity is expressed. It does not explicitly focus attention on the dynamic nature of population health—i.e., on the relation between influences at one point in time, and their expression in health status at another, perhaps much later point—the general phenomenon of *latency*.

A Spectrum of Latencies

All causality unfolds through time. The critical question is, how much time? At one end of the spectrum are processes that involve such short response times as to appear almost instantaneous. The sources of heterogeneity in health status would then be contemporaneous with the observed heterogeneities themselves. For example, the Great London Fog of 1952 was followed within days by large increases in mortality from a number of different causes, not just cardiorespiratory diseases. Similarly, a recent study of mortality of persons with "unambiguously Jewish surnames" found lower-than-expected numbers of deaths (again from a variety of causes) in the week before Passover, a decline that did not appear in persons of other religious/ethnic groups (Phillips and King, 1988).[5]

These are clear demonstrations of phenomena with immediate effects on health. When we study heterogeneities in health status among subpopulations and attempt to correlate these with *contemporary* differences in the other circumstances of these populations (income, class, education, etc.), we are implicitly assuming either that these other circumstances have instantaneous effects or that they or their effects are strongly persistent through time.

Most health effects are not instantaneous. In particular, most relationships between social class and health status are likely to unfold over time. But this time may be of the order of fifty years or more. Barker, Winter, Osmond, Margetts, and Simmonds (1989) have shown that male birth weight and weight gain before one year of age, measured between 1911 and 1930, are powerful and independent (negative) predictors of coronary death in mid-to-late adult life. Some might argue that these findings do not necessarily imply an intraorganismal, biological causal pathway. Rather they may merely reflect the extraordinary persistence over time of the health effects of early socioeconomic deprivation—i.e., both weight in early life and subsequent heart disease are themselves associated with poverty—operating through a variety of mechanisms of varying latency, over a lifetime.

Against this view must be set the tight, stepwise gradient in heart disease risk with infant weights found by Barker et al. (1989), a "dose-response relationship" strongly suggestive of causation. As well, the study failed to find adult lung cancer mortality to be related to infant weights, suggesting that the well-known social class gradient in smoking did not contribute much to the heart disease/infant growth relationship observed. These authors' previous papers also provide strong evidence of long-lag-time effects of deprivation in early life (Barker and Osmond, 1986, 1987), albeit at the less convincing ecological (i.e. aggregate, not individual subject) level of analysis.[6]

The possibility that there may be very long latent periods between the origins of illness and its expression will be less problematic if those origins themselves are strongly persistent over time. Unfortunately, one cannot make this assumption. In a separate study, Barker and Osmond (1987) looked at three Lancashire towns essentially similar in their current socioeconomic profiles, but very different in their mortality rates from all causes between the ages of fifty-five and seventy-four. They find the explanation of these differences in the very different social circumstances that prevailed in the towns in 1911, when these persons were infants. Investigators of heterogeneities in health status who attempted to explain these differentials by examining recent differences in social circumstances would be searching for a cause that had long since vanished, and would accordingly find nothing. Yet, for most work done in this field, even twenty years is a long time. Indeed, for many disciplines five to ten years of follow-up is ambitious.

There is, however, one measure of socioeconomic status that is strongly "persistent" over time: educational level. Education, as measured by highest level of schooling attained, is determined relatively early in life, and then remains more or less constant for the subsequent decades. Thus "concurrent" educational levels *do* reflect social conditions several decades ago. Those who find strong correlations between education and health status, and particularly those who argue that education is the best or even the only *determinant* of health, with all other measures of "social class" serving as proxies, may simply be picking up the important effects of other variables, less easily measured retrospectively, with very long latency.

Indeed, even the long latency periods found by Barker and Osmond may understate the length of time over which such effects operate. The health status of individuals in later life can be shown, on the basis of the above work, to be affected by factors operating on the health of their parents in early life. This is particularly true for the mother. For example, birth weight is strongly related to maternal size, which is in turn related to the mother's growth in early life. Social conditions, or any other factors influencing health, may as a result have effects traceable across generations. It follows that attempts to understand heterogeneity in current health status may conceivably force us to consider circumstances up to and beyond one average human lifespan before.

Four Kinds of Time

Apart from the large variance in time over which latent effects can operate, we believe that it may be useful to distinguish four different types of latent effects, and corresponding roles of time. These may be termed *elapsed, biological, cumulative,* and *historical time.*

Of these, *elapsed time* is the simplest. It refers to the fact that "causes" have delayed effects. Infection today is reflected in the emergence of disease some days, weeks, months, or years later ("incubation periods"). The overall distribution of delay times for a population, however, is specific to the illness, and not primarily related to the circumstances of the individual. Time enters in the form of the difference between point of influence and point of expression, but apart from the length between these two points, plays no other role.

Biological time, by contrast, is embedded in the life cycle of the individual. The point in that cycle at which certain events occur is critical to their subsequent expression. For example, in Barker and Osmond's findings on weight gain (Barker et al., 1989), it seems to be the weight gain in the first year of life that is critical. Once this age-related "window of vulnerability" has been passed, subsequent fluctuations in weight do not have as powerful long-term effects.

Another example is provided by tuberculosis, illustrating a "window of expression" rather than a window of influence. A child infected with TB early in life often does not develop the disease, but remains vulnerable to its expression both in young adulthood (for unknown reasons) and again late in life (presumably in response to a decline in immune competence). Between these windows, the individual, while infected, is much less likely to develop the disease.

Cumulative time is the concept that underlies many well-known chronic disease processes in industry, such as silicosis, occupational cancer, or the atropine-like effects of certain pesticides. Here, time is necessary for small, sublethal doses of a toxicant to accumulate to a point at which disease will express itself. For silica, the effect is simply one of an accumulating proportion of scar tissue in the lung with increasing lifetime exposure to respirable aerosols—leading ultimately to breathlessness even at rest. For occupational cancers, it is thought that increasing time of exposure increases the probability of multiple discrete injuries to a particular cell, which will ultimately give rise to cancerous cell lines. The latent effect here is so well established that no negative occupational cancer study is credible without a statistically powerful sample of workers available for analysis who have been followed at least twenty years since first exposure to the putative carcinogen.

Finally, *historical time* is related to the epidemiological concept of cohort effects. Latency effects may depend on the point in history of the society, as well as the organism, at which particular events occurred. An individual infected with, or exposed to, the tubercle bacillus in 1900 had a much smaller chance of developing the disease, and a fortiori of dying from it, than an individual exposed in 1840 (Lilienfeld and Lilienfeld, 1980). A variety of explanations might be and have been offered. (The increased efficacy of medical treatment for those with disease, however, is *not* among them. No effective treatment was available before World War II.) The point is that the subsequent course of events, the unfolding through time of each individual's response to particular circumstances, can be influenced by when, in the course of evolution of the population, these events occurred.

Another example may be the evolution of socioeconomic gradients in mortality by age group. It may be that the persistence of early life effects in birth cohorts exposed during another era is the explanation for socioeconomic gradients in later life even in those societies that have most energetically pursued equalizing policies in recent times.

The failure to take account of the full length of time over which such latent effects can operate, might thus result in serious misinterpretations of the effectiveness of interventions. In the informative case of tuberculosis in particular, the residual burden of geriatric illness in industrialized populations is clearly a result of long-delayed effects of high rates of infection, early in life, among the populations who are now elderly. In this case, the biological characteristics of the illness itself (specifically its long latency and window of expression late in life) are interacting with the historical factor of much higher rates of exposure among the current elderly population.

These latency periods imply the existence, under at least some conditions, of a very substantial degree of "epidemiological momentum" in the health status of populations. If current observations reflect factors operating over as long as a century, it follows that attempts to change observed trends will be successful only over a long period of time, if at all. Present patterns, either of improvement or deterioration, will tend to persist for a number of years, more or less regardless of intervention. Everyone is now familiar with a negative aspect of such momentum in the case of the HIV epidemic. Much of the projected morbidity and mortality, over the next five or even ten years, has already "occurred" (in the sense of now being predetermined, barring a treatment breakthrough), in those persons who are already infected with the virus. Similarly, demographic momentum has been understood for decades to limit the short-term impact of fertility declines on *overall* population growth rates, in countries where the age structure itself must continue to cause high birth rates as a result of past levels of fertility.

What is suggested here, however, is a much more general kind of momentum that may pervade health-related processes at the population level. This momentum, or inertia, may explain some part of otherwise apparently inexplicable heterogeneities in health status—at least inexplicable in terms of more proximate exposures, whether positive or negative.

IMPLICATIONS

Research Agenda

One obvious implication of the preceding discussion is the need for more, and better quality, longitudinal studies of health, function, and illness extending across the life cycle, and if possible, across more than one generation. Furthermore, our discussion implies that the range of "exposures" and "outcomes" studied should be extremely broad. This would permit the testing of hypotheses regarding protean, rather than simply disease-specific, causal pathways. For example, birth weight and its interactions with early childhood environment have been linked with a variety of health outcomes up to decades later.

As a result of the farsightedness of some investigators in the immediate pre- and postwar period, there are several cohorts, some of them population based, of middle-aged individuals for whom detailed information on their early childhood circumstances is available. It is only now that these cohorts are entering the age range in which they are at sufficient risk of serious chronic disease, such as heart disease and cancer, to allow a search for associations with early exposures. This gives us an historically unprecedented opportunity to test hypotheses of health effects with very long latencies.

As an example, long-term follow-up of the randomized controlled trial of children enrolled in the High/Scope Early Childhood Enrichment Program, from the 1960s in Ypsilanti, Michigan, suggests that the intervention group has continued to do better than the controls in a wide variety of ways. These involve improved educational attainment, reduced criminality, and reduced teenage childbirth—all of which ultimately have implications for the health status of the study subjects and their offspring that cut across many disease outcomes (Schweinhart et al., 1985).

Some may counter that a research strategy of searching for associations in historical cohort data will simply be "fishing expeditions"or "data dredging" in relation to a multiplicity of exposures and outcomes. However, several hypotheses regarding the long-term effects of specific early life exposures already exist. These beg for more rigorous testing.[7]

Funding for following such invaluable cohorts beyond an initial limited time frame is, however, very difficult to obtain. There are logistic as well as scientific hurdles to be overcome here, but there is also a fundamental lack of awareness on the part of granting agencies of the importance of this work, which often does not fit the classical epidemiological model of disease-specific etiological investigation over shorter time spans. Typically, most epidemiological research into illness causation is funded by government or voluntary agencies with a mandate to examine risk factors for only one disease (e.g., Parkinsonism), organ system (e.g., the National Heart, Lung and Blood Institute in the United States), or pathologic type (e.g., the National Cancer Institute of Canada). There are few sources of funding for studies of the determinants of overall health. No doubt it is harder to raise funds with which to investigate the basic determinants of health than to fight the specific and labeled "villains" that rob friends and family of their loved ones.[8]

Another implication of the concepts presented above is the need to identify strategic windows of vulnerability in the life cycle, where fundamental determinants of health status tend to embed themselves in human biology. For instance, the 1970 British longitudinal follow-up of children to age five years suggests that behavioural problems are the first to manifest themselves in children living in relatively deprived circumstances, but that excess medical problems may initially be absent. The crucial question, which could now be answered by follow-up, is whether these behavioural problems are portents of future failure at the all-important juncture of childhood and adulthood—a time of crisis for individuals growing up in modern Western (and increasingly, Eastern) societies.

It would not be surprising to find that criminality and drug-taking were strongly correlated with adverse early childhood environment and related behavioural dysfunction. In fact, such beliefs are already a part of conventional wisdom concerning contemporary life patterns. This conventional wisdom does not, however, generally recognize the prospect that subsequent "hard" health effects of very long latency might occur, in persons with childhood risk factors, along a gradient of severity that includes diagnosable chronic disease in later life.

For instance, Marmot and Theorell (1988) have shown that blood pressures among the lower ranks of the British civil service do not follow the pattern seen in the upper ranks, of declining after the work day is over. And Barker, Bull, Osmond, and Simmonds (1990) have recently gone on to show that midlife blood pressure is closely related to birth weight and placental size at birth. Moreover, these differences parallel the current social-class pattern of mortality from heart disease. Might such long-term patterns of differential health status begin with relative deprivation in early life, leading to missed opportunities in adolescence and young adulthood, and the chronic stress of alienating, boring work in midlife?

Might not these social factors, operating at crucial times in individual development, embed themselves in the biology of an individual in a way that leads to increased risk of many different diseases? The phenomenon of daily blood pressure changes is only one example of such a mechanism. Much exciting work has been done in animals regarding the effects of psychological stimuli on the functioning of the neuroendocrine and neuroimmune axes (Dantzer and Kelley, 1989; Henry, 1982; Sapolsky, 1990). These insights add to our emerging picture of the full range of determinants of population health.

Research Strategies

The overriding strategic problem raised by our emphasis on longitudinal studies is the tremendous time lag from study inception to usable results. But this is only true if *longitudinal* is taken to mean entirely prospective. There are research strategies for shortening the time required for study completion. The first of these has been outlined above: the extended follow-up of cohorts assembled decades ago by farsighted social scientists. Second, we can draw upon the extensive experience with the "historical cohort design" in occupational health. These studies, which form the backbone of our knowledge of occupational cancer causation, are based on the fortuitous existence of employment records, containing detailed work histories.

These records are often kept for several decades by large employers. They allow epidemiologists to reconstruct exposure-based cohorts and "follow them forward in time" to ascertain health outcomes of interest—usually through computerized linkage to routinely collected mortality or morbidity databases. Twenty years of experience with this methodology has clearly demonstrated its utility and provided a range of powerful design and analytic tools for overcoming the problems inherent in the usual cohort design.

This methodology can be applied to a broader range of exposures and health outcomes to investigate the basic determinants of population health status. An example is provided by the work of Wolfson, Rose, Gentleman, and Tomiak (1990) relating socioeconomic status, as measured by preretirement income, and subsequent mortality risk. Utilizing only data routinely collected over the last few decades for the purpose of calculating pension entitlements, they found steep mortality gradients after age sixty-five across a range of annual incomes many years earlier.

If this data set could be linked to the Canadian National Mortality Data Base (containing cause of death), or to a comprehensive linked database recording use of all types of health care services, one could obtain a much richer understanding of the ways in which the health of Canadians is related to income. Furthermore, after such linkages had been accomplished once, it would be both feasible and useful to repeat them on an ongoing basis, with relatively small recurrent costs. This is critical if, as recent epidemiological work suggests, such health gradients are changing over historic time as successive birth cohorts, with very different childhood experiences, age.

Another strategic concern is how one creates a comprehensive picture of the broad determinants of health status throughout the life cycle. Here we must consider ways to overlap the results of prospective and historical cohort studies that are, individually, confined to a segment of the cycle. At present, there are several longitudinal studies that can provide a picture of the first thirty–forty years of life. Similarly, innovative exploitation of occupational cohorts could provide much useful information about the period between the ages of twenty-five and sixty-five. Marmot's first cohort of British civil servants is but the best of many examples of this (Marmot, 1986). Finally, a generation of long-term follow-up studies of elderly groups is emerging from the gerontology literature that, when supplemented by studies such as Wolfson's, will provide similar information about the final decades of life. When these various studies are considered together, they cover the life cycle in an overlapping fashion and represent a first iteration in the creation of a comprehensive picture of health status—portending, eventually perhaps, a kind of overarching "meta-analysis" of what makes (and keeps) people well.

Researchers interested in documenting health effects of long latency should be particularly alert to changes over time in age-specific patterns or other gradients of disease. For example, Frost's ground-breaking work on cohort effects in tuberculosis in the 1930s began from the observation that the disease had previously been most common among young adults, but was rapidly shifting toward becoming an affliction of later life (Lilienfeld and Lilienfeld, 1980). A similarly rich source of insights is the observed reversal of the socioeconomic gradient for coronary heart disease during this century. Relatively rapid changes in the descriptive epidemiology of any disease (or of overall longevity itself) can provide important clues to causal pathways that transcend specific pathologic processes. However, it is only within a very broad framework for analyzing the determinants of health, such as that presented here, that researchers are likely to take full advantage of opportunities to investigate the processes prior to specific diseases that may be critical to the determination of population health status.

NOTES

1. But genetic factors alone are not necessarily determinative either; see the discussion by Baird in Chapter 5.

2. In short, observations of heterogeneity have the form "X correlates with Y," from which we are led to consider what it is about characteristic X that influences health status Y. Differential susceptibility suggests that some other factor Z causes both X and Y. In contrast, reverse causality or selective drift claims that Y causes X.

3. At the turn of the century, infectious diseases were the principal causes of death, whereas today cancers and cardiovascular diseases are predominant. Despite this fact, the socioeconomic gradient, as expressed in standardized mortality ratios across social classes in Britain, has not shrunk. It is true that in the past certain infectious diseases such as polio were more prevalent among the upper classes, as are malignant melanoma and breast cancer today. But, with the exception of these few diseases, there has been a consistent socioeconomic gradient of mortality during a time of profound change in major causes of death.

4. There may, of course, be contributing factors, osteoporosis, for example, or inebriation. But these too are identifiable, and are in any case not sufficient "causes."

5. In both cases, the perturbation in mortality was followed almost immediately by a compensatory shift in mortality in the opposite direction. This has led epidemiologists to think of the initial perturbation as "precipitation" rather than causation per se. In other words, people "destined to die" have their date with destiny changed, but not by much. While perhaps true, this is only a quantitative distinction. We are all destined to die; postponement is the only possibility on offer.

6. A more recent ecological analysis of similar data across British geographical units suggests that virtually all association between infant death rates a half-century ago and current CHD mortality rates disappears when current SES of these units is properly controlled for (Ben Shlomo and Davey Smith, 1991). This rebuttal of the ecological evidence of long latency effects of early childhood deprivation does not, however, refute the tight individual-level association demonstrated by Barker et al. (1989) birth weight/infant weight gain and CHD rates in midlife.

7. For example, Forsdahl (1977) suggested that "great poverty in childhood and adolescence *followed by prosperity* is a risk factor for [all-cause mortality and] arteriosclerotic heart disease" (p. 91). Although Elford et al. (1991) rightly call for

a more specific and biologically rooted framing of this general hypothesis, this is more to enable its testing by feasible epidemiologic designs than a criticism of Forsdahl's thinking per se. We found it striking that Forsdahl excluded his findings about all-cause mortality from the title and abstract of the paper, even though these showed a stronger and tighter relationship with birth weights more than fifty years earlier than did CHD deaths. Could it be that Forsdahl downplayed this more protean result because of the emphasis on disease-specific causation prevailing in the academic research environment?

8. Apart from the difficulties of obtaining support, the reward structures that govern an academic career do not encourage the long-term commitment of major effort to the establishment and maintenance of such cohort studies.

4

The Social and Cultural Matrix of Health and Disease

E. CORIN

I. "NO MAN IS AN ISLAND": SOCIOCULTURAL ENVIRONMENT AND INDIVIDUAL RESPONSE

In Chapter 2 we introduced an analytical framework portraying the multiple and complex determinants of health and disease. This chapter focuses on the relationship between the social and cultural milieu, and the individual (host) response, in the production of health and disease. It emphasizes the extraordinary complexity of the concepts and causal pathways sketched out in Figure 2.5.

The importance attached to host response reflects, among other things, a growing awareness that individuals cope in a variety of ways with many different forms of external stress. The health effects of these different forms of stress are powerfully shaped by the social and cultural milieu in which individuals are embedded. The influence of sociocultural variables on health and disease has been repeatedly documented in large-scale cross-cultural studies. Yet epidemiological studies in Western industrialized societies generally assume that host response mechanisms—coping style, individual biology, social resources available to the individual—operate only at the level of the individual. By contrast, cross-cultural research suggests that these mediators also have an important collective dimension, a dimension that will be illustrated in this chapter through a few examples of well-known studies. Less well understood are the ways in which sociocultural factors affect the production of health. Bits of evidence, generally from smaller scale in-depth studies of particular communities, are nevertheless available. Some of these are also reviewed below.

These studies illustrate the mutually informing power of epidemiological and anthropological perspectives. They have been chosen to show the mechanisms of action of a few key sociocultural variables. The examples are organized around two major health problems: blood pressure and hypertension (exemplary of stress-related problems), and schizophrenia and depression (illustrative of the complex interactions between collective and individual determinants of health and disease).

II. THE EVIDENCE

A. The Alameda County Survey: Sex-Related Differences

The Alameda County Survey in California (Berkman and Syme, 1979) is a landmark study of the influence of social and community ties on health status. Individuals without social ties were found to be more likely to die from various causes than those with more intensive social contacts. This observation held even after controlling for potentially confounding variables such as self-reported physical health status at baseline, socioeconomic status, and health practices.

The results indicated that the collective experience of individuals, in particular the different socialization of males and females, powerfully influenced the way in which community ties affect health status. Marriage, for example, was more important for men, while contacts with friends and relatives and membership in community groups were more relevant for women. These sex-related differences have been repeatedly confirmed in other studies.[1] They can only be understood in light of the cultural norms and values associated with sex roles, and the different constraints and opportunities faced by men and women during their life histories.

B. Cardiovascular Diseases: The Impact of Culture Change

Cardiovascular diseases and blood pressure disorders are thought to be especially sensitive to stress. They are often used as indicators of the degree of stress experienced by groups and individuals under specific conditions, such as culture change.

One of the classic studies in this area (Marmot et al., 1975) investigated the health circumstances of Japanese living in three settings representing varying degrees of exposure to Western influences: Japan, Hawaii, and California. The United States has a high rate of coronary heart disease (CHD) while Japan has a very low rate. It was therefore of interest to see if the Americanization of Japanese was followed by an increased rate of CHD.

Almost twelve thousand men of Japanese ancestry living in the three settings were compared on prevalence of CHD at comparable levels of blood pressure and cholesterol. There was a significant gradient of increasing CHD from Japan to Hawaii to California, with relatively smaller differences between Japan and Hawaii than between Hawaii and California. Conventional individual risk factors (i.e., cholesterol, blood pressure, smoking differences) were not sufficient to explain the observed trend. Among the risk factors identified as likely contributors to this gradient were several "life-style" factors with an obvious collective dimension: diet, occupation, and patterns of social interaction.

Assuming that aspects of Japanese culture act as buffers against stress, Marmot (1981) attempted to quantify the subjects' relationship to Japanese culture. He estimated the degree to which respondents had been exposed to traditional Japanese culture during upbringing. People were classified by how much they sought personal contacts and social support among Japanese rather than non-Japanese. The more traditional men had a lower CHD prevalence rate than their nontraditional counterparts. This held even after controlling for dietary preferences and other known individual risk factors for heart disease.

Such differences in prevalence rates are difficult to interpret, and one should be careful not to jump too fast to the conclusion that traditional Japanese culture has a protective value. Higher prevalence rates could result either from an increased risk of getting the condition, or from improved survival. The only firm conclusion is that different patterns of prevalence and survival correspond to different degrees of Westernization. This correlation deserves further study, particularly of the mechanisms of influence of collective, cultural variables. Marmot was able to capture the role of culture only incompletely through a proxy measure of acculturation and assimilation.

C. International Pilot Study on Schizophrenia: Cross-Cultural Differences in Disease Evolution

Several long-term studies on schizophrenia have shown the extent of individual variation in the course and severity of this disorder. Current research is attempting to identify characteristics of individuals that are associated with differential outcomes. But cross-cultural studies have indicated that there are also significant differences in outcome depending on cultural setting. These differences suggest the influence of collective variables. In particular, a number of studies have suggested that prevalence rates or outcomes may be more favourable in third-world countries (Eaton, 1985; Littlewood, 1990; Murphy, 1982; Torrey, 1987; Warner, 1983). Some analysts have disregarded these data because of nonuniform diagnostic criteria; indeed, one of the main difficulties in psychiatric epidemiology is the assessment of the validity of prevalence rates and agreement on common definitions and disease criteria.

In the 1970s, the World Health Organization (WHO) undertook a pilot study to assess the feasibility of developing standardized instruments and procedures for psychiatric assessment that could be applied reliably in a variety of cultural settings. The study also hoped to explore the possibility that the course and outcome of schizophrenia differ from country to country. The International Pilot Study on Schizophrenia (IPSS) was conducted in nine developed and developing countries. At each field research centre, all patients contacting a psychiatric service during a one-year period were screened and assessed with the Present State Examination (PSE), a standardized semistructured interview guide. Patients were evaluated after two and five years on the basis of several clinical and psychosocial indicators.

Two main results emerged from the IPSS. First, similar schizophrenic syndromes were found in all eight participating centres. But second, the course and outcome of the disorder *did* vary significantly among countries. On virtually all measures, a greater proportion of schizophrenic patients in Agra (India), Cali (Colombia), and Ibadan (Nigeria) had a more favourable, and nondisabling, experience of the disease than in the other centres (Aarhus, London, Moscow, Prague, and Washington). Standard sociodemographic and clinical predictors did not account for the differences among the centres.[2]

Predictive factors specific to the individual, identified in European and North American cultures, may not be sufficient, or even relevant, to explain prognosis in other cultures. "A large part of the variance in the course and outcome of schizophrenia may be due to factors that have not yet been identified" (Sartorius, Jablensky, and Shapiro, 1978:108). These unidentified factors may well be the collective ones neglected by the IPSS.

D. Depression: The Relativity of Risk Factors

Also in the 1970s, Brown, Harris, and their collaborators undertook population surveys of female psychiatric disorders in several settings—

458 women aged eighteen to sixty-five years living in Camberwell (a working-class South London borough; Brown and Harris, 1978); two traditional Gaelic-speaking rural populations in North Uist and Lewis in the Outer Hebrides (Brown and Prudo, 1981, 1987); and in the early 1980s a longitudinal one-year study on 303 symptom-free women in Islington (a borough in North London; Brown, Craig, and Harris, 1985; Brown, Andrews, Harris, Adler, and Bridge, 1986; Brown and Harris, 1989). Psychiatric symptoms were measured through a shortened form of the PSE.

The comparison between Camberwell and the rural Outer Hebrides revealed two interesting features. First, the overall rate of psychiatric disorders in Camberwell was higher than in North Uist. The Londoners had a higher prevalence of depressive cases while the prevalence of other diagnoses, especially anxiety, was higher in the Outer Hebrides. Second, social class (however measured) did not account for variations in prevalence in the rural setting, although it did in Camberwell.

The psychiatric disorder rate in the Outer Hebrides is associated with a two-factor index of women's involvement in traditional island activities (regular churchgoing and crafting). The most integrated women had lower rates of depression but, quite unexpectedly, also displayed much higher rates of anxiety or phobic disorder. This suggests that a traditional way of life is a significant but complex influence on health in rural communities, simultaneously protective and debilitating. The effects of an "individual" behaviour such as crafting or churchgoing may depend on how it is embedded within a larger collectivity, a phenomenon that is as yet not fully understood.

III. THE CULTURAL DIMENSION: METHODS AND MEASUREMENT

A. The Epidemiological Vantage Point

Current methodological and conceptual approaches give epidemiology its strength but are also the source of its limitations. The authors of the Alameda County Survey, for example, acknowledged that their measures of social and community ties were very crude, and that a broader conceptualization of social variables was needed. In fact, most current epidemiological research suffers from a similar, if sometimes less pronounced flaw. Most of the social and cultural determinants considered in these studies are measured using a few discrete variables that are treated as if they were properties of individuals rather than of groups.

There are several reasons for this pattern. First and most obviously, large-scale studies face inevitable cost and feasibility constraints. More substantively, the epidemiological approach to social and cultural determinants of health reflects its origins in the conceptual framework of medicine portrayed in Chapter 2. The main aim of epidemiological research is still to document and explain systematic differences in the distribution of health problems, as medically perceived. The preferred explanations are those derived from traditional medical reasoning. Thus epidemiologists focus first and most intensely on plausible biological hypotheses; only when these cannot account for observed differences do they consider social, psychological, and cultural influences. As a result, there is often a great discrepancy between the detail and care with which genetic or physiological hypotheses are formulated and tested, and the loose and crude treatment accorded to social and cultural hypotheses.

At a still deeper level, this "categorical" approach to sociocultural factors fits comfortably within the prevalent scientific paradigms, which strip human realities of much of their social context. Other approaches to social and cultural realities tend to be disregarded and dismissed. As emphasized in Chapter 2, the (implicit or explicit) conceptual framework powerfully conditions the set of possible pathways and hypotheses. Young's (1980) critical review of stress research documents this tendency very clearly. The current discourse on stress "effectively subverts sociological reasoning" by displacing the human subject from his or her place in society to a "desocialized and amorphous environment" (Young, 1980:133).

This displacement mirrors conventional North American beliefs about human nature and society: The individual is the basic unit of society, and is conceived as the bearer of fixed psychological dispositions. Society is an epiphenomenon, the sum of the dispositions, beliefs, decisions, and actions of the individuals who "belong" to it. The power of this conventional knowledge lies in the fact that people regard it as self-evident, but it also conditions the way data are collected and interpreted. These conventions identify, organize and highlight particular objects and events, while leaving others as unconnected and irrelevant. Much of the research on stress, according to Young, proceeds from, and therefore can only confirm and reproduce, "conventional knowledge". It is incapable of taking seriously alternative ways of thinking.[3]

The IPSS—and its sequel—illustrate the way in which the medical frame of reference, combined with an excessive concern for "instrument reliability," can severely limit the research questions posed and the methods used to gather and interpret evidence.

Following the IPSS, the WHO undertook a second cross-cultural study (the Determinants of Outcome Project, or DOP) designed to test a number of hypotheses about how social and cultural factors affect the course of schizophrenia. Rather than starting with well-founded cultural hypotheses based on available cross-cultural research, however, the investigators limited themselves to variables that they could more easily and reliably measure. Their aim was to account for variation among countries on the basis of well-identified individual-level measures that are predictive of the onset and relapse of schizophrenia in Western societies.

The study focused on two main categories of determinants: major life events, and "expressed emotions" in the family (hostility, criticism, overinvolvement). It employed measures and methods established in studies of Western societies. Rather than taking advantage of cross-cultural comparisons in order to enrich existing knowledge of schizophrenia, the WHO team instead tried to confirm the universal validity of individual predictors associated with the course of illness in Western societies.

The study's implicit bias toward universality was vividly revealed in the chief investigators' comments about the difficulty of applying the Life Events Scale in three centres (Agra, India; Chandigarh, India; Ibadan, Nigeria), and about the differing results from developed and developing countries (Day et al., 1987). They interpreted the similarity of major life event rates across the six developed-country centres as evidence of validity, while differences in the Indian samples were dismissed as probably due to methodological problems. (No parallel methodological scrutiny was applied to data showing similarities.)

The Indian coinvestigators were suspicious of the applicability of the study instruments in an Indian context and the validity of data collected in this way. Nevertheless, the chief investigators chose to apply their standard methodology and to include data that the Indian coinvestigators found intuitively unacceptable. Confronted with the fact that their data were of limited value for explaining observed differences between developed and developing countries, they limited their conclusions to the suggestion that one should concentrate on the "combined effects of multiple stressors," i.e., the combined impact of life events and family atmosphere. They did not reconsider the validity of the "life event" concept itself, or the relevance of Western scales to developing societies; nor did they consider the possible impact of larger collective variables.

This study illustrates the dangers of an inappropriate transfer of intellectual constructs from one culture to another.[4] The challenge, for both epidemiologists and anthropologists, is to combine generalizability and cultural validity.

The authors of the related study of expressed emotions (EE) appear more sensitive to the cultural limits of their conceptual and methodological apparatus (Leff et al., 1990). Faced with the limited predictive value of the EE measurement for their Indian sample and with the fact that the pattern of association and evolution of the various emotions rated in the EE index is different from what has been documented in the West, they concluded that the meaning and impact of "emotions" cannot be assumed a priori. They underscored the need for another, more anthropological investigation exploring the basic cultural context governing the expression and meaning of specific emotions in an Indian context.

The methods chosen by the WHO's DOP study reflect in part real constraints imposed by the need to collect comparable cross-cultural data. But they also reveal less interest in cultural variation, and a bias toward universality. This bias is inherent in the medical (Kraepelinian) frame of reference, which dominates present-day psychiatry.

Kraepelin, who was one of the fathers of psychiatric classification, was in fact a strong advocate of the contribution of "comparative psychiatry" to the development of psychiatry as a truly scientific discipline. He assumed, however, that it would eventually be possible to identify the universal, biological causes and correlates of the specific diagnostic categories of mental illness. As a result, he was not interested in the role played by social and cultural factors in psychiatric disorders. From this perspective, the point of cross-cultural research was to test the soundness of Western psychiatry's diagnostic classifications. As the WHO studies show, this perspective continues to place powerful restrictions on cross-cultural investigations.

B. Contrast and Complementarity between Two Approaches

In-depth anthropological studies of a single community are based on assumptions and perspectives very different from those used in epidemiology (Corin, Bibeau, Martin, and Laplante, 1990; Janes, 1986). Such studies consider "the community" as the central unit of analysis and generally adopt a more systemic approach to causality. Data are collected through qualitative ethnographic methods: field work, participants' observations, interviews with key informants. Information is analyzed in sociological and anthropological categories: kinship systems, family structure, power relationships, social roles, beliefs, values, etc. Community studies aim to reveal relationships between cultural, social, behavioural, and psychological processes within a single community or geographic area.

Researchers are also interested in the transformation and adaptability of values, beliefs, and social institutions. One could say that while epidemiological research is mainly interested in identifying at-risk populations and associated factors, community studies seek to identify a system of disease-causing conditions and collective ways of coping with problems.

The way "culture" is dealt with in the two approaches offers a good illustration of their differences. In epidemiological research, culture is defined through one or more categorical variables: ethnicity, place of birth, mother tongue, etc. Marmot, as we have seen, has also constructed a score of "traditionality." By contrast, anthropology considers culture as a web or matrix of collective influences that shape the lives of groups and of individuals. There are variations between anthropological schools and, within those schools, between European and North American traditions. But all define culture to include: ways of life, shared behaviour, social institutions, systems of norms, beliefs and values, and the world view that allows people to locate themselves within the universe and give meaning to their personal and collective experience.

Of course, societies differ in their degree of homogeneity or heterogeneity, in their adaptability to changing conditions, and in their tolerance or rigidity regarding personal or collective differences. One could say that for anthropologists, culture is a perspective on reality, rather than a collection of categories marking differences among individuals.

This approach to culture also has limitations. It is all-encompassing and difficult to study empirically. Its systemic orientation complicates comparisons. As a result, the majority of studies reviewed below have explored different strategies for integrating quantitative epidemiological methods with more qualitative anthropological methods.

One research strategy consists of systematically using epidemiological comparative data in order to formulate and test hypotheses. This has been done most successfully by Murphy (1982) in the area of comparative psychiatry. His work is a rare combination of an approach that is highly critical of existing evidence, with a creative way of considering data and their implications.

In his study of the social and cultural determinants of the onset and course of schizophrenia, Murphy began with a few examples of unusually high (southwestern Croatians and Irish) and low (Hutterites, Tongans of the South Pacific, and Taiwanese aborigines) rates of prevalence. He also considered societies where a shift from low to high rates has been carefully documented (Achinese in northwest Sumatra and Tallensi in northern Ghana). In each case, his approach was the same. First, he scrutinized all the evidence that could indicate a possible bias in available rates. Second, he considered and eliminated a set of alternative plausible explanations in terms of individual differences such as genetics, socioeconomic status, diet, exposure to viruses, and (for migrators) self-selection, as well as differences in diagnostic criteria or rates of institutionalization. Third, he examined the role of collective "more intangible and debatable factors" deriving from culture, the family, and community life.

He paid particular attention to intrasocietal differences and to the categories of people who are especially at risk in a given society. This allowed him to formulate specific hypotheses regarding the social and cultural factors that could be associated with the observed differences. But these "explanations" remained quite speculative and bound to a particular society. Murphy found it virtually impossible to disentangle the various hypotheses when one remains within the boundaries of a single sociocultural group. Therefore, the next step was to compare societies that share exceptionally high or low rates of the disorder. What do they have in common and how are they different? His conclusions are presented in Section V.C.

This approach is very demanding, since the strength of its conclusions depends critically on the validity of the available cross-societal quantitative and qualitative data. A more common research strategy applies a similar method to the study of intrasocietal differences.

Quantitative data allow researchers to identify subgroups or categories of people who seem particularly at risk for a given health problem. Their social and cultural situations are then scrutinized to identify peculiar features that could be associated with their increased vulnerability. The identification of the potentially relevant collective processes is guided by what is already known about the etiological factors associated with the disease. It is difficult to assess, however, how much can be generalized from etiological hypotheses derived from single case studies.

A second research strategy consists of going *back and forth between quantitative surveys and in-depth community studies*. The current approach is to use fragments of life stories or other qualitative data to illustrate the meaning attached to quantitative findings (de Almeida Filho, 1987). A few studies have integrated the two methods further and have given more space to qualitative data about community life. For example, in the first phase of a study of health problems among Samoan immigrants in California, Janes (1986) gathered medical and demographic data through brief interviews with and examinations of three hundred adults affiliated with several churches. Significant differences were observed between men and women; to understand these the author selected a representative community and carried out an in-depth study based on participant observation[5] and informal interviews with community members. These led to hypotheses embodied in scales and instruments to measure potentially relevant social and cultural variables, and to the design of a second survey to test these hypotheses.

Despite the specificity of their methods and objectives, socially and culturally sensitive studies of the determinants of health problems have led to a few common conclusions that will be reviewed in the rest of this chapter. "Cultural" influence is always easier to identify in unfamiliar societies; our own culture is transparent to us like the air we (usually) breathe. Thus most of the studies considered here do not involve western societies. Their conclusions, however, indicate the potential role of cultural phenomena in health and disease—a finding that also applies to "western" societies.

IV. STRESS-RELATED DISORDERS IN A CONTEXT OF CULTURE CHANGE

It has long been believed that culture change (over historical time or through migration) reveals both the damaging and the protective aspects of community life. Studies clearly show that it is not culture change in itself that has an impact on health. Rather, the effects stem from the extent of the change, the degree to which the change affects cultural values and rules of behaviour, and its impact on traditional ways of coping with stress.

The main factors that influence the extent of impact of culture change are illustrated by empirical studies. (One could postulate that similar collective variables play a more general role in mitigating or accentuating the impact of stress on life and health.) The persuasiveness of such studies differs; they reveal the difficulties of studying how social and cultural processes affect health. Nevertheless, they lead to insights and hypotheses that could be further tested through more rigorous designs.

A. Social Differentiation under Economic Constraints as a Source of Stress

Culture change often has a significant impact both on the structure of social relationships, and on access to the material goods and sources and symbols of prestige that contribute to social identity. This has been the focus of a set of studies in various societies by Dressler (1982, 1985; Dressler and Badger, 1985; Dressler, Mata, Chavez, and Viteri, 1987). He favours a "discrepancy model" of culture change, postulating that the adaptation to modern life is not in itself problematic, but becomes so only when the individual has limited access to economic resources.

The notion of "life-style stress" is central in this model. Life-style is defined as the symbolic aspect of social class or of modernity status; life-style stress results from the conjunction of a low economic status and a relatively expensive life-style. Dressler's main hypothesis is that life-style stress undermines social identity. His second hypothesis is that for upwardly mobile persons, life-style stress is less of an issue and that the major source of stress would more likely be a disruption in the sense of control, as described in the classical epidemiological literature on Western societies.

Dressler first constructed and tested this model in a survey of a hundred randomly selected forty- to forty-nine-year-olds in St. Lucia, in the Eastern Caribbean (Dressler, 1982, 1985). People were identified as low or high economic status,[6] and low or high material life-style.[7] Life-style stress was then defined as the association between high material life-style and low economic resources—in short, trying to live beyond one's means. To test his second hypothesis, Dressler also constructed a sixteen-item scale of perceived stress, based on culturally relevant life change events (e.g., death of mother, losing a job, going to court) and a measure of emotional control.

Data confirmed the existence of two pathways in the social production of disease. Neither material life-style nor economic status has a significant main effect on blood pressure. However, the interaction of the two variables is significant: Higher blood pressure is found among persons in the high-material-life-style/low-economic-status category. Since many situations of culture change are characterized by the presence of real economic limitations combined with an increased cultural emphasis on material life-style, one could expect that such life-style stress affects a significant proportion of the populations subject to culture change.

On the other hand, even if higher perceived stress is globally associated with lower socioeconomic status, it is only in the high-socioeconomic-status group that perceived stress and lack of emotional control are in themselves directly related to mean arterial blood pressure, as they are in Western societies. Dressler's study shows that, at least in St. Lucia, the stress process varies according to class. The sources of stress or, in the terms used in Chapter 1, the degree of strain resulting from different stresses therefore change depending on the individual's place in the system of social stratification.

Data collected in a southern black community (Dressler and Badger, 1985) showed the same pattern of correlations. However, other studies clearly indicate that the impact of social differentiation is itself strongly framed by characteristics of the larger social and cultural context. For example, in a Mexican community Dressler et al. (1987) showed that a single index of modern life-style (acquisition of material culture and engaging in cosmopolitan behaviour) is the best predictor of blood pressure, independent of economic status. Dressler explained this discrepancy with other studies by noting that this particular community is characterized by a general absence of upward mobility. In such a context, the mere acquisition of a modern life-style could be considered as culturally at odds with the overall ethos of the community. Therefore, the "discrepancy model" of culture change as spelled out in Dressler's prior studies seems to apply mainly in societies where there have been changes in both the social class structure and in individual life-styles.

Historical and sociocultural change occurring at a macrolevel is thus translated into stress on the individual, and the individual's response to these stresses—the degree of strain—can lead ultimately into disease. At the same time, the symbols and meaning produced by particular social arrangements and cultural values modify the extent of individual responses to these stresses.

B. The Impact of Changing Conditions Varies According to the Significance Attached to Traditional Ways of Life

While culture change can greatly modify traditional ways of life, such change is not always detrimental. Kunitz and Levy (1986) collected data on 279 Navajo men and women sixty-five years of age and older, living on the western end of a reservation in north central Arizona.[8] This area is generally regarded as among the most "traditional" regions of the reservation. They found a marked contrast in the health patterns of men and women.

For women, hypertension is consistently associated with various indices of acculturation, including level of education, attendance at a boarding school off the reservation, and English language fluency. In addition, isolation is also significantly associated with hypertension. But these associations were found only for women. On the other hand, residence off reservation for at least one year is, among men, significantly associated with a *lower* prevalence of diagnosed hypertension.

Cultural data shed light on the meaning of these results. In traditional society, the situation of women appears to be much more secure. The mother-daughter bond is especially significant; women typically remain in their family of origin upon marrying and retain rights of decision-making. For women, involvement in the educational system and wage work might represent the loss of this secure place. Their increased sense of vulnerability might then be reflected in hypertension.

On the other hand, anthropological studies reveal the marginal position occupied by young adult men within a matrilineal, matrilocal society. Earlier studies showed that within the traditional society, the group more at risk for hypertension is that of young adult men [De Stefano et al. (1979), cited in Kunitz and Levy (1986)]. Kunitz and Levy hypothesize that in such a context, migration might be beneficial for men. (This observation of high stress among young males has extraordinary parallels in the matrilinear societies of nonhuman primates.)

C. The Impact of Culture Change Varies According to the Degree of Discontinuity with Traditional Values

Salmond, Prior, and Wessen's study (1989) of a New Zealand community also focuses on the transition between the traditional and the modern worlds, and the associated change in values. For fourteen years he followed a cohort of 654 adult Tokelauans who migrated from a subsistence life-style on a Pacific atoll to an urbanized Western life-style in New Zealand. As part of this study, he measured annual rates of change in blood pressure, adjusting for age, baseline body mass and blood pressure, and rate of change in body mass. The adjusted pressure of the migrant men showed significant increase over the duration of the study.

Increases in age-standardized blood pressure were positively correlated with measures of the degree of assimilation. But this correlation was strongest at the first round of data collection; it was less marked at the second, and only marginally present at the last one.

There is also some evidence from the last round of data collection that men who experience conflict between their status and their private values have elevated blood pressure: Among high-status men (according to the traditional norms), those who ascribed to non-Tokelauan values had significantly higher blood pressure than did those who adhered strongly to the Tokelauan values. Salmond suggests that these men are in a situation of personal dissonance. The traditional society is strongly hierarchical; high-status men would find themselves split between their own changing wishes and values, and collective expectations that they assume various tasks and responsibilities attached to their traditional status.

Similar conclusions can be drawn from studies of various groups of immigrants in Canada and in the United States (Murphy, 1987). In general these show that the impact of present circumstances varies depending on how well those conditions correspond with the expectations and values generated during the socialization process within the immigrants' cultures of origin.

The disruptive effect of culture change on well-being is generally proportional to the degree of discrepancy between modern and traditional values. Similarly, the potential impact of immigration varies according to the degree of discrepancy between what the individual migrant's background had prepared him or her for, and the sources of support and fulfillment now available.

D. Current Mechanisms of Adaptation to Change Can Prolong, or Mark a Break with, Traditional Coping Strategies

Culture change, as it affects social structure and traditional ways of life, does more than introduce potential sources of conflict or stress. It can also undermine well-tried collective coping strategies developed to help confront difficult situations. A study on health problems among Samoans who had migrated and settled in northern California demonstrates the importance of considering traditional patterns of adaptation to different situations (Janes, 1986).

The collective strategies adopted to face harsh conditions in the new environment appear to be a direct transposition of ancient coping strategies. In traditional Samoan society, the local descent group is an important source of support and affiliation; diffuse kinship networks are maintained through a set of exchanges and obligations. Church congregations are also an organizational unit of utmost importance, integrated into all areas of life. This double structure plays a central role in receiving and helping new migrants.

But this support system seems to erode under the pressure of growing socioeconomic constraints, and the acceptance of Western-style values. Samoan institutions are, in California, increasingly monetized. Thus participating in church and kin affairs, and enjoying the prestige they can provide, becomes expensive. Traditional coping strategies thus have paradoxical effects in the new environment. On the one hand, they sustain strong community values and provide individuals with avenues for satisfying their needs. But on the other hand, active participation in collective institutions can become a source of stress, simply because of the expense.

Janes constructed an index of "status inconsistency" to reflect these Samoan peculiarities. The hypothesis that the most severe stress would be experienced by individuals of a relatively high traditional status who have limited access to the resources necessary for demonstrating their prestige, was partially confirmed statistically.[9] For low-income people, high kindred involvement is associated with high blood pressure; for people with greater economic resources, high kindred involvement or high leadership status is associated with low blood pressure. This indicates the protective value of involvement in traditional kinship activities—if one can afford them. If one cannot, they become a source of vulnerability.

This status inconsistency has a greater effect on women than on men. This may be because for Samoan women leadership status is often based on that of their husbands. It may therefore be less of a source of direct satisfaction for women, who may resent the cost of maintaining status at the expense of other concerns for family welfare.

In summary, a group may respond to the stress of culture change by developing coping strategies built on the traditional organization of social relationships and ways of managing difficult situations; it calls upon the key values of the community. But in the new environment, these collective strategies may be altered in such a way that they cease to be protective for individuals, and can indeed be sources of further stress.

V. PSYCHIATRIC DISORDERS: AT THE CROSSROAD BETWEEN COLLECTIVE AND INDIVIDUAL DETERMINANTS

Studies done in a context of culture change consider that change as the stressful situation, responsible for variations in health outcomes. Research has focused on the identification of variables that mitigate or worsen the impact of stress, without paying too much attention to the disease outcome or to the stressful situation itself.

Mental health research, however, has gone further in understanding the influence of social and cultural determinants on particular health problems, and in searching for their mechanisms of influence. On one level, studies show that cultural variables affect the way in which distress and disease will manifest themselves in a particular cultural context. This has significant methodological implications for epidemiologists who plan community surveys. On another level, in focusing on what constitutes a source of stress, these studies show that the impact of a stressful event or situation, the strain it generates in the individual, is affected by its meaning, and that meaning is context (or culture) dependent. On yet a third level, research on mental health problems calls into question the idea that traditional cultural matrices are necessarily protective. As just described, Janes's study of Samoans in California showed how the alteration of cultural practices in a new environment can convert them from protective to harmful; but such practices are not always benign even in their original context.

A. The Interactive Relationships between Disease Manifestations, Illness Experience, and Diagnostic Labeling

Yet the field of mental health is characterized by a particular difficulty in defining the diagnostic borders between disease entities. The history of psychiatry and comparative research reveal marked changes in the incidence of some diagnoses over time and between societies. Dramatic forms of hysteria said to be common in nineteenth-century psychiatric practice have almost disappeared in Western societies, and the diagnosis itself is no longer part of the North American DSM-III classification system.[10] On the other hand, the frequency of "borderline personality" seems to have increased tremendously during recent decades. Depression, once declared missing in African societies, has since been rediscovered under the guise of "masked depression."

Cross-cultural variations in patterns of mental illnesses, "culture-bound syndromes," are now commonly considered as particular manifestations, local variations, of the main DSM-III diagnostic categories. In this way practitioners can preserve the claim that they are working, as good scientists should, with universal categories and concepts. The challenge posed to mainstream North American psychiatry by the observation that its "fundamental" categories appear to be culture-bound is thus blunted or dismissed. Previously alleged differences between European and North American rates of schizophrenia, for example, have been explained away as merely the expression of differences in the use of diagnostic criteria.

In the absence of clear biological correlates for many psychiatric disease entities, however, it is virtually impossible to sort out how much of cross-cultural variation is due to differing diagnostic procedures, how much to differing approaches to mental health phenomena, and how much to differences in the reality itself. Progress has been made in the development of *reliable* diagnostic criteria, but progress in reliability does not equate with progress in *validity*. Conclusions drawn about the social and cultural determinants of psychiatric disorders still largely derive more from the presuppositions of researchers, than from the findings of research.[11] The symptomatic picture is in fact a composite of universal disease-related elements and of culture-specific features.

One of the objectives of the WHO's IPSS was to document the universality of schizophrenia, of its manifestation, and of its rate of occurrence across societies and cultures. As noted above, cases were identified with a standardized diagnostic instrument, the PSE, to assure cross-country reliability in diagnostic procedures. An attempt was made to standardize the diagnostic principles that clinicians seem to use, and to apply them in the form of a computer program to PSE data in order to obtain a completely standardized reference classification. The PSE provides for two alternative calculations of incidence rates: one based on a "broad" diagnostic definition of schizophrenia and another on a "restrictive" definition limited to a subtype of core schizophrenia called S+ (WHO, 1979; Sartorius et al., 1986).

The use of the broad definition reveals significant intercultural differences for the rates of new cases (from 1.5 to 4.2 per year per ten thousand population) and indicates a variation in the relative preeminence of specific symptoms. On the other hand, the range of variation in incidence rates narrows impressively (0.7 to 1.4) when one uses the more restrictive computer-based definition.

At the very least, then, one can say that the WHO study discloses both important similarities and important differences, and that both sets of findings warrant attention. Furthermore it should draw our attention immediately to the problem of establishing diagnostic criteria for schizophrenia. The IPSS findings indicate that the validity of the "maintained hypothesis"—the universality of schizophrenia—seems to turn on which of two definitions one uses. And the two alternatives were apparently regarded as equally plausible a priori by the researchers—since they chose to use both.

The defining criteria of schizophrenia have been the object of long debates through history, so that no single definition can be considered as "the" definition. Culturally sensitive psychiatrists such as Kleinman (1988) have contested the value of excluding from the analysis all the "fringe cases," which seem to be in fact more sensitive to cultural influences.[12] Yet it is striking to note that in their conclusions the investigators chose to focus principally on the "universal" findings, from the narrow definition of the disorder. Implicitly they dismissed the results from the definition that failed to yield the a priori "right" answer. The WHO study does in fact show an influence of culture on the incidence of schizophrenia, but a bias toward universality prevented the investigators from exploring its significance.

There are significant differences in the symptoms that are most commonly displayed by persons in different cultures suffering from "the same" disorder. These differences in prevalent symptom patterns are linked to differences in basic cultural conceptions of the person and of the world. For example, the DOP (Katz et al., 1988), found that Indian schizophrenics tended to show a pattern of depression, morbid jealousy, and a "self-centered" orientation, while Nigerian patients displayed a highly suspicious, bizarre, anxious behavioural pattern. In an earlier study comparing Italian and Irish schizophrenics, Opler and Singer

(1959) found that the Irish expressed more preoccupations with guilt and sin, more systematic delusions, and more drinking problems. The Italians by contrast had a greater tendency toward talkativeness, hyperactivity, excitement, and pronounced mood swings.

Thus, even if disorders share characteristics similar enough to justify the common diagnosis of schizophrenia, their symptoms display a marked variation with culture. The relationship between these culturally specific symptom patterns and the course of the disorder has not yet been sufficiently explored.

Kleinman's (1986) study of depression and neurasthenia in China shows a better grasp of the complex interplay between various levels of determinants in both shaping and labeling the disorder. The author was struck by the high prevalence of a diagnosis of "neurasthenia" in psychiatric clinics in China. In the West this diagnosis has almost disappeared, having been replaced by "depression".

Briefly stated, in the nineteenth-century neurasthenia was defined as a putative "chronic malfunction" of the cerebral cortex associated with weakness, headaches, and dizziness. In China, neurasthenia retains this connotation of a physical illness. It neither conveys the stigma attached to mental illness nor implies personal accountability for the associated physical correlates of an emotional illness (Kleinman, 1987). Kleinman's research in China explored whether observed differences in diagnostic prevalence are a result of different labeling conventions, or of real variations in the expression of symptoms. Such real variations might be due to cultural influences; Kleinman also attempted to identify associated social determinants.

He interviewed one hundred patients with a diagnosis of neurasthenia, collecting systematic data on symptoms, course, illness behaviour, help-seeking, and ethnomedical beliefs associated with the current illness. Each patient also received a standard psychiatric assessment using a modified version of the *Schedule for Affective Disorders and Schizophrenia* (SADS). Open-ended ethnographic interviews attempted to determine the social significance of the symptoms in day-to-day illness behaviour in work, family, and community settings, and the various "uses" made of those symptoms—for explaining or justifying behaviour—by the patient and others.

Kleinman found that patients and their families both interpreted the illness primarily in physical terms. They reported an enormous burden of suffering, but perceived this as associated with physical complaints, in spite of an impressive listing of psychosocial stresses that were also perceived as having caused the disorder. Psychological symptoms were mentioned, but only in response to specific questions based on a symptom checklist; they were not described in spontaneous narratives.

These observations clearly reflect an inconsistency between the complex experience of being ill and the way that sufferers describe their illnesses. Help-seeking behaviour showed a similar pattern, with overuse of medical services for the perceived physical complaints. Follow-up of patients showed that their symptoms were significantly relieved by antidepressant medication, but their social impairments persisted or grew worse.

In his discussion, Kleinman emphasizes the role of "social uses of somatization"—the benefits to patients, families, and others of emphasizing the physical dimension of a complex psychophysiological experience of distress, and of interpreting psychological problems in physical terms—in the Chinese cultural and sociopolitical context. Building on Mechanic's work in North America, he shows how this process of interpretation is promoted by three characteristics of Chinese society:

1. In Chinese society, psychological illness is viewed as to some degree disgraceful or blameworthy. Physical illness, by contrast, is quite socially acceptable and indicates no failing of the individual. This creates an obvious pressure on patients to express and indeed perceive only the physiological component of their distress. The Western concept of neurasthenia seems to have been absorbed within the traditional Chinese idea that weakness of vital essence causes disease; physical complaints are an acceptable way to express distress, demoralization, and unhappiness.
2. The display of physical symptoms may also be an effective way for the individual to cope with excessive stress. Studies within the epidemiological framework defined by specific disease entities typically assume that "becoming ill" is an ineffective way of dealing with difficult situations. But anthropological studies have shown that it can be quite effective, personally and socially. As Kleinman notes, claiming sickness to explain withdrawal from dangerous political situations was an established tradition among Confucian scholar-bureaucrats. His interviews reveal that in modern China chronic illness behaviour can be used to justify repeated failure on the national university entrance examination, or to obtain relief from heavy work obligations or the burden of family separation. The disaffected and potential dissidents may even use chronic illness as an excuse for failure to participate in political life.
3. Since practitioners from the same culture share their patients' ideas regarding acceptable modes of symptom expression, they are predisposed to accept the physical interpretation of symptoms rather than to recognize the psychosocial origins and components of illness behaviour.

Western psychiatric researchers, bringing with them a different set of cultural expectations and assumptions, reinterpret as depression the configuration of symptoms that is experienced by Chinese patients and diagnosed by Chinese practitioners as neurasthenia. Individuals in Chinese society do experience and have some insight into the psychosocial component of their symptoms, but these are treated as less important aspects of the physiological "disease" of neurasthenia.

Thus illness experience is not a simple mirror of the disease process. Rather it reflects personal and collective expectations and values; and social and psychological components of that experience can be more powerful determinants of help-seeking behaviour, and of actual disability, than biological abnormalities.

The present scientific evidence does not support a position of complete cultural relativism regarding psychiatric disorders. Some basic disorders seem to be universal. Nevertheless, even "universal" disorders are always understood and interpreted in a specific cultural context. Some investigators have emphasized the "culture-bound" nature of Western psychiatric diagnostic categories, which, they argue, goes beyond simply international differences in labeling conventions and reflects a certain culturally-specific conception of the person.

Fabrega (1984), for example, notes that the identification of the so-called "first-rank symptoms" of schizophrenia depends to a large extent on the prior assumption that people are independent beings whose bodies and minds are fundamentally separated from each other and function autonomously. This in turn presumes "a highly differentiated mentalistic self, which is highly individuated and which looks out on an objective, impersonal, and naturalistic world" (p. 56). Such a conception of the person is far from being universal, either across cultures or over time within our own culture. It is quite specific to the current stage of Western culture, and indeed is held with quite variable degrees of conviction even there.

B. The Impact of Stress Is Not an Objective Characteristic of a Situation

Brown and Harris, in the studies referred to above (1978, 1989), were concerned with the accumulating evidence that "major life events" provided relatively weak explanations of health problems. In their study of depression, therefore, they attempted to refine the way of characterizing provoking agents. They used a "contextual measure" of life events: Each event was scored according to twenty-eight dimensions describing the objective impact of that event on the person's life.

In the Camberwell survey, they found that events that posed a long-term threat, and focused specifically on the person, were most likely to lead to depression. These aspects were therefore used to score the general severity of each event. But the content of the event also influenced its impact: Events that involved a "loss" placed people at greater risk of illness. About one-third of the women experiencing a severe event involving loss later developed depression, compared to only 11 percent of those affected by another severe event.

Interestingly, the notion of loss went beyond a material or relational loss, to include the loss of a "cherished idea." This might include loss of faith in the commitment, faithfulness, or trustworthiness of others, or indeed in oneself—a challenge to one's identity. Over half (twenty-five out of forty-five) of the loss events recorded in the Camberwell study were of a cherished idea, such as to threaten a woman's sense of self-worth; only one-third of the events involved actual loss of a person.

A subsequent longitudinal study undertaken in Islington (Brown and Harris, 1989) yielded the striking result that the impact of an event depended directly on its association with prior events or difficulties. Thus, a particular type of event had a different impact on different individuals, according to its significance in the context of their lives. A particular type of event was much more likely to be followed by depression if it affected a part of life the individual considered important, or one in which the person was already experiencing a marked difficulty, or if the event was connected with a role conflict identified at the first interview. (These were labeled, respectively, C-events, D-events, and R-events.)

Most North American studies postulate that the degree of stress varies according to the number of life events experienced by a person. But the Camberwell findings challenged this assumption of "additivity" by showing that for the most part, just one event of sufficient severity is sufficient for the development of psychiatric disorders. And this severity is determined not just by the characteristics of the event itself, but also by its relationship to the situation of the individual experiencing it.

The Islington study takes this insight further, and replaces the notion of "additivity" by that of "matching," which measures the association between the event and the particular circumstances of the life of an individual. This matching defines the meaning of events for individuals.

An event could "match" on one or more of the dimensions identified above—C, D, and R. The study showed that each additional matching dimension doubles the risk of depression—27 percent for one, 50 percent for two, 100 percent for all three. Thus life events per se are not additive in their effects; but those events that match the circumstances of the person can have strongly additive effects on the probability of developing depression.

The additivity between severe events can take a second form. In the

Islington study, two measures of event "linkage" were developed: the number of linked severe events in a cluster, and the length of time between the first and last severe events in the cluster. The "link index" turned out to be associated with an increased risk for depression even when the number of matching dimensions was taken into account, but only for clusters involving a D-event.

The studies by Brown and Harris are the most detailed attempts, in current epidemiological research, to account for the fact that the impact of a particular event will vary depending upon its meaning to the person experiencing it. Since that meaning will depend, at least in part, on the individual context, they provide operational ways to represent these circumstances and measure their influence. One could apply a similar approach to studying the way cultural norms, values, beliefs, or strategies can mitigate the impact of a major event, or can tremendously accentuate the stress associated with what in another context could appear as a minor incident (like "losing face" in Mediterranean cultures).

Such measures, however, are at best indirect, since "meaning" is essentially defined at the level of each individual life. The impact of an event derives from its specific position within the person's life, in a matrix that is a composite of objective occurrences, and of the individual abilities, fragilities, strengths, and expectations that are both personally and culturally framed.

Brown and Harris (1989) speculate that life events tend to be organized around some key or nuclear scenes, a basic "script" that sets the individual rules for predicting, interpreting, and responding to future scenes, and thus determines the impact of later events. They identified in the Camberwell data a key factor that significantly increased vulnerability to later life events: death of, or separation from, parental figures during childhood. They suggest that this may generate a feeling of helplessness that influences future reactions to stressful events and circumstances. But they do not pursue the study of the cultural dimension of this process.

C. The Social and Cultural Environment Can Itself Be a Source of Stress

Studies on culture change reveal the potential for stress associated with changes at the societal level. But it would be wrong to assume traditional or stable societies always constitute a protective nest. The social and cultural environment in such societies can by itself accentuate the impact of stressful events in individuals' lives, or can generate stresses whose impact goes beyond that of individual life events.

Brown and Prudo's study (1987) of the social determinants of mental health disorders in the Outer Hebrides illustrates the inadequacy of crude indices of social phenomena. Faced with data indicating that "traditionality" is associated both with a lower rate of depression and with a higher rate of anxiety, Brown and Prudo turned to sociological theory, in particular to Durkheim's influential distinction between those aspects of traditional society concerned with *regimentation* (social regulation) and those concerned with *integration* (social cohesiveness and supportiveness). They hypothesized that integration has a protective value against depression, but that the repressive component associated with regulation is linked to anxiety.

To disentangle these two components of traditionality, Brown and Prudo assumed that the degree of involvement in traditional crafts could serve as an index of social integration, while churchgoing, in this Calvinist society, might represent a combination of integration (social support) and regulation (threatening references to hell; strict rules governing day-to-day organization of religious practice). The authors hypothesized that both churchgoing and crafting would be associated with low rates of depression, but that churchgoing would be more closely associated with high rates of anxiety.

These hypotheses were only partially confirmed. Participation in traditional crafts and churchgoing were both associated with a lower rate of depression, but in fact participation in crafts turned out to be *positively* correlated with anxiety. This suggests that some aspects of integration (insofar as that is in fact represented by craft work) appear to contribute to anxiety even as they protect against depression.

The investigators then looked at the correlation between their chosen social integration indices and other potentially relevant variables. These suggested that the protective value of integration, as they measured it, is due in part to the fact that their measures are associated with lower probabilities of both adverse life experience and isolation. In addition, content analysis of individual interviews showed that in this society, women perceive that religious beliefs give them ethical guidance for worldly activities and provide support, purpose, and direction in the wake of adversity.

The potentially damaging effects of integration become easier to understand when one considers that a substantial proportion of chronic anxiety and phobic disorders develop following the death of a close relative, most often the death of a parent. Moreover, these disorders affect primarily women who have shared the dead relative's household.

Brown and Prudo hypothesize that, in this traditional rural society, the early social environment fosters dependency among women and loyalty to the family of origin. It discourages women from emphasizing their own individuality and separating themselves from the group, and undermines their confidence in doing so. This is reinforced at a cultural level by the limited availability of social roles for women in the traditional society of the Outer Hebrides, and by the women's intense commitment to their family of origin. Women are thus caught up in axiomatic relationships that cannot be broken except at the greatest cost. This tremendously accentuates the degree of stress associated with the loss of a close relative.

In this example, cultural values are clearly intermeshed with social rules of behaviour. They produce a certain type of vulnerability associated with a feeling of hopelessness, at the same time as they offer a protection against the hazards of life.

Brown and Prudo's analysis is especially sophisticated, at both the conceptual and the methodological levels. In his study of neurasthenia in China, Kleinman relied more on a general content analysis of patients' and key informants' narratives. But he also concluded that the stresses bearing on individuals are part of a larger social context that has a critical role in determining their impact. The stress of work and that of separation from spouses at different and distant work sites were frequently mentioned by individual patients. But it was clear that the frequency and the significance of these problems can only be understood within the larger context of China after the Cultural Revolution.

On the one hand, the "microdepressogenic" system revealed through individual interviews has origins in the larger society that can lead to demoralization, distress, and despair. Both illness narratives and discussions with Chinese colleagues showed that the impact of these larger social forces in the day-to-day life of those studied was influenced by power relationships in the interpersonal and microsocial environment: family, social networks, work, and community settings.

On the other hand, the influence of this microcontext on sociophysiological processes appears to be influenced by a set of broader cultural meanings and values that determine what support is available, how it is regarded and mobilized, and how loss should be responded to. For example, the importance attached to family life or to the interpersonal dimension of the Chinese conception of self are likely to influence the amount of strain associated with separation or with the self-criticism sessions promoted by the Chinese government. They will also affect the way other people react to individuals placed in this type of situation.

The stresses on individuals are part of a larger framework that moderates or amplifies their potential effects. This larger framework influences the likelihood of experiencing stressful life events, but it also shapes their meaning and it can undermine individual coping reactions through the creation of a more global feeling of hopelessness. Cultural norms, expectations, and values can be paradoxical and contradictory, and can under certain conditions trap vulnerable individuals within a stressful path from which escape is difficult or impossible. As a matrix of life and meaning, culture is not a homogeneous protective nest.

Murphy's (1982) comparative analysis of societies characterized by an unusually high rate of schizophrenia offers an example of just such a pathogenic cultural complex. He identifies certain common cultural features that these societies share: centuries of resented domination by a neighbouring power, massive overseas migration, and intergenerational tensions partly linked to emigration, land shortage, competition for inheritances, and envy.

The most striking of these shared characteristics is a feeling of envy of and resentment toward family members who have gone overseas, and the impossible choice between retaining the emotional advantages associated with the home culture, and gaining the material advantages associated with migration. Whether they have migrated or stayed at home, people in these cultures seem to reproach themselves—and be reproached by others—for having made the wrong decision.

A parallel analysis of societies showing a drastic increase in rates of schizophrenia reveals they have two things in common: a rather stressful contact with a foreign culture, and the need for a change in role or life-style in a context where no satisfying model is available yet it is impossible to return to the former life.[13]

On the basis of these data, Murphy constructs a model of the possible social factors affecting risk of and chronicity in schizophrenia:

- strict and/or contradictory (internalized) social expectations,
- obstacles to attaining rewards implied in those expectations, and
- absence or excessive complexity of roles and guidelines for action.

The stressful impact of this set of circumstances arises from the conjunction of several factors: The stress arising from the situation is perceived as important, it is chronic, and there is no simple solution or escape. According to Murphy, this conjunction of features can provoke schizophrenia in suitably predisposed people. More generally, schizophrenia-prone people are known to be especially vulnerable to an overload of information or stimuli. Problems or contradictions at the cultural level can then precipitate disorders in people whose vulnerability results from genetic, developmental, or other nonspecified predisposing factors.

VI. THE SOCIAL AND CULTURAL MATRIX OF HEALTH PROBLEMS

The foregoing examples of in-depth studies of health determinants illustrate that social and cultural variables are not reducible to a few discrete indices. Social and cultural environments have to be seen as systems of interacting variables variables and processes. The impact of objective stresses will be aggravated or mitigated by a variety of factors, such as collective norms, values, and strategies. Similarly, the effects of stresses are manifested in ways that are related to the social and cultural environment. Figure 4.1's schema is a nonexhaustive illustration of this matrix of influences.

In this chapter, cross-cultural studies have been used to reveal the complexity of the social and cultural matrix surrounding health and disease. Some of this research, like that of Brown and his collaborators, involves rural-urban comparisons within Western societies. In different parts of the world, people create different environments of human interaction and values, which lead to different diagnoses of behavioural problems and to different kinds of responses, coping styles, and social support systems. Cross-cultural studies reveal the larger influence of culture and social structure that shapes the daily lives of individuals and collectivities.

We must be very clear, however, that "culture" or "social processes" are features not only of "other" societies, but also of our own. As long as one remains within one's own cultural boundaries, the ways of thinking, living, and behaving peculiar to that culture are transparent or invisible; they appear to constitute a natural order that is not itself an object of study. But this impression is an unsupported ethnocentric illusion.

VII. IMPLICATIONS FOR RESEARCH AND POLICY

In addition to enhancing our general understanding of the collective shaping of daily life in all societies, cross-cultural studies possess a special significance in view of the increasing cultural diversity of Western societies. Concepts and methods attuned to this social and cultural heterogeneity must be developed for epidemiological and health research, along with more sophisticated methodological and analytical designs. Otherwise, strategies for action derived from epidemiological studies

MACRO
POLITICAL
FORCES

ECONOMIC
CONSTRAINTS

SOCIAL ENVIRONMENT
- social differentiation
- community social life
- social structures of power

manifestations, symptoms
- illness experience
- help-seeking experience
- availability of support system
- diagnostic labeling

CULTURAL STRESSES
- acceptability of traditional ways of life
- continuity/discontinuity with traditional values
- internal consistency/inconsistency

CULTURAL MEDIATORS
- norms and values
- expectations
- coping strategies
  survival and adaptability of traditional coping styles
- social support regulation

Figure 4.1. Matrix of influences of stresses.

will remain disconnected from the reality they are intended to influence. Taking culture into account is not an abstract or academic issue; it can be essential for effective action.

Thus the social and cultural reframing of the "determinants of health" has research and policy implications within our own society. How can research designs be improved in order to address the complexity of health and disease production? What are the implications for policy?

A. Methodological Challenges

First, we must learn to encourage and exploit the complementarity between epidemiological and in-depth studies. The methods of epidemiology are better suited for revealing variation and its correlates than for explaining their meaning. But complementary community studies can be developed to shed interpretive light on some epidemiological findings.

For example, the population survey Santé Québec reveals (among many other things) that in the Abitibi region there is a high degree of psychopathology among women forty-five years and older, that young women (fifteen to twenty-four years old) tend to express psychological distress, and that for men, marriage is very protective against ill health. But to understand the way in which social factors operate to yield these observations, they have to be linked with the typical forms of family organization and of sex relationships in this region.

An in-depth study conducted in six communities in this region (Corin et al., 1990) compares lumbering, agricultural, and mining communities in order to examine the influence of macrosocial forces on local cultures, beliefs, and behaviour. This study reveals that in one of them, a "successful" lumbering community, the protective value of marriage seems to be especially strong for men. This is indirectly revealed through the high rate of suicide and violence among divorced and separated men. The ethnographic study of the two lumbering communities suggests that the main challenge they have to confront as societies is to cope with the rapid social differentiation related to the development of local entrepreneurship and with the split and the coexistence between two normative universes (the traditional rural and the modern). In the successful community, the present feeling of success is always overshadowed by fears of forest disappearance and of the multinational "giants" of the lumbering industry.

Personal narratives indicate that this impression of menace is translated at an individual level into a feeling that social and cultural benchmarks are being eroded, and a strong sense of personal fragility.

The family appears as the locus where larger social tensions and transformations are concentrated and revealed; divorce and separation seem to echo for men the more general fragility of their position within society, and they have a devastating impact. The situation is very different in agricultural and mining communities where tensions take another form and affect other categories of people.

Janes's study of urban Samoans in northern California, referred to above, illustrates the use of methodological complementarity in the reverse direction. On the basis of an intensive community study, the author formulated hypotheses as to the stressful meaning of a given constellation of features. Key concepts were then translated into operational measures, and a subsequent survey collected more extensive quantitative data to test these hypotheses.

Murphy's studies provide another example that clearly demonstrates the merit of a systematic and purposeful utilization of cross-cultural comparisons to formulate and test hypotheses on the influence of culture on health.

In spite of its potential, this integrated two-level approach is still surprisingly rare. This is largely due to the "two solitudes" in which quantitative and qualitative researchers carry out their work—solitudes reinforced by their reciprocal distrust. But understanding of the social and cultural determinants of health problems would be enhanced if both epidemiological and anthropological studies took certain basic principles into account.

a. Toward Socially and Culturally Sensitive Large-Scale Studies

If they are to provide better information on the social and cultural determinants of health and disease, epidemiological studies must meet some basic requirements. Most obviously, sample data must be disaggregated by those descriptors that are potentially relevant for testing the impact of social and cultural variation.

The difficulties encountered in attempting to disaggregate data from the Santé Québec survey provide an illustration. Investigators have collected data to test the relationship between physical and mental health problems, and to test the influence of several psychosocial variables—life events, a measure of social support, a measure of satisfaction with social roles, life-style, service utilization—potentially relevant for an understanding of the social determinants of health. In spite of their crudeness, these indices could have shown the social framing of health and disease in different environments or communities. The sampling methods chosen in the Santé Québec survey, however, place severe constraints on the possibility of clustering data from areas that are socially or culturally homogeneous.

Thus the in-depth anthropological studies that have been carried out in the Abitibi region of Quebec (Corin et al., 1990) have, as described above, been used to interpret some of the findings from Santé Québec. But it is difficult to move in the other direction, and use Santé Québec data to confirm hypotheses derived from intensive qualitative and quantitative studies in a few communities. The Abitibi studies suggested that the different socio-historical contexts associated with lumbering, agriculture, and mining each generate characteristic cultural orientations that translate into different patterns of mental health problems and associated help-seeking behaviour. Some reclustering of the Santé Québec data to test these hypotheses should be possible. But this will come at the price of an important loss of statistical significance, because the importance of such clustering was not recognized when the sampling frame was chosen.

The secondary analyses of the impact of ethnicity in Santé Québec offer an example of another problem with large-scale epidemiological studies: inadequate descriptors for capturing social and cultural variation. The population were categorized as "francophones," "anglophones," or "allophones," without any further qualification. Such a crude descriptor is useless and potentially dangerous, because it creates a seemingly homogeneous category of persons that does not exist in reality. It is not surprising that such a measure should fail to show any correlation with mental health problems. What *is* surprising is that investigators should then draw the strong conclusion that culture has no influence on the basis of such an inadequate descriptor.

More generally, Kleinman notes that aggregate national data mean little if they are not interpreted in local contexts, because there are commonly great differences within and among local communities and social groups. Investigators planning surveys must therefore consider several possible ways to disaggregate their data. A first strategy would be to oversample certain well-defined and potentially significant communities. This would provide "community-specific" data that could be compared to the overall data set, and complemented by more intensive studies. A second strategy would be to do a preliminary selection of neighbourhoods, areas or villages to provide examples of a few categories thought to be relevant to the collective shaping of health problems. Both of these approaches require that "random sampling" be complemented by "selective sampling" guided by social theory. In this way crude cultural and social descriptors can be complemented by data relevant to some specific hypotheses concerning social and cultural variables.

The complex position of individuals within the social and cultural spheres is not captured well, and perhaps not at all, through a single indicator such as "ethnicity." One has to be equally suspicious of simple indices such as "acculturation scores." For example, in an exploratory study of Haitian families, Sansfacon and Corin (1990) used a classical scale developed by Cuellar and Harris for measuring acculturation. Paradoxically, the more educated and long-term immigrants tended to score very low on acculturation, while the much less educated, more recent immigrants scored high. The resolution of the paradox appears to be that intellectuals feel an ideological commitment to "Haitian" culture, while more deprived people, struggling for integration within the host society, prefer to present a "Westernized" self-image during the interview.

Individuals usually participate simultaneously in several social and cultural spheres (family, religion, work, leisure, associations, etc.). These may be connected with each other, and interacting, or they may be mutually isolated. And their interactions, if any, may be complementary or in opposition. Surveys, or the in-depth studies complementing them, should provide some indication of the different reference groups that form the background to individual responses and behaviour, and at least attempt to describe the person's position within these different spheres.

Murphy's data on "European offshoots" illustrate the interesting potential of such information (Murphy, 1978, 1980). He identified inter- and intracultural variations in rates of admission to hospital for mental illness and in lengths of stay. These variations were then compared with detailed data on the religious affiliation of immigrants and their degree of participation in church activities. These comparisons led him to hypotheses as to the protective or constraining influences of the specific religious perceptions and practices of people from different ethnic origins.

The empirical study of key variables must respect the cultural meaning associated with a given concept in a given milieu. It should enable disclosure *of variations in meaning that are associated with different cultural environments*. A general tendency among Western researchers is to take for granted the universality of our own understanding of concepts such as "social support" or "coping." On the other hand, culturally sensitive authors have drawn attention to the error of "category fallacy," which consists of taking a concept developed for a particular cultural group (that of the researcher—usually Western) and applying it to members of another culture for whom it lacks coherence and where its validity has not been established (Kleinman, 1987). Even if the concept can be "reliably" identified in the second group, reliability in measurement does not guarantee validity.

Kleinman's study on neurasthenia in China illustrates how the cluster of signs and symptoms identified as depression in the West lacks cultural validity in Chinese culture, even if depressive symptoms can be identified by Western investigators. Similarly, a study of coping in a southern black community (Dressler, 1985) showed that what is generally considered a "positive" style of coping for white men in the West is counteradaptive for black men, who are not supposed to appear as too assertive in the whites' world.

Studies of social support networks offer additional examples of the way in which different cultural contexts can change the meaning and the influence of an apparently universal concept. Dressler, for example, found that contrary to common expectation, in some black communities greater "support" from the extended kin network is associated with a larger number of mental health symptoms for women seventeen to thirty-four years old. Ethnographic research revealed that in this community young women are closely watched and expected to follow strictly the advice given by important kin. The "support" received from the extended family represented not real help, but rather the imposition of controls and burdensome obligations.

A study of social support and help-seeking behaviour among the elderly in the province of Quebec (Corin, 1986) suggested that regardless of the pattern of social support actually available, individual and collective norms and expectations determine the specific types of others on which people prefer to, and feel entitled to, rely for support. People from different backgrounds differ in their "preferred supporters." Rural elders look to the other spouse when present; privileged, urban elderly in the city of Quebec look to their children. Women from deprived urban areas expect help from their family and neighbors, while men from those areas prefer to rely on friends and neighbours.

Biegel, Naparstek, and Khan (1980) have shown that both for the elderly and for respondents from particular ethnic communities, the feeling of belonging to a given neighbourhood is more important for mental health than more specifically identifiable interpersonal support. Although social support is typically assumed to be provided by family and friends, its meaning and scope can vary considerably in different cultures. Looking across cultures, key elements of a global feeling of support can include the feeling of being blessed by the ancestors, of being supported by a maternal uncle, the opportunity to interact with a "compadre," or the sense of having respected all the precise rules of a complex mourning ritual.

Thus while "social support" is widely accepted as a factor mitigating the impact of stress and promoting mental (and physical) health, the precise meaning associated with various social links, with the social environment, and with cultural rules and values will vary with the cultural context. One has to be sure that the instruments used for collecting data will identify and respond to the main components of social support in a milieu. In order to interpret measures of support, one has to be sure that all that was measured does in fact indicate support, and that all important dimensions of social support are well included in the scale. This is of more than conceptual interest; it is also important for planning any action to strengthen the social support network in a given setting.

The challenge for epidemiologists is to construct instruments that are simultaneously culturally sensitive and capable of collecting data that are comparable across cultures. Dressler's solution was to begin with a general definition of social support and to use open-ended interviews with key informants and all available ethnographic data as a basis for drafting culturally appropriate questions. Others have used a combination of standardized, well-established instruments, carefully translated, along with questions based on categories or notions taken from within the studied culture that seem to be close to the concept of interest to the investigators (Manson, Shore, and Bloom, 1985). Still others (Brown and Harris, 1989) take care to collect verbatim, as well as more standard, responses, so as to be able to reexamine and recategorize items such as "conceptualization" and "understanding progress." There is then an ongoing dynamic relationship between data collection, hypothesis formulation, and the return to data to confirm or modify an hypothesis.

b. Toward Intensive Studies Comparable across Cultures

Even if it is possible to define measures of key variables that are more sensitive to the influences of different cultural contexts, some cultural variables or dimensions are simply not defined at the level of the individual. They must be identified and described at the collective level. Ecological variables, which describe objective features of the individuals' environments, can be included in epidemiological studies. But in-depth community studies are more appropriate for the analysis of collective systems of values, meanings, and behaviour.

An exclusive focus on in-depth analysis of small communities, however, presents two major risks. The researcher can be trapped in a web of complex interactions without being able to draw any general conclusions at all from the data. The study is then limited to descriptive research. Alternatively, the author may achieve a coherent but untestable vision of the data, leading to the formulation of post hoc hypotheses reflecting that vision. Community studies should include a systematic documentation of specific features or processes that are believed to be significant within some more general theoretical model of the social and cultural determinants of health and disease. These "significant" features and processes will, of course, vary according to the precise research focus.

The Stirling County Study (Leighton, 1959), a classic in psychiatric epidemiology, has opened avenues in this direction. Intensive studies of the various communities, supplemented by general quantitative data, allowed the researchers to classify them according to their degree of integration and disintegration. Parallel psychiatric epidemiological data revealed that the prevalence of mental health problems is directly related to the degree of social disintegration.

In the Abitibi study, investigators tried to systematize the collection of ethnographic and qualitative information, and to gather culturally sensitive data that were also amenable to comparison. The general research objective was to examine the "cultural accessibility" of mental health services, e.g., their degree of fit with local modes of perception and behaviour.

The ethnographic data on these collectivities could be compared, because they were organized around three main axes (integration/disintegration, collective competence/dependence, opening/closure toward the outside world). These three axes directed the observations and interviews.

Data on perceptions and behaviour in the area of mental health were collected from illness narratives of actual reconstructed cases identified on the basis of fourteen "behavioural descriptions" corresponding to mental health problems that seem to be universal. The analysis of illness narratives indicated that individuals' identification and description of their mental health problems are organized around a few key notions that parallel the important social and cultural characteristics derived from the ethnographic study of the communities. Analysis of the use of mental health services revealed the practical relevance of this kind of qualitative analysis for understanding the patterns of use characteristic of each of these communities.

VIII. CHALLENGES FOR POLICY AND INTERVENTION

Previous chapters have emphasized the socioeconomic gradient in health. Socioeconomic status (SES) is, however, only one aspect of the social context. Such status, however defined, is very far from encompassing all the ways in which the social environment may influence health, or focusing all the possible strategies for remedial policy and action. An exclusive emphasis on SES could have the perverse effect of enforcing a purely objective and deterministic conception of environmental influences on the health of individuals and groups.

A narrow focus on SES promotes an essentially passive picture of deprived people and communities. [This picture is easier to accept if one ignores the important message of Marmot's *gradient* (Chapter 1). The relationship between health and hierarchy is *not* simply a correlate of deprivation; it holds all the way up the scale.] Entire groups of the population are in need of "assistance" from professional services or governmental agencies. This appears to be a most peculiar way to remedy what may be the health consequences of powerlessness.

A more global understanding of the social determinants of health, and of the characteristics of the collectivity that aggravate or mitigate their influence, might lead to much more targeted and interactive interventions involving the various groups and communities as partners.

In Abitibi, for example, data on the use of mental health services reveal interesting intercommunity variations. The analysis of both the overall utilization data and the categories of people with unusually high or low rates of utilization clearly indicates that the use of services is influenced by (differing) collective values and strategies. It seems obvious that this information should be used for health services planning.

But the use of such information must also be culturally sensitive. People in the more "fragile" communities tend also to be the more reluctant to use mental health or social services. If these communities are simply targeted as "at risk," the labeling effect could destabilize the collective survival strategies that the community has developed to maintain its social identity. The potential "gatekeepers" through which it is necessary to pass in order to reach and mobilize the community will vary from milieu to milieu, as will their degree of openness toward outside intervention.

There are analogous constraints on and dangers in attempting to intervene in certain urban areas, in particular cultural communities, or in "target groups" such as teenagers. "Helping" programs, if they are to be effective, must take these factors into account. This should help avoid two main risks: noncompliance or rejection of programs that would, as a result, remain irrelevant failures, and further undermining of vulnerable groups or communities.

Progress in this direction will require us to distinguish issues of content from those of process. It is clearly unrealistic to try to design policies and actions individually adapted to the special circumstances of each local group. It should be possible, however, to build into general programs both a concern for flexibility and mechanisms to achieve it. If one cannot provide "ready-made packages" adapted to each group's dynamics, it is nevertheless possible to draft some principles that can guide local service administrators, service teams, and individual practitioners to adjust their actions to local conditions.

The following are offered as examples of such general principles:

- Programs have to be culturally and socially acceptable and appropriate; they must respect social definitions of privacy frontiers, of the rules for giving and receiving support, and of appropriate channels for action.
- Programs must build on a community's strengths and insights, and try to reinforce them; they must not contribute to a collective sense of inadequacy or fragility by well-intentioned but culturally inappropriate actions.
- Attempts to modify attitudes and behaviour should be based on an understanding of their cultural origins and significance, their present functions, and their central or peripheral position within the life of the community.
- Outreach programs should take account of the relative importance, the degrees of tolerance or intolerance, accorded to various problems in a given community. For example, a certain degree of violence might be well accepted, and even valued as a male attribute, in a community based on hazardous and precarious occupations. In a rural community valuing conformity and decency the same events might cause great concern.[14]
- The concept of "at-risk groups" should be complemented by that of "target conditions." Attention should be focused on the way in which specific or general health problems arise from a complex web of social and cultural determinants in a given environment, a web which may extend well beyond the identified "at-risk group."[15]

The real challenge for culturally sensitive policymaking is to open practitioners' minds to the importance of these principles. Community intervention has to proceed in step with progress in interdisciplinary knowledge and understanding. Present trends in the province of Quebec toward the decentralization of health services planning and administration could, in principle, support this kind of approach.

The growing social and cultural heterogeneity of Western societies makes it imperative to understand the nature and influences of collective processes in order to develop and adapt effective strategies for intervention. As Peter Glynn, then assistant deputy minister of Health and Welfare Canada, noted: "services and activities will have to be dramatically altered to recognize the role of culture in human health and disease" (cited in Beiser, 1990:6).

NOTES

1. Men have been shown to rely significantly more on their spouses for support and intimacy, while women tend to rely on a larger span of social resources (Corin, Tremblay, Sherif, and Bergeron, 1984). The greater protective value of marriage for men is confirmed by epidemiological data. For example the matched-records study of deaths for the period 1959–1961 (Mechanic, 1978:162) showed that mortality rates for single, widowed, or divorced men, relative to their married counterparts, were higher than the corresponding relative rates for women. Similarly, Perrault (1990) cites Statistics Canada (1978) data on the rate of first admissions to inpatient psychiatric care, which show a rate for divorced and widowed persons that is double that for married persons. But the rate for widowed or divorced *men* is much higher than that for their female counterparts. She also cites U.S. data on suicide in the age range forty to sixty, showing that the relative rate for separated or divorced men is over three times that for women. Similar large differentials are found between widows and widowers.

2. It is striking that the only variables documented as potential predictors in the IPSS were specific to the individual: sociodemographic characteristics, past personal and family history of mental disorders, and predictors related to characteristics of the initial psychotic episode. While engaged in a cross-cultural study, the WHO employed a conceptual framework essentially similar to that represented in Figure 1.1.

3. Similar critical analyses have been applied to the evolution of the concepts of life-style (Coreil, Levin, and Jaco, 1985), type A behaviour pattern (Helman, 1987), and social support (Jacobson, 1987). Coreil et al. trace the evolution of the life-style concept from Marx, for whom life-style was economically determined; and Veblen and Weber, for whom life-style was more related to the social status order; to Adler, who used the concept to refer to the individual as a purposive actor in life, and to design a certain "personality style." Common to these various notions was the idea that life-style is a unifying concept linking various parts of a whole personality and connoting uniqueness and creativity expressed in action. The current intellectual tendency, by contrast, is to consider life-styles as discrete and independently modifiable personal habits— risk factors, in the jargon of the epidemiologist. The concept has been transformed into its antithesis, so that today "behaviors are treated as isolated elements, divorced from their social context and bereft of the meaning which derives from the larger cultural frame" (Coreil et al., 1985:431).

Helman (1987) rejects the conventional interpretation of type A behaviour as an individual personality trait. Instead he suggests that this behaviour pattern literally and figuratively embodies the contradictions among the values of modern Western capitalist societies. Type A behaviour, by this formulation, is extreme conformity with Western capitalist values, to the point of deviance. The use of the concept to explain the incidence of coronary heart disease in non-Western societies would therefore be without meaning.

Jacobson (1987) emphasizes that social support is not an objective reality, but is part of an interpretive framework. It cannot be dissociated from its cultural foundations—from the factors that influence the making and the breaking of social relations, from the meaning attributed to relations, and from the conceptions regarding who should give and get support. Norms on reciprocity, autonomy, and helping behaviours are always relative to a given context.

4. Indeed, to the extent that these Western-developed constructs exclude *by design* competing collective hypotheses, they will also fail to reveal any similar phenomena that might be present in Western cultures.

5. Participant observation is based on sharing the daily life of people and communities one wants to study. It includes formal and informal questioning, as well as the observation of behaviours, relationships, naturally occurring events, etc. It permits the observer to comprehend the general social and cultural context necessary for understanding the specific topic that constitutes the object of the research.

6. The occupational scale was constructed with St. Lucian informants and reflected both income and prestige.

7. Indices considered were house ownership, home construction material, and presence of electricity, plumbing, toilet, livestock, radio, stereo, gas stove, refrigerator, settee, and car. These measures were closely correlated with each other, and were combined in a unidimensional scale.

8. The study population was a 50 percent random sample from a list of people who had been treated at least once in an Indian Health Service Clinic or hospital in the previous ten years. Two sources of data were used: an extensive interview and a review of inpatient and outpatient medical records.

9. Three scales were constructed: rank of per capita income; a leadership scale consisting of different items for men and women; a scale of kindred involvement. Each scale was divided at the median into high and low categories. Two pairs of status dimensions (economic resources/leadership, and economic resources/kindred involvement) were cross-tabulated and mean systolic and diastolic blood pressures were calculated for the individuals within each of the cells in the resulting two-by-two tables. There is a fairly substantial difference between the "consistent" and "inconsistent" groups in the high-leadership and family involvement categories, suggesting that inconsistency is an important source of stress. Differences between high- and low-income categories, however, were only significant for people with high kindred involvement.

10. *Diagnostic and Statistical Manual of Mental Disorders* (3rd.), published by the American Psychological Association.

11. The scientific status of the discipline (and of its members) requires, however, that its basic elements be universal. Ideally, such universality would emerge from consistency of observation. But if the data are uncooperative, an imposed consensus of interpretation can serve almost as well.

12. As Kleinman (1988) observes, the DOP's investigators do not address the question of the epistemological significance of scrapping most of a sample that shows heterogeneity in order to work with the most homogeneous subsample: "The restricted sample is artifactual since it places a clinical template on the original population that excludes precisely those cases that demonstrate most cultural heterogeneity" (p. 21). By contrast, the broad sample includes all first-contact cases of psychosis meeting the diagnostic criteria and is therefore the valid one from a cross-cultural perspective.

13. Achinese men, for example, have to abandon the role of warrior, and take up roles associated with cultivation and trading. These were formerly regarded as undignified activities, suitable only for women and the conquered. In this changing environment, they are especially at risk for schizophrenia.

14. Programs should take account of these differences, but not necessarily be guided by them. Each local community is embedded in a larger society, which also has cultural norms and values that must be respected. A particular cultural

community may regard assaults of various forms against women, for example, as of no great significance. But such cultural values must not be permitted to interfere with the full enforcement of the laws of the wider society; each member of every cultural group is entitled to their protection.

15. For example, young women of low socioeconomic status (and their children) have become the most significant "at-risk group" for smoking and diseases caused by smoking. Yet policies to reduce tobacco-induced disease may be more effective if they are not targeted solely at this group—for example, a general ban on advertising, or serious efforts to prevent sales to minors.

5

The Role of Genetics in Population Health

P. A. BAIRD

INTRODUCTION

Many people have difficulty considering impartially and objectively the application of genetics to human beings. There are at least two important reasons for this lack of receptivity.

The first is the emotional legacy of Nazi Germany. The gross misuse of genetics in social policy—the devaluation and brutal treatment of selected groups, not only in Nazi Germany, but in North America and parts of Europe—has left a lingering suspicion. At some level, many still equate genetics with inhumane control.

Second, if something is determined by genes, it appears to be predestined, and to leave no scope for individual choice. This undermines the cherished notion that individuals are self-determining agents with free will. Further, genetic determination appears to preclude acceptable social remedies—"it's just in your genes." We cannot expect these threatening ideas to be embraced with alacrity.

Yet genetics is a critical determinant of health, as indicated in the framework developed in Chapter 2. Measuring the precise frequency of genetically determined disease or of the genetic contribution to disease in a population is, however, very difficult. The onset of genetic disease may occur at any time in the life cycle, and results from a complex interaction between the genetic endowment (genotype) of the individual and the environment. Some diseases are the direct consequence of genes that do not permit normal function in any environment. In others, a genetic predisposition is only expressed under certain environmental conditions.

We can think of health as a homeostatic balance between individuals and their environments. The genes we have are the product of a long evolutionary history; they have survived because they permit maintenance of homeostasis within our usual range of environments. Disease results when:

1. the individual has genes that do not allow adaptation to ordinary environments (e.g., phenylketonuria, cystic fibrosis, hemophilia);
2. the environment is so hostile that it overwhelms the adaptive capacity of normal human mechanisms, whatever the genetic endowment (e.g., inadequate diet, toxins, viral infections);
3. there is some combination of environmental insult and genetic predisposition (e.g., diabetes, heart disease).

Genes set the limits of our possible responses, not only to physical and biological environments, but also to our psychological and social experiences. There is evidence (Chess and Hassibi, 1986) that humans come into the world with certain personality attributes and "styles" set, and in the normal range of social environments these persist.

The relationship between genetic endowment and environment can be illustrated by a simple genetic model of disease determination in individuals with early heart attacks due to high cholesterol. There will be a range of variation in this group. At one extreme are individuals whose genetic makeup will not allow homeostasis on a normal diet. At the other are individuals whose metabolic machinery is fine, but whose particular environment is so extreme—very heavy cholesterol intake—as to overwhelm normal homeostatic mechanisms. If dietary cholesterol is low in the whole culture, then "genetic" cases will constitute a greater proportion of those with early heart attacks.

Environmental and genetic aspects can be separated conceptually, but in reality interact in a complex, subtle, and pervasive way whereby the genotype may in fact influence what particular kinds of environmental exposures an individual receives. For example, there are genetically determined differences in the experiences to which individuals are attracted, and also in the experiences they evoke from their environments (Scarr and McCartney, 1983).

The diseases now common in developed countries do not have just an environmental or just a genetic cause. They are due to interactions between the individual's genetic makeup and his or her particular experience. With more prosperity and better living conditions it is probable that the relative contribution of genetics to disease has increased in the last century. But a rigorous assessment of the frequency of genetic disease is not easy.

EVIDENCE

The Measurement of Genetically Determined Disease

Population statistics are usually only available for such events as mortality by cause, or hospital admission by disease coded to the International Classification of Diseases (WHO). Neither of these allows an estimation of the prevalence of genetic disease as they are not etiologic (causal) classifications. Rather they are a mixed bag. Some diseases/events are classified by anatomic site affected, some by nature or timing of onset, and some by etiology. For these reasons, it is not at present possible to specify quantitatively the contribution of genetic factors to death and disease.

Despite these limitations, it is clear that genes significantly affect health status and disease at all stages of life.

Data from Different Life Stages

Conception to Birth. Over half of fertilized eggs in healthy women fail to produce live-born babies. Losses occur at the preimplantation stage, at the postimplantation stage prior to the woman recognizing she is pregnant, as well as later losses recognized as spontaneous abortions. Preimplantation loss is difficult to measure in humans, but by extrapolation from other mammals is likely to be substantial (Hendrick and Binkerd, 1980). Dominant lethal genes are likely to play an important role here.

There is good evidence from biochemical studies of women at risk for becoming pregnant that between 40 and 60 percent of zygotes that implant are lost before the woman realizes she is pregnant (Miller et al., 1980). Finally, about 15 percent of *recognized* pregnancies in humans end in spontaneous loss prior to twenty weeks gestation. In nonhuman primates the figures are of the same order of magnitude as those for humans, with estimates of recognizable loss (spontaneous abortions) from 7 to 22 percent for various species (Hendrick and Binkerd, 1980).

Genetic causes are a major factor in these failed pregnancies, most strikingly during the first three months after conception. For example, demonstrable chromosomal abnormalities are found in over half of early spontaneous abortions (Hassold et al., 1980; Carr, 1977). These defect rates among early spontaneous losses do not appear to be changing. For example, data collected over the last twenty years in Seattle (Shepard, Fantel, and Fitzsimmons, 1989) show approximately a fifth of embryos and fetuses have a localized defect in form or structure (morphology) or an identifiable set of defects (syndrome). There is no clear trend of change over time.

In the case of stillbirths and neonatal deaths, the results of several surveys show that between 6 and 7 percent have a chromosome abnormality.

From Infancy to Young Adulthood. At least 5 percent of live-born individuals in a large population of over one million consecutive births were found to have disease with an important genetic component before age twenty-five years (Baird, Anderson, Newcombe, and Lowry, 1988). These represent individuals with severe enough problems to require medical services prior to that age.

The impact of genetic disease on the use of pediatric health care is substantial. For example, a sampling of over twelve thousand admissions to a pediatric hospital found that 11.1 percent were for "genetic" causes (that is, listed as being of Mendelian inheritance in McKusick's [1988] catalogue), 18.5 percent were for congenital malformations,[1] and 2 percent were "probably" genetic. Thus over 30 percent of all admissions represented the effect of genetic disorders and birth defects (Scriver, Neal, Saginur, and Clow, 1973). It is particularly noteworthy that the majority of pediatric patients with multiple admissions fall into one of these three groups. The contribution to use of medical resources by individuals with genetic disease is out of proportion to the percentage of the population affected by them. These findings have been confirmed in several other studies, and in recent decades about a quarter of children admitted to pediatric hospitals have had disorders strongly influenced by genetic factors (Day and Holmes, 1973; Hall, Powers, McIlvaine, and Ean, 1978).

The relative importance of genetic causes of disease in our population has increased markedly in this century for many disorders. In the early 1900s, for example, the infant mortality rate in the United States was about 150 per 1,000 live births. About 5 of these 150 (3 percent) were thought to be wholly or in part genetically determined. The infant mortality rate is now below 10 per 1,000 live births in most developed countries. However, the incidence of genetically caused deaths is now believed to represent over one-third of all infant deaths (Kaback, 1978), as other causes have dramatically decreased.

By the mid-1980s the perinatal mortality rates in the United States and

Great Britain had also fallen to about 10 per 1,000 live births. Most of these deaths occur in the first few days of life. The two main causes, congenital anomalies and prematurity, may have a genetic background. Approximately 7 percent of infants that die perinatally have demonstrable chromosomal abnormalities.

The decline in the contribution of infectious disease and nutritional deficiencies has thrown genetic disorders into greater prominence. Emery (1983) reports that the proportion of childhood deaths in U.K. hospitals from genetic causes increased from about 15 percent in 1914 to about 50 percent in 1976. He also found that in Madras in the latter year the situation was very different, with less than 5 percent of childhood deaths in hospitals being due to genetic causes.

As another example, Scriver and Tenenhouse (1981) have noted that rickets was an endemic disease in industrialized Western nations in the nineteenth century. Its main cause was deficiency of vitamin D, because of inadequate diet and poor exposure to sunlight. In the 1920s the role of vitamin D was elucidated and food supplementation on a population basis was initiated. The incidence of rickets declined dramatically. While cases still continue to appear, they are no longer environmentally caused. Most individuals with rickets now have inherited genes resulting in a disorder of mineral metabolism even when normal amounts of vitamin D are present. The proportion of genetically determined rickets cases is now much greater. This is yet another example of several thousand genetic diseases (McKusick, 1988). For many diseases, the proportion attributable to heredity is likely to have increased as the environment has changed.

From Middle to Late Adulthood. We have very limited knowledge about the effects of genetic factors on the overall health of people after twenty-five years of age. The incidence of disorders of late onset, with multiple and complex causes (multifactorial) in which genotype is implicated, may be up to 60 percent if such conditions as diabetes, hypertension, myocardial infarction, ulcers, and thyrotoxicosis are included (UNSCEAR Report, 1986). If certain cancers are also included, this figure would be even higher.

Age-specific mortality rates show a characteristic U-shaped curve over the human life span, with rates highest at each end of the age spectrum. The causes of death at the two ends of the spectrum are not, however, the same (Childs and Scriver, 1988). Deaths in early life are characterized by abnormal development and difficulty in adaptation to life after birth. Mendelian disorders are typically diseases of prereproductive life (Costa, Scriver, and Childs, 1985), with over 90 percent apparent by the end of puberty. They reduce the life span and usually cause psychosocial handicaps. The diseases of the elderly, in contrast, are mainly associated with sociocultural, economic, and physical environments, and increasing senescence.

As a cohort moves through the life span, its genetic variability decreases. The least adaptive genes are the first to be lost, along with the individuals that bear them. After puberty the genes that remain are likely to be maladaptive and contribute to disease only in some particular environmental circumstances.

In contrast to the decreasing genetic variability, the variability of environmental experience must increase throughout life. The genetic contribution to the diseases that affect the cohort is likely to diminish as it ages. For disease categories with a wide range of ages of onset, monogenic forms are more likely to be found among early-onset cases. Multifactorial cases should be found more frequently in middle age; in the very old, the disease will likely be due primarily to environmental determinants.

Childs and Scriver found that the available evidence with regard to nine disorders [Alzheimer's, celiac, Crohn's and Parkinson's diseases, duodenal ulcer, gout, non-insulin-dependent diabetes mellitus (NIDDM), rheumatoid arthritis, and systemic lupus erythematosis] was compatible with a decline in the impact of genes on disease with increasing age. This may provide some insight into both the determinants of disease and the potential of preventive efforts aimed at environmental factors.

Single-gene disorders of early onset carry heavier burdens than those of later life (Costa et al., 1985) and are also relatively resistant to treatment (Hayes, Costa, Scriver, and Childs, 1985). Those cases in which genes are an important determinant may be more difficult to prevent. There must be an irreducible minimum of genetic contribution to disease and death that feasible environmental manipulation cannot prevent. The genetic variation in the population will determine the limits to what can be achieved by any environmental measures, and this should be taken into account in evaluating what is possible.

Treating a population as if all members were at uniform risk, and then attempting to improve their environment, cannot eliminate all disease and will certainly have diminishing returns. There will always be individuals with a monogenic origin for their disease. For this group a different strategy is indicated. Although the proportion with a very strong genetic component will be relatively small, these cases, being "early onset," will have a greater impact. For example, the overall contribution of monogenic causes to deaths from heart disease is small. But genetic factors account for a high proportion of deaths from heart disease prior to age forty-five. Greater understanding of genetic pathophysiology may make it possible to tailor "microenvironments" to fit particular genotypes.

Assessing the Genetic Component

Determining the role of genetics in disease will require better methods of classifying disease and processing health data. Computerized record linkage will be increasingly important (as Chapter 11 particularly emphasises), not only to build longitudinal health histories on individuals but to link these into family groupings and sets of individuals with common parents (sibships). Administrative and other health data sets that already exist can be brought together to detect familial clustering. If such clustering is found, various methods may be used to disentangle genetic from shared environmental factors, or more likely, to identify the interaction between the two (King, Lee, Spinner, Thomson, and Wrensch, 1984).

Twin Studies

Monozygotic (MZ) twins are genetically identical as they result from the splitting of one fertilized ovum, whereas dizygotic (DZ) twins are only as genetically alike as any two siblings. This allows comparison of genetically identical and genetically different individuals who are usually raised in a similar environment. It therefore makes possible an estimation of the degree of genetic influence on a disease. It is also possible to look at identical twins reared apart or together to help estimate the effect of environmental factors.

If a disease were completely determined by gene(s) then the concordance rate in MZ twins should be 100 percent and the concordance in DZ should be the same as in pairs of siblings who share the same parents. Studies of many common adult disorders in MZ and DZ twins show much higher concordance in MZ than in DZ pairs. This is true for schizophrenia, multiple sclerosis, alcoholism, affective disorders, epilepsy, the neuroses, NIDDM, and allergies, clearly demonstrating that there is a genetic component to these diseases. The concordance rate in these studies in MZ twins is, however, less than 100 percent, equally clearly demonstrating the presence of other determinants (Gottesman and Shields, 1976; Spielman and Nathanson, 1981; Hrubec and Omenn, 1981; Allen, 1976; Newmark and Perry, 1980; Pyke and Nelson, 1976).

Heritability Studies

It is important to note that estimates of heritability of a trait relate to the particular population and particular conditions in which it is measured. For example, if the environment changes, an estimate will no longer be valid. Estimates of heritability have been made for many human traits. They should be interpreted only as indicators of whether the role of genes is relatively large or small in the population and circumstances in which the condition is measured (Cavalli-Sforza and Bodmer, 1971).

Estimates of the heritability of traits measurable as continuous variables (e.g., blood pressure, serum lipids) can be derived, if certain assumptions are made, from observations in MZ and DZ twin pairs or in parent-offspring or sib-sib pairs. The estimation of how much of the variation in the population is due to genes is complex. However, such estimates help us understand the contribution of genes to a particular trait.

Adoption Studies

Individuals raised by adopting parents provide the opportunity to examine given traits or disorders in adopted individuals for resemblance to the biological and the rearing families. They provide a window on "nature-nurture" issues. This approach has been followed for a number of traits such as blood pressure and for disorders such as schizophrenia (Kety, Rosenthal, Wedner, and Schulsinger, 1976; Mednick and Gabrielli, 1984; *Lancet*, 1983; Guze, 1985) and alcoholism (Goodwin, 1981).

The Danish adoption studies are excellent models for how genetic aspects of complex disorders can be elucidated. For example, an interesting recent study of adoptees shows that premature death in adults, especially death due to infections and vascular causes, has a strong genetic background (Sorensen, Nielsen, Andersen, and Teasdale, 1988).

Early adoption also enables one to compare the concordance rates in MZ twins reared together and apart. The concordance rate is similar, whether the MZ twins are reared together or apart, for both schizophrenia and affective psychoses (Slater and Cowie, 1971; Price, 1968). This suggests that the usual range of adopting environments has little impact on the occurrence of these conditions; any environmental factor must either have its effect very early or be ubiquitous.

Numerous studies designed to elucidate whether there is a genetic component to various psychiatric disorders have taken advantage of the excellent records kept in Denmark. For example, in one study, registers of individuals with schizophrenia were searched for those who had been adopted in early infancy. The biological and the adopting relatives of these individuals were then traced and interviewed by a psychiatrist unaware of whether or not they were controls. The incidence of schizophrenia in the biological relatives was three times that in the adopting relatives, where it had the usual population incidence. If schizophrenia is learned behaviour this should not be the case (Kety, 1983). For the disorder under study, a greater resemblance to the biological family than to the family of rearing has been found in adoptees who exhibit schizophrenia, affective psychosis, criminal convictions (Mednick and Gabrielli, 1984) and alcoholism (Goodwin, 1981), thus clearly demonstrating a genetic causal component. Of course, these approaches do not elucidate the nature of the particular genetic mechanism.

Adoption studies can help clarify the importance of familial/cultural components relative to genetic components. It is obvious that alcohol must be available to someone to become alcoholic, whether or not a genetic predisposition is present. Social and familial factors interact in determining the frequency of the outcome "alcoholism" in a population, although genetic factors may be important in determining who becomes alcoholic. This illustrates the point that the causes for sick individuals and sick populations are different (Rose, 1985).

Associations between Genotype and Disease

Humans differ in an identifiable way in their HLA (human leukocyte antigen) system and their ABO blood group systems, and different genotypes within these systems have been found to be associated with the occurrence of any one of a variety of diseases. Increasingly, differences between people in recombinant DNA polymorphisms will be evaluated and correlated with a variety of disease outcomes in the same way. There are now a number of well-documented examples where having a particular identifiable genotype is associated with disease susceptibility (or resistance). Within the HLA system, for example, having the gene for B27 is associated with approximately ninety times the usual risk for ankylosing spondylitis. Having the gene for DR4 is associated with six times the risk of insulin dependent diabetes, but having DR2 on the other hand has only one-fifth the usual risk of this disease (King et al., 1984, Tables 5 and 6).

There have been a large number of studies of ABO blood groups and it has been found that individuals with a given disease have a particular blood group significantly more often than an appropriately matched group without the disease. Early studies were not always appropriately done, but nevertheless it appears that there are some real associations between ABO blood group and some diseases. For example, blood group O individuals are at risk for gastric and duodenal ulcers, but blood group A individuals are at risk for stomach cancer, rheumatic disease, and pernicious anemia (King et al., 1984, Tables 5 and 6).

Another example of how genotype is related to disease is that people carrying one gene for a particular type of hemoglobin—hemoglobin S—are more common in areas of the world where malaria has been endemic. It has been shown that these individuals are more resistant to malaria infection than those without the gene (Paszol, Weatherall, and Wilson,

1978). This advantage has led to natural selection keeping this gene at a higher frequency in these populations, even though it is lethal in those individuals where both genes in the pair for hemoglobin are genes for hemoglobin S (that is, they are homozygous). A similar situation exists for a gene on the X chromosome. Several different forms (alleles) of this gene have been found, each of which causes an enzyme deficiency (glucose-6-phosphate dehydrogenase deficiency; Beutler, 1978). Males with one of these genes on their X chromosome develop hemolytic anemia if they are exposed to fava beans and some pharmaceutical agents. Females who inherit the gene are unlikely to be affected as their second X chromosome carries the normal form of the gene—females may therefore be healthy carriers. Geographic distribution of high frequencies of carriers is again correlated with areas where malaria was previously endemic. Having the gene must have provided an advantage in terms of less susceptibility to malaria.

There are a number of statistical techniques that can be used to clarify whether familial clustering is due to genetic cause—for example, segregation analysis, linkage analysis, path analysis on pairs of relatives, and sib-pair methods. To summarize, the accumulation of evidence demonstrates conclusively that genetics is an important factor in determining health.

How Do Genetic Determinants Relate to Socioeconomic Determinants?

How then does this evidence for genetics as an important determinant of ill health relate to the evidence in previous chapters? Health is also clearly related to social class and to psychosocial determinants. Any attempt to ascertain relative causal importance should bear in mind Rose's (1985) thoughtful analysis of the distinction between the causes of cases and the causes of incidence. He rightly points out that the question, Why do some individuals have hypertension? is quite different from the question Why do some populations have a high rate of hypertension? The answer to the latter has to do with the causes of incidence: What determines the population mean? What influence acts on the population as a whole? The answer to the former must explain differences among individuals within a given population. The determinants of incidence are not necessarily the same as the causes of cases. For example, strong associations between mean values for sodium intake in different *populations* and their mean blood pressures are easily demonstrated. Yet it is very difficult to show any relation between diet and blood pressure for *individuals*.

If it is assumed that several genes for vulnerability exist for each of the common adult diseases (and this is very likely the case), these genes must be distributed similarly over the different social classes. This must be so because the gene pools of these classes are not separate in most Western countries. There is significant social mobility and intermarriage, enough that over several generations the gene distribution would be similar in the different social classes. If 20 percent of individuals in each class have such vulnerable genotypes, but in a particular social class only one in ten individuals is exposed to the environmental "trigger" (such as stress, poor diet, poverty, lack of self-esteem), then only 2 percent of individuals in that class will suffer from the illness (Holtzman, 1988). If, on the other hand, almost all individuals in a class experience the relevant environmental factor, then 20 percent of them will become ill with these disorders.

Since most common diseases today are likely due to interaction between the genotype and environmental factors, it is not surprising that most studies show a clear relationship between illness and social class. But the connection to genetic predisposition is masked in these studies. The important point is that genes determine *who* may get sick within a class, but environmental factors determine the *frequency* of sickness among susceptibles. Progress in understanding how illness is distributed in the population will be made by studies that control for one set of influences (genetic or environmental), while investigating the other.

It would be rewarding if we could identify those individuals who have the environmental factor present, then compare the genetic makeups of those affected and unaffected. The development of DNA markers and new genetic methods may facilitate this approach.

POLICY IMPLICATIONS

Should We Try to Change Gene Frequencies in the Population?

The documented role of genetics as a disease determinant raises the question of whether we can or should try to change the frequency of some genes in the population. The answer is no.

Genetic manipulation of the population seems unwise for a number of reasons. In most cases there is far more to be gained, and in less time, by environmental manipulation to promote health than by genetic manipulation. To try to manipulate our genotypes given our primitive state of knowledge of an incredibly complex, exquisitely coordinated and regulated genetic system would be showing hubris with regard to our future as a species. Furthermore, any involuntary program would violate widely held values of individual autonomy with regard to reproduction.

What then is the place of genetic knowledge in health care? What should we advocate or propose? Is a knowledge of the genetic aspects of health determinants merely of curiosity value?

Again, no. Our increasing knowledge makes it possible to take advantage of some specific opportunities for intervention. But before addressing these, it is worth specifying the context within which this investigator believes any genetic program should be offered.

Genetic services should be offered in a noncoercive, fully informed context. This means real choices should be available and services for individuals who have genetic disease, as well as diagnostic and preventive services, should be supported. The primary goal should be to provide help and choice to individuals and families, not to decrease genetic disease from a population point of view.

Fears have been expressed that preventive programs for genetic disease and birth defects will make us a less caring society. There is a concern that genetic testing would increase the pressure to make sure individuals at risk for having such children underwent testing and did not carry an affected individual to term. There is also the claim that increased testing would lead to fewer handicapped individuals, and that this would increase discrimination against them.

What is the likelihood of these outcomes? We will never eradicate genetic disease and birth defects: They are an inextricable part of our complexity and will always be with us. Humans have about one hundred thousand different structural genes. For most genetic disorders it is only after the first individual has been born with a specific genetic disorder or birth defect that a family is in a position to take advantage of programs for further avoidance.

Genetic variation is what gives us our reservoir to deal with future environmental change and to continue our evolution as a species. Some genes that cause disease in double dose are advantageous if people only have one copy. It is well recognized that all of us carry several genes that, if they were present in double dose, would cause disease or disability. None of us is "genetically pure" and we would not wish to eradicate this genetic variation.

Moreover, becoming a fully formed and functioning human being is an extremely complex process and there are bound to be some developmental errors along the way (Kurnit, Layton, and Malthysse, 1987). Most often these cannot be predicted and thus will continue to occur. And even if screening programs reduce the birth incidence of genetic disorders, the increased survival which results from improvements in the treatment of chronic congenital disease and the provision of social support may increase the prevalence of affected individuals (Baird and

Sadovnick, 1988; Bamforth and Baird, 1989). Many birth defects are of unknown cause but some may be related to "life-style" factors (diet, alcohol, cigarette smoking) that are difficult to change without changing many social aspects of society, including poverty. The main point is that as a society we simply will not be able to avoid having some of our citizens be handicapped from birth.

We must take seriously the concern that the availability of prevention will lead to pressures on people to make particular choices. These decisions are complex, and depend (among many other factors) on how grave is the view that an affected couple takes of a potential genetic disease. The desire for prenatal diagnosis definitely does not imply devaluation of the handicapped. Many families seen in genetic centres wish to avoid the birth of a second child with a disorder, while caring deeply for the handicapped child they already have. It is essential, however, that counseling be objective and that the couple not be pressured in any way.

Even objective information can be dangerous; individuals can potentially be harmed as well as helped by genetic information about themselves. Programs should be introduced only after appropriate evaluation for their psychological, ethical, and social implications. The mechanisms that should be put in place before genetic programs are implemented on a widespread basis are discussed below.

Genetic Programs: How and Where

Modern advances in knowledge now provide a number of opportunities to incorporate genetic services into appropriate health care. Unlike traditional health care—the diagnosis and treatment of disease in particular individuals—these services also offer a real chance to avoid the occurrence of disease. A given individual may be spared the development of disease in the future, or it may be possible for parents to avoid giving birth to affected individuals.

Genetic screening programs can serve several objectives. Individuals with a particular genotype may be identified and offered intervention or treatment—screening newborns for phenylketonuria, for example—or programs may identify individuals at risk of having children affected by genetic disease. Genetic screening falls into several different categories:

1. *Screening for Single-Gene Disorders*

As a species we have a long evolutionary history, and natural selection has ensured that most of our genes are useful and advantageous. However, certain deleterious genes cause major problems for their possessors.

Except for those on the X and Y chromosome in males, for all genes there are two copies of each gene in each cell of an individual. If both members of a gene pair code for fully functional gene products, the individual will be normal. If both copies code for defective products that normally are essential for life, the individual will have a lethal disease. If one member of the pair is normal and the other defective, the fate of the individual will depend on whether there is sufficient normal product to allow healthy function.

Disorders determined by single genes (Mendelian disorders) are caused by a defect in a single pair of genes. They may be transmitted in a dominant, recessive, or X-linked way. In dominantly inherited disorders only one member of the gene pair is abnormal, but the normal gene is unable to cover for its malfunctioning partner. An affected person has a 50 percent chance of passing the abnormal gene on to a child, so that the pattern seen in families here is for the disorder to pass from generation to generation, affecting males and females equally. Some examples are familial polyposis coli and Huntington disease.

For recessive disease to occur, both genes in the gene pair—one received from the mother and one from the father—must be abnormal. Having only one abnormal member in a pair, as each parent does, does not cause difficulty. Usually an affected child is the only affected individual known in the family, although there is a 25 percent risk for each sib to be affected. Some examples of this category are phenylketonuria, cystic fibrosis and Tay-Sachs disease.

In X-linked recessive disorders the problem gene is located on the X chromosome. Since males have only one X, if this has the X-linked disease gene they will be affected. In these families females may be healthy carriers of the gene but half their sons will have the disease. Some examples in this group are hemophilia and Duchenne muscular dystrophy.

Over four thousand of these simply inherited diseases have been identified in humans so far (McKusick, 1988). Some such genes can now be detected through programs screening high-risk groups. Particular deleterious genes may be concentrated in some population subgroups. Several historical mechanisms—for example, genetic drift, founder effect, or selective advantage—can produce this pattern. Because different population groups have different histories, a particular group may exhibit "clustering" of a disease associated with a particular gene.

This clustering is helpful in targeting screening programs to particular population subgroups such as immigrant groups within the composite North American population. There are a number of such subgroups where particular genes occur in higher frequency. One such gene is that for Tay-Sachs disease in Ashkenazi Jews. Symptoms appear in affected individuals in the first year of life and cause nervous system degeneration with blindness, severe mental retardation, seizures, and paralysis, with death usually occurring by the age of five. Active community prevention programs based on carrier screening have resulted in a very significant reduction in the birth incidence of Tay-Sachs disease in North America (Kaback, Zeigler, Reynolds, and Sonneborn, 1974). Prenatal diagnosis is available for this disorder, and the birth of many affected infants has been avoided. This has been a well-accepted and successful initiative, which was voluntary, community-based, and included educational and counseling components (Kaback, 1983).

Now that the gene for cystic fibrosis has been located, screening for carrier detection is likely to develop rapidly (Kerem et al., 1989). This disorder is common (1 in 2,500 births) in individuals of northern European extraction. Such population screening programs should permit those couples who wish to do so to avoid the birth of affected individuals. "At-risk" parents can be identified before they have the first affected child. If carrier tests are not available or not done, then the only way carriers are identified is by having an affected child. The proportion of couples who would choose termination for affected fetuses is likely to differ from society to society.

The frequency of the gene defect for thalassemia in people from southeast Asia and China is similar to that of the cystic fibrosis gene in northern Europeans. In North America these groups from Asia are offered screening. Similarly, populations of Mediterranean origin may be screened for β thalassemia, and the birth incidence of thalassemia, especially in southern Europe, has been very significantly reduced (WHO/Mediterranean Working Group on Hemoglobinopathies 1986, 1987). Obviously the families of affected individuals and carriers should always be offered testing, as they are more likely to be carriers.

2. *Chromosomal Disorders*

Another category of genetic disorders are those due to extra or missing chromosomes or parts of chromosomes. These abnormalities can be visualized through a microscope when cells from the affected individual are examined.

The main opportunity for avoiding chromosomal disorders is through testing high-risk pregnant women. Some chromosomal defects have well-defined and predictable mental and/or physical manifestations (phenotypes). These phenotypes are predictable within a known range of expression, for example, Down syndrome, Trisomy 18, Cri du Chat syndrome. Although all chromosomal abnormalities of microscopically detectable size are theoretically detectable early in pregnancy, in fact there are identifiable subgroups of mothers at increased risk because of older age or family history. It seems appropriate to offer prenatal detection to such subgroups.

3. *Congenital Anomalies*

Some congenital anomalies (abnormalities present from birth) are due to single-gene defects, or to chromosomal defects, but many are multifactorial, that is, they result from interactions between environmental factors and the individual genotype in ways we are only beginning to understand. A common example is neural tube defect (spina bifida and anencephaly), which occurs in about one in seven hundred births in British Columbia (Trimble and Baird, 1978a), and with similar frequency in most Western countries. This condition can be identified prenatally with a high degree of accuracy, and prenatal screening is available in a number of countries. Although many other birth defects may also be detected through prenatal tests, either by biochemical tests or imaging techniques such as ultrasound, screening is not done on a population basis. At present the identification of those women who should have prenatal testing comes only with the birth of an affected child for most congenital anomalies. Genetic programs can at best offer the opportunity for avoidance of the birth of a second affected child in these families.

4. *Family Testing Following Patient Identification*

Among those with most common disorders (e.g., heart disease, diabetes mellitus, colon cancer) are subgroups in whom there is a monogenic contribution to the occurrence of the disease. For example, most "early heart disease" is probably the result of a multifactorial vulnerability that, in conjunction with the usual distribution of environments, puts some individuals over the "threshold." However, there are some individuals whose early heart disease is the consequence of a single dominant gene. Because genes cluster in families, it is likely that the same gene will be found in their relatives. If there are ways to prevent expression of the gene (e.g., diet for familial hypercholesterolemia; venesection for hemochromatosis), then services offering genetic identification of family members should be available. Such services afford individuals the chance to avoid serious health consequences by changing their "microenvironment."

It is important to note the difference between *testing* of families of persons identified as having a specific disease, and *screening* of unaffected individuals in a population. The former is likely to be much more cost-effective as it will yield a much higher rate of case finding.

5. *Prenatal Diagnosis*

Prenatal diagnosis may be used to detect any of the conditions discussed in the above four categories, but it has aspects that are best discussed as a separate category. Prenatal diagnostic techniques are used to diagnose genetic disorders and birth defects that result in marked disability or death early in life. In most cases the only possible intervention is termination of the pregnancy. For a few disorders, however, diagnosis permits therapy *in utero* or special management during pregnancy and delivery to minimize further damage to a vulnerable infant. For example, for a fetus with methylmalonic acidemia the mother will be given vitamin B_{12} to minimize damage to the fetus; for a galactosemic infant the mother may go on a low-galactose diet. Thus, even those couples who find abortion unacceptable under any circumstances may still benefit from prenatal testing. Most will be reassured by negative findings, some will learn of conditions that are remediable, and the rest will at least be afforded an opportunity for preplanning.

Since there are many different possible indications for prenatal diagnosis, the specific test will be determined by the particular risk group of the mother. For example, a mother with a previous child with Tay-Sachs disease will have hexosaminidase A measured in the amniotic fluid sample; a woman who is at risk because of increased age will have chromosome analysis of a sample of fetal cells. The decisions to undergo prenatal testing and the use of the information in choosing a course of action will also depend on the cultural and religious beliefs of the couple.

Currently the main indications for offering prenatal testing (in order of frequency) are:

- Increased maternal age: As the age of the mother increases, so does the risk of Down Syndrome (Trimble and Baird, 1978b) and other trisomies. Many jurisdictions offer prenatal diagnosis to women who will be thirty-five years or older when the child is born. This can decrease the birth incidence of Down Syndrome by approximately 25 percent in most North American populations (Sadovnick and Baird, 1982).
- Neural tube defects (NTD): Although the precise pathways to this common anomaly are not clear, we can identify those at increased risk in one of two ways. First, testing the blood of all pregnant women will show that a few have a high level of serum alpha fetoprotein. This is associated with occurrence of NTD in the fetus. Second, women with a previous child with NTD, or a history of NTD in their or their partner's family, also have an increased risk. Accurate diagnostic evaluation of these identified higher risk fetuses is possible with ultrasound (and, if necessary, amniocentesis).

• Family history of specific disorder: A previous child may have had a Mendelian disorder, chromosome anomaly, or birth defect, or the family history may be such that the woman may be a carrier for an X-linked disorder. If a prenatal test is available (either biochemical, cytogenetic, or DNA) or it is possible to evaluate for abnormal morphology indicative of the diagnosis (e.g., skeletal abnormalities on X-ray) then this testing is offered.

In single-gene disorders that are recessive, most couples at risk can be identified only after diagnosis of an affected child has shown both parents are carriers. This "retrospective" identification and counseling allows families to avoid birth of further affected children, but has little effect on the total birth rate of affected children. Population screening is the only approach that would have a significant impact on the incidence of recessive inherited diseases.

All available studies show that most couples wish to know of and avoid the risk they may run of having children with a serious congenital handicap. Furthermore, fewer than 10 percent reject termination of pregnancy under such circumstances (Rothman, 1988). Prenatal diagnosis is used by at-risk couples to achieve a healthy family (Modell, Ward, and Fairweather, 1980). Counseling is an important aspect associated with identification of those with particular genes, and has been shown to decrease affected offspring in the next generation. Reproductive decisions made after counseling are related to the magnitude of risk (Carter, Roberts, Evans, and Buck, 1971).

• Other special circumstances: Maternal disorders (e.g., diabetes mellitus) or maternal exposure to an agent or factor, resulting in defects in the embryo and malformation in the offspring, may justify offering prenatal diagnosis.

There are obvious social and ethical implications to prenatal diagnosis. It is important that there be ongoing societal discussion of the issues so that culturally appropriate use is made of this technology. It is also important to remember that in most prenatal diagnostic programs approximately 96–97 percent of test results will be normal. Furthermore it has been shown that having such programs available means that more normal fetuses are carried to term (Hook and Willey, 1981). In their absence some high-risk couples would simply abort out of hand. Thus prenatal diagnosis gives many couples who would otherwise not feel they could have a family the option to have normal children.

There are two main avenues by which people come to be offered genetic diagnosis and counseling. They are identified, by their physicians or by themselves, either because a family member has had a genetic disorder, or because they have been identified as at risk by a population screening program.

The process of genetic consultation and counseling is complex and time-consuming and has not yet been well integrated into the clinical practice of medicine. Funding mechanisms for provision of this service differ from place to place, having grown up in an ad hoc fashion. If the rapidly escalating new insights into human diseases being made in genetics are to be brought to practical use, a cohort of trained individuals will be needed to deliver these services in the coming decades.

The Potential of Gene Therapy

The rapid advance of genetics, particularly DNA technology, will offer new potential uses of this knowledge. Gene therapy has been suggested, for example, to treat some severe genetic diseases. New genetic material could be inserted into affected individuals' body cells to perform the functions that their faulty inherited gene is unable to carry out. But this is likely to have negligible impact on disease prevalence in the population for the foreseeable future.

In the first place, the incidence of such single-gene disorders is low. Moreover, practical difficulties limit the range of genetic disease that might be treated by this approach. For example, the disease outcome must be due either to changes in a protein or metabolite that circulates (so that its level could be affected by the action of a gene inserted into an accessible tissue), or to changes occurring in a single accessible tissue (e.g., blood, bone marrow, liver). If a "disease" gene only expresses locally in inaccessible tissues such as brain or bone, it is not at present possible to see how a normal gene could be delivered to those tissues.

In addition, any normal gene inserted must not only be delivered to the relevant tissue, but it must express (make its product) at normal times and in normal amounts for long periods of time. At present our understanding of gene regulation is still in its infancy. Gene transfer may enable an affected individual to make a previously missing protein, but that protein may then be treated as foreign by his or her immune system. Even though the rapid growth of molecular biology makes it likely that many genes will soon be identified and obtained in a pure form, these practical difficulties mean that few inherited diseases are likely to be suitable candidates for gene therapy for many years.

Gene therapy as usually proposed is analogous to most other "medical" treatment. It affects only the body cells, not the gonads. This means that treated individuals will pass on the genes that they received from their parents. They will not pass on the inserted genes because only their body cells—not their germ cells—have been changed. Successful gene therapy will affect the phenotype but not the genotype; it will not influence the prevalence of the defective genes in populations any more than other medical treatments.

It is worth reemphasizing that human characteristics such as intelligence, appearance, and kindness are determined by the complex interactions of the effects of several genes with the social and physical environment. The possibilities of being able to modify such characteristics by changing the DNA of an individual are now so remote as to merit no more than distant speculation—science fiction. The difficulties to be overcome even to correct the DNA of an individual with a well-studied monogenic disorder are formidable (Medical Research Council of Canada, 1989).

Identification for DNA "Risk" Markers

A less remote scenario may result from the elucidation of the genetic components of such common disorders as atherosclerosis, rheumatoid arthritis, and diabetes. It is likely that many people have a gene (or genes) that determines whether external influences will precipitate one of these illnesses. Whether the disorder develops depends on the additive combination of genes and environmental effects exceeding a threshold. If particular genotypes are exposed to particular experiences, the threshold may be passed and the disease emerges—that is, these diseases are multifactorial in etiology (Falconer, 1965). Although several genes may contribute to the genetic vulnerability, they need not all have the same impact on the final outcome.

Identification of "risk" genotypes through recombinant DNA approaches may allow earlier intervention in the cascade of events leading to overt disease and clinical manifestation. But there are serious dangers. The idea that certain genotypes, detectable by recombinant DNA probes, make individuals more likely to develop particular diseases, fits immediately into "body as machine/doctor as mechanic" modes of thinking. In this way of thinking, the triggering or enabling influences of a variety of environmental determinants can easily get lost. A simple causal sequence from gene to disease is more easily grasped than the complex notion of a web of social, economic, and personal factors interacting with individuals' different genotypes.

Population-based programs of detection using DNA probes also have powerful economic attractions. The biotechnology industries can see enormous profits in the development and marketing of a range of test kits. Private insurers have a strong interest in identifying high-risk individuals so as to minimize their own exposure to risk. Employers may also find such capabilities attractive; healthy employees are more productive and less costly.

There are, then, a number of dangers in proceeding too quickly into implementation of "identification and prevention" programs, however well-intentioned. It is possible to do great harm, and waste considerable resources, because of failure to weigh carefully the ramifications and pitfalls of such an approach to human illness.

Currently, there are two main camps with regard to the place of genetics in health care. One camp (often geneticists and other scientists who are not practicing clinicians) tends to overestimate the potential contribution of genetics to human health, and is rather naive about the role of human nature and social interaction in determining health and behaviour. This naiveté is shared by the media, for example, in reporting the recent discovery of the "gene" for alcoholism.

The other camp includes many sociologists, philosophers, and historians concerned about the central importance currently given to genetics in the world of biological and medical research (e.g., the multibillion dollar Human Genome Project described below). They fear a possible reprise of mistakes made earlier this century when genetic concepts were misused in the service of political and social goals in Germany and the United States.

Is there perhaps something to be learned from both views?

Genetic approaches are essential if some individuals are to be given appropriate care and real choice. It is very clear that for some diseases, the genetic contribution is so critical that the role of the usual range of environments is trivial (e.g., severe recessive disorders). For these there is a real place for genetics programs as outlined above.

However, genetic approaches may not be a high priority for disorders of multifactorial origin. For example, in the last several decades mortality from cardiovascular disease has fallen by more than 40 percent, although there has been no change in the genetic constitution of the population. For the many disorders where environmental factors are important, it may be less important to discover who is at genetic risk than to put our societal resources into changing the environment for all.

An appropriate implementation of genetic principles and technology would respect the power of genetics, and its potential to give choice to individuals and families, in some situations. But it is important that we do not overestimate what genetic technology can do and so apply it inappropriately with resultant expensive harm.

Need for Pilot Studies before Wide Implementation

The dangers inherent in premature and uncritical implementation of programs for genetic identification suggest that some "hurdles" might usefully be put in place. A program should be expected to meet certain criteria before implementation. Most obviously, no identification program should be offered on a population basis unless a rigorously proven disease avoidance or treatment strategy is available. This will require well-designed pilot research studies *before* implementation at the population level (Baird, 1990).

These pilot studies would have to address the issues of full disclosure, autonomy, informed consent, and confidentiality. It would also be important to evaluate the psychological effects of being identified and/or of following a preventive strategy. The use of predictive genetic diagnosis creates a new category of people who are not ill but who know that they may develop a specific disease. How will this knowledge affect them?

There are also a variety of methodological problems to be overcome in such pilot studies. There may be difficulties in mounting randomized controlled trials, especially if the media have prematurely publicized some technology as beneficial so that citizens do not want to be randomized (e.g., chorionic villus biopsy trial, vitamins, and NTD prevention trial). In addition, several different genotypes may predispose to a given disease and the clinical endpoint may be reached in more than one way. The magnitude of the attributable risk may be different for each of several genotypes (Kolata, 1986). The environmental codeterminants may be different for these different genotypes. Some individuals may have more than one genetic risk marker. To add to the methodologic complexity there are protective genes as well, as has been seen for coronary artery disease (Kessling et al., 1988) and for diabetes mellitus.

Pilot studies must also adjust for the effect of cultural and economic factors that interact with the genotype to determine disease. As noted in earlier chapters, the nature and quality of human interaction is an important influence on health that may promote or mitigate genetic vulnerability. Ways of measuring and evaluating these complex interactions are still very primitive. The meaning of a given genetic identification may be different depending on the social class of the individuals identified. It may be necessary to follow the study group over several decades to obtain the needed information on outcome.

Even if an efficacious strategy exists, individuals (or their parents) may not comply with the recommended "avoidance" strategy. Compliance in taking antibiotics, even if prescribed for acute illness, is well under 100 percent (Becker, 1985), and for antihypertensive treatment only half comply with at least 80 percent of the drug regimen (Sackett et al., 1975). Compliance with a regimen that needs to continue for years, in the absence of any illness as a motivating factor, would probably be even less. But unless compliance is high, a targeted genetic program may be a less useful application of health funding than, for example, a broad social campaign to decrease the level of a known environmental hazard.

Some Specific Criteria to Be Met before Wide Implementation

Before wider implementation, the preventive "strategy" should have been followed by a large enough group of individuals for long enough that its safety and benefit in avoidance of the disease can be judged. In this context it is sobering to realize that effective interventions have been discovered for relatively few genetic diseases, even in the single-gene category.

It is also essential that before implementation on a population basis, the personnel and facilities to provide appropriate counseling and follow-up are identified and funded. Conveying risk information effectively is a complex undertaking. Large numbers of individuals will be identified by any population screening programs. Thus nonspecialists will have to do much of the screening and counseling. Education and training of these personnel (e.g., general practitioners, nurses) will therefore need to be addressed.

There should also be good information available regarding the relative value of the program compared with other measures for improving the health status of the population, that is, the "opportunity cost" must have been assessed. This information is needed by decision-makers in allocating funding across many competing priorities.

Also, before wide implementation, quality control mechanisms must have been established for the laboratories that will do the testing, since it is essential to minimize the transmission of erroneous information (Holtzman, 1989). Regulation of new DNA tests, whether in public or for-profit laboratories, should be established, along with appropriate guidelines governing access to the test results.

We cannot close Pandora's box. Programs for genetic identification will start: The technology is available, the concept is appealing to many, the product will be pushed by commercial interests. DNA testing for "risk" markers is here before we have thought through its implications. There is a real danger that screening for "risk" genotypes will not be carried out as a unified, well-planned public health program but on an opportunistic ad hoc basis. Premature application, hastily embarked upon, may discredit *any* potential benefit, and so risks stimulating Draconian across-the-board prohibition of *any* DNA risk identification.

The eventual identification of genetic differences in risk for common disorders from one person to another will have profound legal and ethical implications. How do we avoid creating a population whose members are continuously concerned about their own particular genetic predisposition and their risk of becoming ill? How can we protect from discrimination individuals who do not wish to have testing but who later become ill or disabled from potentially remediable disease—"it's their fault"? How can we prevent employers from excluding the genetically predisposed instead of reducing harmful environmental work exposures? We must make sure the law and our social values prevent the coercive use of tests.

Unless it is possible to deal with the potential pitfalls and dangers of genetic testing in a considered and considerate way so that it does not become stigmatizing or socially disabling, we may not be able as a society to take advantage of the potential for avoiding disease. Citizens simply may not participate, or the whole approach may be outlawed.

Newgenics?

Eugenics has been defined as improvement of the human species by selective breeding. It continues to be held in general disrepute for good historical reasons; it is associated with coercion or interference with reproductive choice in most people's minds. But the concept continues to emerge in one form or another because the idea of improving humankind genetically has a continuing appeal. What do we have to learn from the last forty years of advances in genetics?

The obvious success of agricultural breeding programs depends on *very* strong selection methods. In humans, even a modest change in a quantitative trait (e.g., height or intelligence) would require overwhelming social change. For example, the tallest half of the population would have to produce *all* the children for the next generation to have even a small impact on average height (Friedman, 1991). Such a change could instead be achieved by social policies that enriched the environment and nurtured the socially disadvantaged. The latter would enhance the quality of citizens' lives rather than restricting options for half of the population.

Selective breeding in humans is simply not possible without unacceptable public programs of intense coercion. In addition, any initial rapid "improvement" would not continue over many generations. The rate of improvement would slow dramatically as variability in the population was decreased by the selective breeding (Dalton, 1985; Stern, 1973).

There would also be an increase in the frequency of single-gene and multifactorial genetic diseases. This would be due to the greater genetic homogeneity (decreased variation) in the population because of the strong selection.

In essence, the more we know about genetics the less likely we are to recommend an imposed eugenics program—it simply would not work. Not only would it be ineffective, but it would entail an appalling social cost.

Turning over the eugenic coin, concern is sometimes expressed that treating individuals with genetic diseases so they then remain in the breeding pool will mean the human species will rapidly become "unfit." In fact, the frequency of a disease gene in the population depends on its mutation rate (how fast it is formed) and on how strongly the environment selects against it (so it is not passed on to children). Most diseases caused by mutant genes are uncommon because there has been selection against them over many generations.

For recessive genetic disorders—almost all the relevant genes exist in only one "dose" in individuals—such people are healthy, but carriers. For example, for a recessive disease that occurs once in ten thousand births, 1 in 50 people are carriers. If, because of treatment, homozygotes—that is, affected individuals—survive and have children, the extra number of disease genes added to the population gene pool is negligible. It is estimated that it would take one hundred generations of successfully treating all individuals affected by such a disease to bring the disease frequency up to 1 in 2,500 births. Within such a long time span it seems likely that we will come to understand the metabolic pathways and disease processes and be able to deal with them effectively.

The rate of increase for X-linked genes would, however, be faster and for dominant genes, faster still. For a dominant gene with a frequency of one in ten thousand births, the frequency would be one in one hundred after one hundred generations of wholly successful treatment. For diseases with a multifactorial etiology, the impact of relaxed selection is hard to predict because of our lack of knowledge regarding the specific genetic contribution and regarding what will happen to the environmental component in the future.

OTHER SOCIETAL ASPECTS

The field of genetics is a rapidly evolving one: Will our wisdom grow along with our knowledge? Consider, for example, the Human Genome Project—a megaproject administered through the U.S. National Institutes of Health with Nobel laureate James Watson as director. Its goal is to sequence the approximately three billion pairs of nucleotide bases of which the human genome is composed, and in the process to identify the position of the approximately one hundred thousand human structural genes.

This megaproject is discussed and marketed in some quarters as if delineation of the sequence of the human genome will solve all the biological ills of humankind. Yet few would seriously dispute the fact that economic, social, and environmental factors are considerably more important determinants of health and disease worldwide. And in any case, knowing the sequence (and even variation around the "normal" sequence) is of no use unless that knowledge can be correlated with the lifetime clinical findings associated with these variations.

We need much better understanding of the cascade of pathways from the gene through intermediary metabolism and physiology to observable endpoints in human health and functioning if we are to intervene therapeutically. Reaching this stage could constitute the whole task of human biology for the next two centuries. Geneticists may have "oversold" the immediate health benefits of research on the human genome. Obviously, they have a vested interest in promoting this.

Genetic testing and genetic predisposition need to be understood in a larger social context. For example, we live in a time when environmental degradation threatens our opportunity to live healthful lives. The Human Genome Project does not necessarily draw away resources that would otherwise have been used for environmental improvement, but it does raise questions about the breadth (and depth) of consideration underlying this type of decision to make resources unavailable for *any* other use. We need to develop ways of allocating resources so as to better people's lives in the long term.

The glamour and "big science" aspects of new genetic knowledge, especially that acquired by use of recombinant DNA approaches, should not seduce us into using genetic identification prematurely and inappropriately. We may find that for the foreseeable future relatively few such programs turn out to be worthwhile. In the long term, with a considered and careful approach to implementation, and with a legal and social context that preserves social justice, it may be possible to use our increasing genetic knowledge to enhance our own and others' lives.

CONCLUSIONS

Since genetic factors are among the determinants of health, they must be taken into consideration if we are to have a deeper understanding of the pathways to health and illness. There are some disorders where the inherited metabolic machinery of the individual will not allow normal functioning in the usual range of environments; the associated diseases will usually burden the earlier part of the human life cycle. These provide a real and appropriate place for genetic service programs to contribute to population health.

The complexities of the web of causation for most common afflictions in adult life are likely to limit the contribution of DNA identification of at-risk genotypes. The potential for wasting resources and causing harm is real and serious. There is thus a need for pilot studies and careful evaluation before population screening programs are implemented. But the simplistic model of disease causation that is currently prevalent in our culture (Figure 1.1) puts us at risk of foolish and precipitate action.

If we can avoid this danger and tread carefully, we may eventually be able to apply our increasing genetic knowledge to the enhancement of people's opportunities for healthy lives. This will require interventions to change the environmental factors leading to the common disease outcomes, rather than the genetic predispositions. Such interventions must be based on a more complete picture that also contains the social, economic, physical, and cultural factors that interact with our biological makeup to determine health.

NOTE

1. Congenital malformations refer to abnormalities at birth, regardless of cause.

6

If Not Genetics, Then What? Biological Pathways and Population Health

R. G. EVANS, M. HODGE, and I. B. PLESS

Earlier chapters have explored the common observation that there are marked differences in health status not only among human populations, but particularly among subgroups within populations. They have presented evidence arguing that such "heterogeneities" are linked to various aspects of the socioeconomic and cultural environment, past and present. In particular (but without restricting the generality of the foregoing) *something* associated with social status is inversely related, presumably causally, to poor health.

Although this evidence is compelling, it would be even more convincing if one could picture plausible biological mechanisms or processes producing such effects. Clearly demonstrated causal linkages would be better still.

Some of the biological pathways to heterogeneity in health status are quite obvious. Malnutrition or undernutrition, for example, may be a consequence of low income. The connections between poor nutrition and both infections and some chronic diseases have been extensively documented. But nutritional derangement must be quite extreme for these mechanisms to result in premature mortality. Although poor nutrition is now believed to contribute to many more causes of ill health than was recognized even a decade ago, it cannot explain all the gradients in health status among populations.

Another common and well-established biological pathway is through "crowding," in the home, school, workplace, or neighbourhood. Mechanisms of transmission for infectious disease, especially when microbial spread is airborne (e.g., influenza), are well documented and beyond dispute.[1] History records a number of particularly virulent epidemics whose spread and impact were both faster and more severe in poorer, more crowded communities. Both the proportion of people contracting the disease (the attack rate) and the proportion with disease who died (the fatality rate) were higher.[2] Similarly, both the poor-quality housing and hazard-strewn neighbourhoods in which poorer people live are associated with higher injury rates among children and adults (Dougherty, Pless and Wilkins, 1990).

But there are remarkably few linkages between illness, and either the "environment," variously defined, or patterns of consumption behaviour, for which the underlying biological mechanisms are clearly understood. Even smoking, a behaviour strongly correlated with ill-health and premature death, offers (as yet) only partially understood biological pathways. The effects of "tars" on lung tissue and nicotine on the circulatory system are understood. But some smokers escape disease, while some nonsmokers also suffer from circulatory diseases and occasionally even from lung cancer.

Considerable evidence is now accumulating that offers an outline, if not a full picture, of some of the underlying biological pathways, not just related to smoking or crowding, but for the much more subtle effects of social and cultural environments. This chapter reviews the current understanding of relevant phenomena at the cellular or subcellular level within individuals.

STRESS AND COPING

Keys to understanding the biological pathways through which environmental and social factors have their effects may be found in the ways in which humans and other primates respond to stress.[3] Particular sources and forms of stress may be surmountable or overwhelming in different individuals, or in different circumstances.

The body's reaction to stress is determined by the interplay of several physiological systems. These include complex elements of the immune, neural, and endocrine systems. Over the last few decades, advances in immunology and neuroscience have led to a clearer characterization of the connections among these systems, shedding light on possible mechanisms by which the host response to environmental insults and stresses is mediated.

Selye's work in the 1930s (Selye, 1976) pioneered a new understanding of the body's response to stress. Moving from studies of animals to studies involving humans, he demonstrated that similar stresses have different effects determined by how an event is perceived. Moreover, he was able to show that some forms of stress produced positive responses.

In the early 1960s, research on the role of families in the occurrence of disease began to appear. Invariably, these studies focused on the tension between the external stresses faced by individuals, and their "coping" responses. Stated simply, it was postulated that stressful events result in strain, but that this can be reduced or reversed when effective coping mechanisms are brought into play.[4] Coping could include ways of accepting, tolerating, avoiding, or minimizing stress as well as its more traditional sense of mastery over the environment. It is not limited to successful efforts, but includes all purposeful attempts to manage stress regardless of their effectiveness.

Coping mechanisms can be conceptualized as inherent characteristics of the individual (coping styles) or as skills that are acquired (coping strategies). Or they could be viewed as external buffers either naturally available (e.g., supportive families) or purposefully introduced to provide support (e.g., self-help groups or similar social support networks).

Viewed historically it appears that the concepts of stress and coping became prominent at about the same time that many, especially medical sociologists, were focusing increasingly on the role of families in influencing the health of their members (Antonovski, 1979). While neither concept met the great expectations that greeted it initially, they have stimulated a generation of investigators to study the role of families in the processes of disease occurrence. And the continuing interest in the effects of stress may be just beginning to yield significant results.

Prompted by laboratory work involving rats stressed by crowded quarters, Meyer and Haggerty (1962) postulated that similar mechanisms might be at work to explain why some children with streptococcal infections became ill, while other similarly infected children remained asymptomatic. The study that followed, often referred to as the "stress and strep" project, supported the hypothesis that children who had experienced some form of stress were more likely to become symptomatic within two weeks than children similarly exposed to the infectious agent but not to stressful experiences. Despite the evident importance of these findings, both clinically and at a more fundamental, biological level, this work has never been precisely replicated.

Nevertheless, more recent reports from several laboratories provide equally convincing evidence that stress increases susceptibility to the common cold. It is not yet clear whether this now well-established association is due to reduced host resistance making the subject more likely to become infected or more likely to become clinically ill once infected.

The latter appears to have been the mechanism found in the stress and strep study, whereas Cohen, Tyrrell, and Smith (1991) attributed the dose-response relationship they found between reported stress and respiratory illness to increased rates of infection. On the other hand Stone et al. (1992) report on seventeen subjects who were experimentally infected and had confirmed rhinovirus infection. Only twelve had clinical symptoms, and among these the average number of self-reported major life events (assumed to be stressful) was significantly greater than among those who remained asymptomatic. Earlier studies of the common cold offer less clear-cut results. Totman, Kiff, Reed, and Craig (1980), for example, attempted to predict experimental colds using five measures of recent life stress, only one of which yielded a significant association.

A similar line of enquiry was launched by Cassel (1975). Like Meyer and Haggerty, he was led from intriguing observations on the responses of animal colonies to stress, to work on families. In his introduction to a monograph summarizing the results of epidemiological studies linking family features to health, he states:

> In the most general terms, the theory that has guided these studies has been that susceptibility to a wide variety of diseases and disorders (including somatic as well as emotional and behavioral disorders) is influenced by a combination of exposure to psychosocial stressful situations and the protection afforded against these situations by adequate social supports. (p. 2)

Thus, although the family in general was the ostensible focus of these studies, the family as a mediator (or generator) of stress emerged as a prominent subtheme.

Kaplan and Cassel (1975) note that the most impressive feature of the studies in their volume was their having come to similar conclusions despite having been conducted independently, using diverse populations, varied research designs, and different measures of health outcomes. They concluded that "certain elements of family structure and functioning, (however measured), were found to be related to the different aspects of health status of the family member" (p. 3). The details of this work are less noteworthy than the observation that achieving or avoiding certain health states is in some way dependent on aspects, real or assumed, of family behaviour. However, the mechanisms through which physiological effects might emerge in response to such behaviour remained elusive.

A slightly different perspective on the same issue is introduced in a recent review of the relationship between "Control and Health" (Syme, 1991). Control is defined as "a property of individuals or of situations; a quality of individuals as well as . . . a function of training and opportunities or of social and cultural circumstances" (p. 20). The family may serve as the conduit through which a sense of control is transmitted and thus becomes the property of individuals, as opposed to circumstances. Syme (1991) and Thompson and Spacapan (1991) review a number of studies that demonstrate that perceived control is positively related to better health outcomes. However, it is still far from certain what accounts for the relationship. As Thompson and Spacapan state, "a great deal of empirical evidence suggests that beliefs in control are associated with better health outcomes. This relationship may be due both to a direct physiological link between control and health and to an indirect pathway mediated by health-promoting behaviors" (p. 4).

Studies focusing on health and resilience bear out the findings of those addressing control. Just as some health workers (and polemicists) dislike repeated references to disease and prefer to emphasise "positive health" (a worthy notion, but not one that is readily measurable), so some prefer to focus on health and resilience, rather than maladjustment or disease (Garmezy and Rutter, 1983). In a recent review article, Masten, Best, and Garmezy (1990) define resilience as "the process of, capacity for, or outcome of successful adaptation despite challenging or threatening circumstances." They examine three resilience phenomena in studies of the mental health of children:

- good outcomes in high-risk children,
- sustained competence in children under stress, and
- recovery from (mental and physical) trauma.

Although the evidence they cite is based on a variety of studies whose methods are not described in detail, the conclusion they reach seems tenable: "human psychological development is highly buffeted and . . . long lasting consequences of adversity usually are associated with either organic damage or severe interference in the normative protective processes embedded in the caregiving system." But they then add:

> Children who experience chronic adversity fare better or recover more successfully when they have a positive relationship with a competent adult, they are good learners and problem solvers, they are engaging to other people, and they have areas of competence and perceived efficacy valued by self or society.

(Recall from Chapter 1 the characteristics of the "vulnerable but invincible" children of Kauai studied by Werner.) What remains unanswered is the question of how this comes about.

The review by Masten, Best, and Garmezy (1990) begins by restating that many studies have shown that poverty, low maternal education, low socioeconomic status, as well as family instability, low birth weight, and schizophrenia in a biological mother, may all be viewed as risk factors for a variety of untoward psychosocial outcomes (e.g., lower academic achievement, more emotional or behavioural problems, lower work achievement, trouble with the law). They also note that there is some evidence that the risks associated with multiple adverse factors may be additive, or even multiplicative. Nevertheless, they emphasise that even in the face of all such factors, many suffer few or no adverse consequences.

Clearly there is much truth in these observations. They parallel the conclusions of others who have studied what appear to be inherently stressful situations only to find that the consequences are much less adverse than they expected. For example, Pless and colleagues have repeatedly examined the psychological effects of having a chronic physical disorder during childhood (Pless, Roghmann, and Haggerty, 1972; Pless and Pinkerton, 1975; Nolan and Pless, 1986; Pless and Nolan, 1991). Although these studies clearly demonstrate an excess risk of psychosocial disturbance in early adulthood related to chronic disorders during childhood, it is striking to discover how relatively small these risks are. Accordingly, the important question becomes not why the emotional problems follow but why they are not much greater. How is it possible to live with diabetes, epilepsy, or arthritis throughout childhood and *not* experience severe psychological and emotional consequences? One popular answer is that the family serves as a mechanism to enhance coping or to buffer the effects of stress (Varni, Wilcox, and Hanson, 1988).

While almost all of the evidence for resilience can be seriously criticized in terms of study methods, the cumulative weight of the findings is persuasive (Garmezy, 1985, 1991). It is, in effect, the other side of the coin of the equally convincing (though often equally flawed) evidence showing how often socioeconomic disadvantage or other forms of stress do, indeed, appear to lead to adverse health states. But the central question remains: How, in biological terms, do these effects come about? By what means are ostensibly "external" factors able to have such a profound influence on mental and physical well-being, culminating in the marked differences in longevity and various measures of morbidity that we observe across social hierarchies and other population groupings?

In general, investigators pursuing these lines of enquiry have noted the considerable difficulty of identifying and measuring the degree of external stress separately from the organism's response. Without an independent marker of stress, the process of investigating any posited stress-strain relationship has a tendency to become circular. How can we know if a particular event or experience is in fact a stress? Because it has certain effects on the organism—what we are here calling strain—that are believed to be responses to stress. Thus stresses tend to be defined by their effects, and vice versa.[5]

It is clear, however, that known stresses do not all produce measurable responses in all individuals. Thus coping mechanisms, styles or strategies that mitigate the effects of stress, are hypothesised to vary among individuals. But here too, circularity emerges because of the difficulty of measuring "stressful" events. The presence of coping cannot be conclusively demonstrated by the fact that a stress has failed to evoke the expected response; it is possible that what is assumed to be a stress is not, in fact, stressful (or is much less so) in some persons or situations than in others.

The death of a spouse, for example, is usually considered to be a highly stressful "life event." For one person, this might in fact be so, but for another—an abused wife—it might be a blessed relief from the stress of the marriage. It is sometimes argued that unemployment, another commonly identified external stress, is in fact much less stressful in societies where it is a common and widely shared experience, than in those where it is an unusual occurrence, suggesting personal failure. The "same" event can represent a very different degree of external stress.

On the other hand, two people who lose spouses might experience what for each of them is in fact a very stressful event, but might have very different resources for coping with that stress. One is supported by a large family or circle of friends, for example, while the other is now left alone. The same stress might then generate very different strain responses in these two—but how would an external observer in fact know that the stresses were the same? At best, one can observe only the response of the organism.

There *is* in this case a conceptual distinction between the external stress and the strain response, but this will not help the investigator who is trying to measure the relationship when there is in fact no independent measure of the external stress, and where the strain responses to the same external event may vary. One would need to know the surrounding social and cultural context, the story, in order to interpret accurately any biological or behavioural markers—which appears to be precisely the point made by Corin in Chapter 4.[6]

To add to the confusion, investigators have constantly to keep in mind the important distinction made by Selye and his colleagues between "stress" and "distress." As noted above, Selye showed that the results of stressful situations may not always be bad. He found that under some circumstances stress may stimulate a variety of useful, constructive behaviours—which should be no surprise to anyone who ever sweated to meet a deadline or rose to any other stressful occasion. Just as the parts of a machine may operate within a certain range of normal "working strain," so biological organisms require a certain degree of external challenge to keep them fit—again, no surprise to any trainer of animals or humans. One cannot blithely assume that all stresses yield negative responses.

Indeed, the same idea is implicit in Cannon's original formulation of the responses of the adrenal glands to stressful stimuli: Adrenalin release serves either to help the organism "fight" or to launch it into "flight" (Cannon, 1939). Under the conditions in which most of us evolved, one or other response was highly conducive to short-run survival, for ourselves or our offspring. Since circumstances demanding this response were not unusual, it would be surprising if evolution had not equipped us with a certain tolerance, or even taste, for external challenge. (Consider, for example, the teen-age male.)[7] But too much fighting or fleeing has never been good for one's health.

As noted above, the response at the cellular level to environmental insults appears determined by the interplay of several physiological systems, including the immune, endocrine, and nervous systems. The classic "fight-or-flight" response, for example, for all its apparent simplicity and directness, relies on an exquisite balance among several body systems. Such a balance could hardly be expected to arise by chance.

Recent research has identified a number of connections among various physiological systems previously thought to be essentially self-contained.[8] Over the last decade, advances in immunology and neuroscience have begun to characterize more clearly the connections among these systems and thus to shed light on possible mechanisms involved in the response to environmental challenge. In the process, it is becoming increasingly clear that the Cartesian zeal for compartmentalization that has dominated Western medicine is, in this field at least, unhelpful and potentially misleading.[9]

It now appears that the population-wide environmental determinants of disease and the different responses of individuals may be linked through the body's nervous system. Perceptions of the external world, detected and interpreted by that system, lead to electrical and chemical responses that in turn trigger responses in other systems.

Particular attention has been paid to linkages between the nervous and immune systems, both because of the central role played by the immune system in warding off various threats to health and because earlier orthodoxy had held so firmly that that system was independent of influences from other body systems. In contrast, one of the most striking recent findings in immunology and neuroscience is that cells in the immune system contain in their membranes receptors that are identical to those found on cells in the nervous system. In addition, cells in both systems produce similar peptides, which can thus interact with the receptors on either type of cell. Thus cells of the two systems can communicate directly with, and presumably influence, each other.

Cells of the immune system communicate among themselves by means of cytokines, soluble substances produced by various types of immune cells. Cytokines, in turn, affect a variety of immune cell types, including in some cases, the class of cell from which they originate. In addition, cortisol, released under the direction of the pituitary gland in the brain as part of the hormonal cascade in the "fight-or-flight" response, has also been shown to affect cytokine production.

The relationships among immune system components have yet to be fully elucidated. In general terms, however, the human immune system acts both to prevent invasion by environmental pathogens, and to clear those that gain successful entrance. This includes the role in which most of us picture that system: as a microscopic army fighting against invading microorganisms. But some of the components of the immune system play roles in noninfectious disease processes. Through a series of related functions, the immune system also directs the repair of damaged tissue, again not necessarily limited to tissue damaged by microbes, and this opens possible connections with many other diseases.

The multistep hypothesis of tumour induction, for example, is compatible with greater cancer risk among individuals whose repair machinery, including cells with immune or inflammatory roles, is less able to clear potential carcinogens or to repair the damage they cause. And indeed it is now recognized that the immune system can contribute to controlling cancer. Although still far from clear, this role is believed to be important for certain types of cancer such as melanoma. Conversely, increased cancer incidence is associated with suppression of the immune system as, for example, in organ transplantation therapy.

There is also evidence that immune pathways influence the development of atherosclerosis. Macrophages, for example, whose immune role is primarily one of processing and presenting foreign material to effector cells, are also involved in the accretion and consolidation of fatty deposits in blood vessels that are causally linked to atherosclerosis and ischemic heart disease (Kaplan, Pettersson, Manuck, and Olsson, 1991; see also Chapter 7).

All of these diverse effects can for our purposes be subsumed under the general heading of immune system functions. They form part of the larger host defense system, the crucial set of mechanisms whereby the organism responds to external challenges and prevents or limits the effects of processes that threaten its well-being or survival. Successful prevention of damage depends on a prompt, complete response by the host. If the individual is unable to respond optimally, tissue damage may be sustained and incompletely repaired and the affected individual will be placed at greater risk of future injury or deterioration.

Having demonstrated the existence of linkages between the nervous and the immune systems, workers in the field began to use the term introduced by Solomon and Moos (1964), "psychoneuroimmunology" or PNI. The relationship is an interactive one: The brain affects the immune system and the immune system affects the brain. Favourable physical and social environments apparently strengthen the organism's immune defenses, while a lowering of these defenses often but not invariably leads to depression, sadness, or other negative affective reactions (House, Landis, and Umberson, 1988; *Newsweek*, 1988; *Consumer Reports*, 1993).

Thus, the previously mentioned "fight-or-flight" response represents a physiological reaction to a situation perceived by the brain. The gross, anatomical components of the body's stress response, such as sweating and increased heart rate, are controlled by the autonomic nervous system (ANS)—so named because it has classically been viewed as beyond conscious control. But there are also "microlevel" responses to stress; both ANS impulses and hormones derived from the nervous system produce immune responses that, while less dramatic than "fight-or-flight," are nevertheless essential to the body's defenses against infection or inflammation. Fibres of the ANS innervate the lymphoid tissue of the spleen, bone marrow, and lymph nodes, and are in close proximity to the immune system cells concentrated in these tissues. Neurotransmitter substances released by these fibres may direct the migration of cells from lymphoid tissues, or may bind to immune cell surface receptors and thus affect the production of key immune system signals or effectors (Snow, 1990).

Thus "information" transmitted from the nervous system can have a range of effects that stimulate or dampen immune responses. But the term *psychoneuroimmunology* itself may now be unduly restrictive in that it implicitly focuses attention on one particular pathway from the nervous system. Current research in neurophysiology, as well as data presented elsewhere in this volume, invites one to consider a number of pathways that begin with sensory stimuli perceived by the organism—things seen, heard, or felt (or presumably smelled or tasted), which are then interpreted by the brain and directly transmitted at the molecular level to other biological systems.

The demonstration of linkages at the cellular level between the nervous and other body systems obviously provides an important link in the chain from social environments to biological effects. But the existence of a communications system tells us little about the nature or the extent of the information passed along it, the impact of that information, or most importantly, why that impact seems to vary across groups or individuals. In what ways do individuals' perceptions lead to physiological changes that influence health, for good or ill?

TALK TO THE ANIMALS

Answers to this question often emerge most clearly from experiments and other studies involving rather invasive procedures. A good deal of the evidence thus comes from research on animals. Some of the most striking recent findings are those showing the powerful influence of sensory stimuli on the development of components of the nervous system itself. Experimental work with cats, for example (Kalil, 1989), has shown that normal binocular vision depends upon the development of appropriate neural connections within the visual cortex in response to visual signals at about four to twelve weeks of age.

If one eye is sutured shut during this critical period, so that the brain receives signals only from the other, neuronal processing capacity will not be assigned to the closed eye. If that is later opened, the cat's vision remains monocular. Signals from a perfectly healthy eye are not "seen" by the brain, because at the critical stage, when the "wiring" of the brain was being completed, no neural connections were developed to process then nonexistent signals.[10] The presence or absence of externally generated sensations has a permanent effect on the "wiring" of the neural system (Teller and Movshon, 1986).

Experimental demonstration of similar processes in humans is understandably restricted by ethical considerations. But clinical observations of patients with long-term visual defects, corrected later in life, provide confirmation. Restoring "sight" to the eye may create only confusion for a brain that has not developed or has lost the neuronal connections required to interpret visual information (Sacks, 1993). And certain focusing defects, correctable with artificial lenses, must however be corrected before the early teens. If the correction is too late the eye will "see" normally, but the brain and the person will not. If a critical stage in development is missed, the resulting perceptual defects cannot later be compensated.

Such effects are not confined to the visual system (see also Sacks, 1989); it may be that all the sensory functions in the cortex develop in response to external signals at critical stages. During the process of growth and development, complex systems of linkages are established among the neurons of the central nervous system. Organisms, including us, begin life with a vast oversupply of neurons; learning experiences lead to the generation of patterns of interconnection among them. In a sense, a complex set of networks is "sculpted" out of the available neuronal raw material by our responses to experience, and repetition of experience and behaviour reinforces these interconnections. On the other hand, neurons that are not integrated into these networks become nonfunctional or die.

It seems plausible that such a process would confer an evolutionary advantage. The organism is born with a substantial degree of flexibility in its neural capacities, and adapts these in response to the external signals it receives early in life. It can thus cope successfully with a wider range of environments than if it were born with all its neural capacity preset. But if the early environment is "information poor" and the signals received are limited or distorted, then the neural development will be also. Unlike mechanical systems (but like other biological systems), neuronal linkages are initiated and maintained by use, and "depreciate" from disuse—"use it or lose it."[11]

The observation that there are particular "windows" in the development of the neural system presumably comes as no surprise to students of language, who have known for some time that there is a critical period early in life during which language is normally acquired, rapidly and easily, along with particular accents and other sounds characteristic of the "native" language. Once that window is passed new language acquisition (or change of accent) may still be possible, but the adult student's impression that the process is increasingly difficult has a biological basis.

Even more interesting, it appears that learning capacity may be affected by the response to stress. Neurons differ in their "plasticity" or ability to change and to form interconnections among themselves.[12] The more "plastic" neurons are critical for the establishment of effective networks, which is part of the process of learning. In a very general sense "learning" consists of changes in one's neurons and in their interconnections, so the more plastic the neurons, the more readily one learns.[13] But the more plastic neurons also seem to be more vulnerable to the hormonal changes that take place during responses to stress, particularly if these are prolonged.[14]

When one is concentrating attention on moving oxygen and sugar to the large muscles, in hopes either of eating or of not being eaten, inessential activities like reproduction, growth and development, maintenance and repair, and learning from one's environment are quite sensibly closed down. Hang the environment—RUN! An increase in the level of glucocorticoids circulating in the bloodstream plays a central role in this process of closing down and concentration of effort.

Functions that are nonessential during an emergency, however, are by no means nonessential over the long term. In the normal course of events there is a feedback system that, upon detection of adequate levels in the blood, signals for a decrease in production of substances stimulating cortisol production. As the emergency passes, the "fight-or-flight" response is turned off and the organism is able to resume normal operations. But the ability to turn off the stress response may be almost as important for the long-run survival of the organism as the ability to turn it on is for short-run survival, because if the syndrome is not properly turned off, and if the level of circulating cortisol remains inappropriately high, the result of prolonged failure to carry out normal maintenance and repair is accumulating damage to a number of different types of cells. And among the cells damaged, or at least rendered more vulnerable to damage from other insults, are the more plastic neurons. Intuitively, those who are most open to learning from new experiences also run the greatest risk of being hurt by them when the weather turns bad; and this seems to be true of neurons as well.

At this point there is a remarkable convergence between the findings of research on the early and the late stages of life. Sapolsky (1992) has shown in studies of rats that there appears to be a positive feedback loop connecting stress, cortisol levels, and the aging process. The feedback mechanism that initiates a reduction in cortisol production seems to become less effective with age. But prolonged elevation of cortisol levels accelerates the aging process. Thus prolonged exposure to stress leads to physiological changes increasing vulnerability to stress—a vicious circle—if one is a rat.

As Sapolsky points out, whether or not such a process also operates in humans represents rather an important question for future research. A "yes" answer, which he finds "nothing short of terrifying," seems to be (tentatively) supported by the limited evidence currently available (1992, p. 390).

Such a conclusion has implications enough. But the remarkable parallel, as Cynader (personal communication, meeting of Programme in Human Development, Canadian Institute for Advanced Research, Toronto, January 1993) has noted, is that at both ends of life, processes are at work that involve the inactivation of neurons. Early in life the "sculpting out" of the functional neuronal pathways, in response to experience and activity, implies the determination of which connections will *not* be made. At this time the more "plastic" neurons, which are critical to the networking/learning process, are relatively widespread in the brain. But as the organism ages they become more concentrated (although not exclusively) in the hippocampus, which is also the location of the feedback process that regulates cortisol production.

Thus a prolonged elevation in levels of circulating cortisol associated with excessive or prolonged stress may have permanent effects on one's capacity to learn, while at the same time reducing one's ability to turn off the response to stress and thus increasing the likelihood of further damage. Sapolsky's choice of the word *terrifying* seems not inappropriate. On the other hand, he also cites evidence indicating that early nurturing can provide long term protection against such effects: "[N]eonatally handled rats . . . had decelerated hippocampal aging. Aged handled rats had more hippocampal neurons . . . and better spatial-learning skills than control aged rats" (p. 100). Supportive experiences at the very beginning of the life cycle confer significant benefits at the other end—for rats.

The finding of a linkage between the exploitation of neuronal plasticity at one stage in the life cycle—through learning—and neuronal survival at a subsequent stage, echoes in a striking fashion a point made in Chapter 3. It was there suggested that the observation of a (negative) correlation between educational level attained and the prevalence of senile dementia or Alzheimer's disease may reflect a real protective effect of education in early life, rather than an interpretation, sometimes offered, that more highly educated persons are better able to "mask" their dementia. There appears now to be a possible biological basis for this suggestion.[15]

Educational level attained is, of course, highly correlated with hierarchical position, at least among human primates. It is possible, therefore, that part of this correlation may result from differences in the effectiveness of neural connections with social rank, which in turn result from differences in either or both early life stress levels and environmental "information-richness."

Interestingly, in studies of free-ranging olive baboons in Kenya, Sapolsky (1990) has found a link between social rank and the consequences of stress (recall Chapter 1). These animals have a well-defined status hierarchy; and dominant and subdominant males differ in, among other things, the effectiveness of the feedback loop that controls the level of cortisol in the blood. When subdominant males respond to stress, their cortisol levels remain higher, longer. In effect, they are on average less able to turn off the "fight-or-flight" response when it is no longer needed; they suffer a greater or more prolonged degree of strain in response to a particular external stress.[16]

Of course such observations immediately bring up the nature/nurture question. Are animals dominant because they are born physiologically superior, or does their position in the dominance hierarchy—however attained—affect the competence of their endocrine systems? Sapolsky's work suggests an answer, and as one might expect in this complex area, it is "both."

On the one hand, disruption of the hierarchy led to physiological changes in the dominant animals. Their responses to stress were more like those of subordinates, until the uncertainty was resolved. This observation suggests that a dominant position leads to more effective physiological functioning. On the other hand, analyses of the dominant animals themselves indicated that some showed the same problems with the cortisol feedback loop that was more common among the subdominants. Others had "dominant personalities," which seemed to be genetically determined.

FROM ANIMALS TO HUMANS—AND BACK AGAIN

In Chapter 1 we noted the possible parallels between Sapolsky's studies of the hierarchies of free-ranging baboons in Kenya, and Marmot's studies of the hierarchies of free-ranging civil servants in London. But there have been a number of other human studies that have focused specifically on the cortisol loop in depressed persons. Psychiatrists continue to be intrigued by so-called "dexamethasone nonsuppressors"—individuals with clinical depression whose cortisol production is not suppressed by administration of a long-acting cortisol analog.[17] In normal individuals, as noted above, the increase in cortisol production in response to an external stress is limited and reversed by physiological feedback mechanisms responding to the level circulating in the blood. But among depressed individuals, there is a (poorly defined) subset, for whom this feedback process is less effective.[18]

This has implications for the effectiveness of the immune system, because there are receptors for cortisol on lymphocytes (immune cells responsible for antibody production), and cortisol-like compounds are used therapeutically in organ transplantation regimens for their immunosuppressive effects. The fact that decreased immune function has been found among people with depression seems to close a neat circle. But this work should be interpreted cautiously, as some findings have been poorly reproduced. Moreover, some investigators have not paid sufficient attention to the characteristics of their subjects. This has led to concerns about the direction of the causal link, if any, between depression and immunosuppression.

On the other hand, observations of nondepressed persons seem to show similar processes at work. Dexamethasone suppression has been shown to be induced temporarily in normal individuals under high stress conditions (Sapolsky, 1992). And psychological stresses, such as bereavement or academic pressure on students during exam time, have been shown to be associated with alterations in immune system function, including reduced natural killer cell activity, decreased lymphocyte proliferation, and reactivation of herpes virus infections.

As noted in Chapter 1, rat and mouse studies have also demonstrated a direct link from sensory experience to the immune system. The immune systems of mice can be "conditioned" by feeding them saccharin-flavoured water and injecting them with cyclophosphamide, a drug that suppresses the activity of the immune system (Ader and Cohen, 1975). If such conditioned mice are allowed to recover from the cyclophosphamide treatment, their immune systems regain competence, but if they are later fed saccharin-flavoured water *without* an injection, their immune systems are again suppressed. The brain receives and interprets the sensation of taste, and somehow converts this to an immune system response.

These studies, greeted with considerable initial skepticism but replicated several times, demonstrate convincingly that how one feels about the world around one, or at least how it tastes, can directly and powerfully influence the competence of one's immune system—again, if one is a mouse or rat. Moreover, the observation that the immune system is "conditioned" implies that these effects can endure beyond the precipitating event. This should perhaps not be surprising, since "learning and remembering" is so important a part of the repertoire of the immune system.

Studies of rats have also shown stress to be associated with diminished ability to fight off viruses and to reject foreign tissue (Dantzer and Kelley, 1989). Thus, virus-infected rats exposed to high-intensity noise have higher mortality than their nonexposed but infected counterparts, and physically restrained rats have a decreased resistance to herpes-like viruses and decreased cytokine production compared to unrestrained rats. However, as in studies of humans under stress, the results require careful interpretation.

What they show unambiguously is, yet again, that sensory impressions processed through the nervous system—perceptions—have biological effects that can be significant for health and even for survival. But the effects of these impressions may depend critically on the situation.

Some investigators have found *enhanced* resistance and immune function in rats under stress. Others have shown that induced tumours grow more rapidly in rats subjected to inescapable electric shock, but not in those subjected to escapable shock. Experiments with dogs have also shown the deleterious effects of and excess mortality from inescapable, as opposed to escapable, shock (Dantzer and Kelley, 1989; see, also, Sapolsky, 1992, p. 100).

The parallel between the extent to which the rat is able to control the stress associated with shock and the notion of "stress and coping" in the literature on humans is most intriguing. It is even paralleled by experiments in which the rat's state may, quite reasonably, be regarded as an analogue of human feelings of "hopelessness." If so, then presumably one can turn that coin over: Perhaps rats, like humans, react positively to the experience of coping successfully with stress. Observations that were "ambiguous" if one naively assumed in such animals a mechanical linkage from external stress to physiological response—a mechanical linkage that we know from our own experience does not apply to humans—are suddenly not only possible but plausible.[19]

Most of the experimental observations are made in circumstances that are highly unnatural, for rodents or for humans. (But what is "natural" for a purpose-bred laboratory rat?) A recent series of primate studies, referred to briefly in Chapter 1, has narrowed the gap between shocked rats and stressed humans. Wild-living rhesus monkeys represent a model of a complex society akin to human society (Suomi, 1991), and they also share over 90 percent of their replicating DNA with humans (Lovejoy, 1981). These monkeys live in matriarchal troops of twenty to one hundred members that are fairly stable over the lifetimes of the monkeys (Sade, 1967). There is a close bond between mother and infant. But this relationship is punctuated by separation when the mother goes into the next breeding cycle, leaving the infant (and the troop) for several days to go off with a chosen mate.

Field observation has shown that this period of separation is very hard on the infants, who display a number of signs of distress. Laboratory studies have revealed a corresponding physiological response, with increased heart rate and cortisol production. But the severity of the response, both physiological and behavioural, is quite variable—as it is in human infants. Most manage to get through the shock, but a small proportion of "hyper-reactive" individuals—about 20 percent—develop symptoms of depression and show long-term immunosuppression (Coe, Rosenberg, Fisher, and Levine, 1987).

These differences among individual monkeys are relatively stable over time. Those with severe separation reactions in infancy will have similarly severe reactions to stress in later life. And these reactions are physiologically similar even though the corresponding behaviour is different at different stages of the life cycle. Longitudinal studies indicate that infant monkeys at risk for more severe separation reactions can be identified by their performance on a standardized neonatal test battery (Becker et al., 1984).

Moreover, the health consequences of such hyper-reactions to stress can be very serious. Adolescent males in particular are ejected from their natal troops and, after a period of time in a "gang" of young males, must win acceptance by a different troop. This is a very stressful time—many do not survive—and hyper-reactivity is not an asset. Yet Suomi (1991) has shown that this trait is inheritable, which would be puzzling if it were unambiguously disadvantageous.[20] In fact, he has also observed that its effects can be buffered by particularly intensive nurturing by either the natural or a foster mother, and that a very supportively reared hyper-reactive infant may in adulthood take on leadership roles.[21] As with Sapolsky's baboons, the answer to the nature/nurture question is "both."

Such observations are quite consistent with modern genetic understanding. Progress continues to be made in identifying deterministic relationships between a single gene and a single condition or illness. But as Baird points out in Chapter 5, it is now recognized that the majority of the afflictions of adult life have a genetic component that is nondeterministic. Particular clusters or networks of genes result in greater or lesser "predispositions" to various illnesses, but the actual consequences of these predispositions for the organism will depend upon its environment and experiences.

Suomi's rhesus studies have focused principally on the psychological response of the animal to stressful events, although there has also been some notice of suppression of the immune system. The separation reaction among rhesus monkeys has been proposed as a "model" for studying depression in humans, depression both being an illness in itself, and potentially leading (in monkeys and in humans) to behaviours with other adverse health consequences. But another extensive series of primate studies has focused more specifically on physical outcomes, in particular on heart disease.

As mentioned in Chapter 1, Hamm, Kaplan, Clarkson, and Bullock (1983), working with cynomolgous macaques under laboratory conditions, fed the animals a "moderate" cholesterol diet (designed to be nutritionally similar to that of the dominant North American primate species). On this diet, the animals developed coronary artery atherosclerosis. But the investigators also observed that there were marked differences in the severity with which the disease afflicted different animals, even though the diets were identical. As emphasized throughout this book, the dispersion around the average response or experience may carry as much information as the average itself—or more.

These animals displayed a distinct status hierarchy, within which the degree of occlusion of the coronary arteries in the subordinate females was *four times greater* than in the dominant ones. Among males there was a two-to-one difference. Overall, males had a greater degree of occlusion on the same diet; among dominant animals the males had nearly four times the degree of occlusion while among the subordinates the difference was again about two to one. Moreover, these effects of status and gender on degree of occlusion were *independent* of differences in other "risk factors" such as the levels of lipids circulating in the blood.

But when this macaque status hierarchy is deliberately destabilized over a long period of time, by introducing "foreign" animals and rearranging the groups, it is the *dominant* males who suffer the greatest degree of occlusion on the moderate cholesterol diet (Kaplan, Manuck, Clarkson, Lusso, and Taub, 1982). This parallels Sapolsky's observations on free-ranging baboons, that the endocrine systems of dominant males functioned less effectively in turning off the cortisol response, when the status hierarchy became ambiguous.

In a subsequent review of these and other studies, Manuck, Kaplan, and Matthews (1986) suggest connections between the animal data and the findings of linkages between human personality types and heart disease. People with the Type A personalities[22] originally identified by Friedman and Rosenman (1969) have in a number of long-term follow-up studies been shown to have higher rates of heart disease than those with Type B—less aggressive and hard-driving. The observation goes back at least to Osler, but the studies are not consistent—several have failed to confirm this finding.

Manuck et al. point out that there are different instruments for identifying Type A personalities, and that these have been shown to give very different results. They suggest that self-administered questionnaires may not elicit the "anger" and "hostility" dimensions of this personality cluster as readily as the structured interviews, which are deliberately designed to be challenging and to stimulate behavioural responses. Subjects may misrepresent themselves in written answers, particularly as to levels of anger and hostility. The studies using structured interview measures do show the linkages to heart disease, suggesting that those based on self-administered questionnaires may simply have misclassified subjects. It may be that the anger and hostility components of personality, rather than the competitive, ambitious, and time-pressured components, are associated with greater risk of heart disease.

Such a partitioning of the Type A cluster of personality attributes is supported by the findings of Howard, Rechnitzer, Cunningham, Wong, and Brown (1990), who have studied the interaction of the Type A personality pattern with an additional personality trait labelled "dependence" or "independence." They note that people with Type A personalities "show greater hyper-reactivity of the sympathetic-adrenomedullary system, as manifested by greater responsiveness of blood pressure and heart rate and heightened levels of circulating catecholamines when under stress," suggesting that this hyper-reactivity may be the link between Type A behaviour and heart disease.

But they also find that this hyper-reactivity, as evidenced in physiologic measures on subjects under both experimental and "normal" job stress, is significantly greater among Type As who show higher "dependence," being "more sensitive to environmental stimuli" and "having a greater need for external guidance."[23] More "independent" persons, who "like to do things their own way," show less physiological reaction to stress. They suggest that it is not the ambitious, striving, time-pressured personality per se that is associated with hyper-reactivity to stress, but the combination of that behaviour with high needs for dependency and support, and the anger and hostility that result from frustration.[24]

These findings may then fit with the macaque studies, since in a stable hierarchy it is the low-status animals that experience frustration and challenge. So long as everyone knows who is boss, life is quite comfortable for the boss. And the subordinates, if they know what is good for them, bottle up their anger. But they are in a cleft stick. The human personality studies indicate that turning one's anger inward is even more harmful to one's health than letting it out. Yet a subordinate who lets out his/her/its feelings also incurs a (more immediate) risk to health. The macaque may be quite badly bitten.

When the hierarchy is disrupted, however, the dominant animals feel even more challenged and must engage in frequent struggles to re-establish their positions. They have little opportunity to enjoy the fruits of superiority. Furthermore, they have more to lose than their subordinates, who are forced to deal with constant frustration. Failure to respond effectively may force them into adjusting to a quite foreign situation—master turned to slave.

The observation that a subpopulation of hyper-reactive individuals is particularly vulnerable to stress also emerges from a recent study by Boyce et al. (1993). After reviewing a number of other human studies showing alterations in immune function following psychologically stressful events, they note "the consistent finding that stress-illness associations are statistically significant, but universally modest in magnitude." Their study measured changes in immune system function in a group of children (in the San Francisco Bay area) before and after entry to kindergarten, and then observed the incidence of respiratory illness during the subsequent twelve weeks.

Their intent was both to correlate immune system responses with illness incidence and to observe the extent of variation in responsiveness among the children. The study was unexpectedly enhanced, however, by the occurrence of the Loma Prieta earthquake at the midpoint of the twelve-week observation period.

Boyce et al. found substantial variability within their study group both in immune response to kindergarten entry and in illness incidence before and after the earthquake. While no clear pattern emerged for the group as a whole, there was a subgroup of children who showed both a rise in illness incidence after the earthquake, and "upregulatory changes in immune parameters" after entry to kindergarten. For this group, increased immune system reactivity was "significantly predictive" of increased illness after the earthquake.[25] Moreover, the incidences of illness and of behaviour problems after the earthquake were both significantly correlated with the extent of distress reported by *the parent* as a result of the earthquake.

The study population was quite small, only twenty children, and only a subgroup of these showed "interesting" results. But the findings seem to parallel those of Suomi for macaques and Howard et al. for Type A humans in identifying a vulnerable subpopulation that is both physiologically hyper-reactive to stress, and at greater risk of actual illness.[26] Moreover, the contributory role of parental distress is at least suggestive of Suomi's observation of the buffering role of nurturing.

Such observations also underline another theme emphasized above. Dominance, or Type A behaviour, or hyper-reactivity, or personality generally, has a significant genetic component. But in men (or women) as in monkeys, how or whether genetic predispositions are expressed depends upon the social environment. The same animals that are least at risk in a stable hierarchy are at greater risk in an unstable one. Moreover, some of the human studies have shown that people with Type A personalities can learn to modify their behaviour in ways that significantly reduce their risk of heart disease—again illustrating the interaction between the genetic and the social determinants of health.

In concluding their review, Manuck et al. emphasize, "Almost without exception, behavior-coronary disease relationships . . . have been independent of . . . other [risk] variables . . . (e.g., serum lipids, blood pressure, smoking, age)." The reader may recall that Marmot's studies of U.K. civil servants, described in Chapter 1, found a (negative) relationship between hierarchical position and mortality from coronary heart disease, which persisted after standardizing for the Framingham risk factor triad of smoking, high blood pressure, and high serum lipid levels. Similarly, Cohen et al. (1991) cited above, found that the relation between stress and colds was independent of other potential "risk factors."

The biological pathways leading to these results could run through the immune or the endocrine system, or both. Reference was made above, for example, to the role of certain components of the immune system in the development of fatty deposits in the arteries. And as noted in Chapter 7, certain of the cytokines produced by the immune system may damage the lining of the arteries, increasing the probability of formation of arterial plaques. But the vasoconstrictor effects of the "fight-or-flight" syndrome influence the fluid dynamics of the bloodstream, which in turn can result not only in wearing of this inner lining at specific foci, but also in changes in the "stickiness" of platelets, so as to increase the tendency to clot formation (again see Chapter 7). There are many more potential pathways known or hypothesized, and likely many more not yet suspected.

CONCLUSIONS

Recent biological research is thus rapidly filling out a picture, some of whose components are in fact very old. That experiences and perceptions can have physiological consequences has been known for as long as humans have been conscious of their responses to fear or anger. And the observation, in very general terms, that some groups of people are systematically healthier than others, goes back not decades but centuries. But the relationships among these phenomena turn out to be extraordinarily subtle and complex. While still a long way from being fully understood, important pieces of the huge mosaic are rapidly becoming clearer.[27]

There is now no longer room for doubt as to the existence of a complex web of linkages, having important implications for health, between the nervous system and other body systems. While the immune system has received particular attention, it appears to be only one component of the network of physiological systems responding to—and in turn influencing—the electrical and chemical output of the nervous system that is triggered by perceptions of the external world.

Moreover, it is now understood that some, at least, of these processes have an important time dimension. They are not just stimulus-response events at a point in time after which the organism returns to (its own version of) normal. As outlined in Chapter 3, biological processes can be time-dependent in several different ways; two appear to be of particular importance in this context. First, the processes initiated by the nervous system to respond to short-term emergencies can have long-term effects, particularly if unduly prolonged or frequently repeated, and these can be damaging to health. The immune system can be "conditioned," or elevated hormonal responses to stress may for a variety of reasons not be turned off properly.

But second, there are critical stages in the life of the organism in which normal development of the nervous system depends upon the receipt of particular external stimuli or the performance of particular activities. If these are lacking, the "wiring" of the nervous system may take a form different from what it would have been if properly stimulated. Alternatively, the ability of the nervous system to respond to external stimuli—to "learn" in the most general sense—can be impaired if the external environment has triggered other physiological responses that differentially disable the more "plastic" neurons crucial to the development of neuronal pathways.

Nor is the nervous system the only one in which the external environment may play a critical role in normal development. The immune system, too, may "learn" responses at an early stage in development, for good or ill. And there may be others—the fields of research are in a state of rapid flux.

The growth in awareness and understanding of these processes is beginning to put in place the biological substructure to support the observations, some of long standing, many others more recent, of the positive and negative health effects on individuals of aspects of their social environments. Widespread findings of the health-enhancing influences of "social supports," variously defined, or the virtually universal observation that health is positively correlated with hierarchical position, also variously defined, quite apart from the more intuitively understandable effects of material deprivation, are now explicable, at least potentially.

The gradient in health status with social position, for example, can be interpreted as the result of a wider array of external stresses bearing on people in lower ranks, combined with fewer resources available to them, on average, to respond effectively to such stresses. Resources for "coping" may be in the form of external assistance; one can call on others either through social networks or with material resources—in the crudest form, money. But they can also include personal resources—material, physical, and psychological. Such a picture underlies an interest in early life experiences as a source of learned coping strategies, or the accumulation of psychological resources, for dealing with external stress.

So humans, like monkeys, baboons, rats, and dogs, may respond to a stressful environment that they cannot control with physiological changes that are harmful to their health. In the absence of such biological pathways, the "natural" explanation for heterogeneities in population health status has been to fall back on genetics—some people, particularly those at the top of hierarchies, are just born fitter. But understanding biological pathways is not in conflict with genetic explanations; it is clear that there are also genetic differences in vulnerability to external stresses. The critical point, however, is that these genetic differences are in *predisposition*, not predestination. The quality of the social and physical environments plays a critical role in determining whether these predispositions will in fact be expressed.[28]

Thus if one asks, Do the biological processes that underlie the correlation between socioeconomic status and health differ among individuals as a result of differences in initial genetic endowment? or in previously "learned" physiological responses? or in the contemporaneous balance between external stresses and coping resources? the answer appears to be yes. "Hyper-reactivity" appears to be hereditary, but early nurturing can have both short- and long-term protective effects, and the combination of these factors influences the resilience or vulnerability with which each of us then confronts and interprets the environment. And that environment, in turn, has immediate and long-term influences on our biological capabilities, influences that trigger positive feedback loops, virtuous or vicious circles. Early advantages and disadvantages are thus self-reinforcing, as they become built into our nervous, immune, and endocrine systems—our selves.

The material presented in this chapter is a limited selection from a vast, highly complex, and very rapidly expanding set of fields of social and biological research. It makes no pretence of being comprehensive or balanced. The intent is to provide a more detailed description and integration of the evidence underlying the themes touched upon in Chapters 1 and 3 in particular.

There *is* a chain that runs from the behaviour of cells and molecules, to the health of populations, and back again, a chain in which the past and present social environments of individuals, and their perceptions of those environments, constitute a key set of links. No one would pretend that the chain is fully understood, or is likely to be for a considerable time to come. But the research evidence currently available no longer permits anyone to deny its existence.

NOTES

1. In addition to the isolated effects of these risks to health, their correlated occurrence compounds their detrimental effects. Consider crowding and poor nutrition; not only are infectious organisms more easily spread in crowded quar-

ters, but their pathological effects are likely to be greater if the susceptible "host" is poorly nourished. The end result is a burden of disease and morbidity that resists corrective action aimed at any one factor in isolation.

2. But wealth may enable a population to protect itself against the threats that crowding poses to health. Two of the most densely populated wealthy societies, Japan and the Netherlands, show the world's best aggregate health statistics. And two other very crowded countries, South Korea and Taiwan, have each shown rapid improvements in recent decades in both health and wealth.

3. It is important to bear in mind the heterogeneity of the different forces that are collectively referred to as "stress." Stresses can be acute or chronic, predictable or unpredictable. Their characteristics may determine the general nature of individual "responses."

4. Coping can be defined as "constantly changing cognitive and behavioral efforts to manage specific external and/or internal demands that are appraised as taxing or exceeding the resources of the person" (Lazarus and Folkman, 1984:1).

5. Indeed, the language in this field has historically been confused; the common reference to external factors as "stressors" results from a tendency to describe the physiological reactions as "stress" reactions. This reflects a frequent lack of clarity as to whether "stress" is inside the organism or outside it.

6. A significant advantage of animal experiments is that one can control and standardize the events to which the animals are exposed, and then measure their physiological responses (see below). If animals respond differently, physiologically, to what appear objectively to be similar events, then these differences can—given enough time and animals—be traced to differences either in their genetic makeup, or in their current or prior physical or social experiences. Thus one can solve the circularity problem . . . but to what extent can one generalize to humans?

7. Humans go to some considerable trouble to expose themselves to situations that generate this adrenal response—"adrenalin sports" such as skydiving or ice climbing, for example, or even skiing or sailing. The key to pleasure—and sometimes survival—in such circumstances seems to be the ability to control oneself and one's environment by channeling the adrenal response into enhanced capability—coping—rather than being overwhelmed by panic. The experience of successful coping with stress—mastery—appears to be a source of considerable pleasure.

8. Surveys of this literature are provided by Dantzer and Kelley (1989) and Biondi and Kotzalidis (1990).

9. A cursory glance at any medical school curriculum or medical directory reveals courses and people claiming expertise over particular components of *homo sapiens*. The result of this compartmentalization of training and practice has been a rather narrow, system-based approach to the diagnosis and treatment of disease. Thus, the idea that the various systems communicate in a highly complex and interactive manner, which is central to the host response to disease, has had some difficulty gaining acceptance. When knowledge and the people possessing and pursuing it are organized into separate compartments, it is difficult to accept that the phenomena themselves may not be.

10. If the cat is reared in complete darkness, however, the critical period can be delayed. When no signals at all are being received, the developmental process may be put on hold. Thus the timing of the allocation of neural capacity, the formation of cellular connections, does not appear to be rigidly determined by

the biological age of the animal. It, too, is sensitive to external signals. But once the critical period is passed, it may be difficult or impossible to go back.

11. This leaves open the question of whether an "information-rich" early environment that was markedly *different* from the one in which the animal was later to live might also lead to the formation not only of inappropriate attitudes and habits, but also of inappropriate neural structures. There is an echo here of studies suggesting that people raised in straitened circumstances, who come to affluence later in life, may be at greater risk of heart disease (Forsdahl, 1977). But this too is uncertain.

12. The ability to modify connections is related to the numbers and types of receptor sites on the cell surface and on dendrites and dendritic spines, which permit it to recognize neurotransmitter substances released by other cells, and to the numbers and lengths of the cellular extensions—axons—with which it can establish contact with other cells.

13. We also speak of "learning" by the immune system, as it develops the ability to recognize and destroy particular forms of "nonself" material—so we develop immunity to particular diseases. And perhaps physical training could be thought of as "learning" by muscle cells.

14. The plasticity of one's neurons is greatest between conception and puberty, which is why it is difficult (though *not* impossible) to teach an old dog new tricks. This suggests that one's learning capacity may be more vulnerable to damage from prolonged stress when one is young.

15. It may be that educational attainment is only a marker for the survival of "plastic" neurons, so that both educational attainment and resistance to (mental) aging might be consequences of (very?) early life experiences. But since learning involves the creation and strengthening of neuronal connections, one should not rule out a priori the possibility of a direct effect. And the hippocampus is once again involved, as a primary site for the degeneration associated with Alzheimer's disease, about half of whose sufferers show some signs of hypercortisolemia (Sapolsky, 1992:337).

16. This raises the intriguing possibility that subdominant males get less benefit out of their "windows of plasticity" or are otherwise harmed because of their lessened ability to control and limit their responses to stress, and therefore that their subordination is reinforced by failure (relatively speaking) to learn and to mature in other ways.

17. Such a substance appears identical to cortisol and so in normal individuals leads to a reduction in cortisol production because the body's feedback system mistakenly believes that a sufficient amount is present.

18. This appears to bear a striking resemblance to Sapolsky's subdominant baboons. (And possibly some of Marmot's lower-ranking civil servants? Or perhaps some in all ranks, but more among the lower ranks?)

19. There appears to be, among some in the scientific community, a distinct resistance to the drawing of psychological parallels between humans and other animals, and a preference for mechanical interpretations of animal behaviour as if these were more "scientific." Anthropomorphizing and projection of human ideas and characteristics onto animals to serve the psychological needs of humans are real dangers, as the more florid expressions of the pet industry make obvious. Yet animal "models" of human disease processes are not contentious. It may well be that resistance to the integration of human and animal observations is also a response to human psychological needs, of a different form.

We still have with us remnants of medieval ideas about the Great Chain of

Being, that animals have no souls, as men and angels do. Descartes gave this idea a modern dress, arguing that animals were simply biological machines without consciousness—considering the treatment that animals receive from humans, this was bound to be a popular view. But the modern researcher, with defensible motives and with compassion rather than cruelty, continues to do things to animals that would be hard to explain to one's children. The more sensitive the researcher, the more likely s/he is to find human/animal psychological parallels distressing. If so, it would not be the first time that the (wholly understandable) psychological needs of the experimenter had influenced the interpretation of experimental results.

20. One would expect that a gene (or perhaps a cluster of genes?) responsible for a selective disadvantage would disappear over time. The genes responsible could, however, be "pleiotropic" having other as yet unidentified effects that *are* advantageous for survival.

21. The chance that a hyper-reactive infant macaque will receive especially good nurturing depends, however, upon the early experience of its own mother. Poorly nurtured macaque females tend in their turn to be less competent at nurturing, thus extending disadvantages across the generations. Such an observation may be highly suggestive for human populations. On the other hand, the observation that protective nurturing can be provided by a foster mother may parallel the findings of some of the studies referred to in Chapter 1 (e.g., Grantham-McGregor, Powell, Walker, and Himes, 1991) showing the benefits of enhanced nutrition and stimulation for high-risk children.

22. People who are highly competitive, are ambitious and have high occupational goals, typically feel under intense time pressure, are aggressive, and readily respond to challenge or frustration with hostility and anger are identified as Type A personalities (Friedman and Rosenman, 1969). But the identification is not always clear-cut. See below.

23. One is reminded of Suomi's hyper-reactive monkeys, with high needs for maternal contact and nurturing; Howard et al. also note that the "dependency" trait has "a high degree of hereditary determination" (p. 149).

24. There is undoubtedly a connection here to the observations referred to in Chapter 1, showing that high job demand and low control are associated with higher risk of heart disease. If certain personality types are more or less vulnerable, one is led yet again to think about the interaction, the "goodness (or badness) of fit," between job characteristics and personality types. As emphasized in Chapter 5, the physical and social environment, past and present, influences the way in which hereditary predispositions will be expressed in health and disease.

25. Strangely, however, the correlation is *positive,* with greater immune system reactivity being significantly correlated with (later) increased illness. The authors offer some possible interpretations.

26. The illness itself is variable—upper respiratory infections among human children, depression-like symptoms among young macaques, and heart disease among middle-aged male humans. Recall the discussion in Chapter 1, that correlations between socioeconomic status or hierarchical position, and mortality or morbidity, seem to be expressed *through* a variety of different diseases, but the particular diseases are not the fundamental phenomena.

27. But the picture may never be complete. It may be beyond the limits of human intellectual capacity ever to understand fully the human organism (and perhaps that was the way it was meant to be). Humans compartmentalize things

in order to understand them, but we ourselves are fundamentally noncompartmentalizable organisms. In any case we should not expect a full understanding of the biological pathways and interactions any time soon.

28. From this perspective, those researchers pursuing highly controversial investigations into the genetic basis of criminal behaviour may be miscasting the question in a misleading and dangerous way. There very probably are genetic variations among individuals that lead some to be more likely than others to engage in criminal behaviour *in particular social settings*. And there do appear to be people who are so abnormal—perhaps in large part for genetic reasons—as to be a permanent danger to those around them. But an understanding of why whole *groups* within populations are much more likely, on average, to engage in criminal behaviour, is *far more likely* to be found in their external circumstances, not in their genes. This is another example of Rose's (1985) distinction between sick individuals and sick populations—the factors explaining the latter cannot be found by investigating only the former. (Such investigations may, however, be an excellent way of *not* finding them, if that is one's objective.)

7

Coronary Heart Disease from a Population Perspective

M. G. MARMOT and J. F. MUSTARD

Coronary heart disease (CHD) is the major cause of death in most developed countries and an important source of illness and disability. Its causes and progress are commonly traced to interacting genetic and behavioural factors. But large differences in the rate of occurrence of CHD both between and within countries, and similarly large changes in these patterns over time, indicate the powerful influence of the social, cultural, and economic features of those societies. As will be recalled from previous chapters, variations in mortality that are associated with income, education, or hierarchical position, are among the most suggestive forms of evidence for the influence of underlying determinants of health that express themselves through particular diseases—including CHD.

In the first half of the twentieth century CHD could reasonably be described as a "disease of affluence." Its increased incidence was associated with increased prosperity in Western societies, where it reached epidemic proportions and tended to strike the more affluent members of those countries. But in more recent years this pattern has completely changed, and the present picture of the disease worldwide is now much more complex:

- The age-standardized death rate from CHD has fallen dramatically, and continues to fall, in the wealthy countries of Europe, North America, and Australasia.[1] It is even falling in Japan, where it has always been very low.
- Within the affluent countries the decline has occurred more rapidly among the higher status members of the community. Thus rates of CHD in these countries are now in general higher among those with lower income, social status, or position in the work hierarchy.
- On the other hand, CHD is emerging as a major cause of death in some developing countries, and CHD rates are rising in the former communist countries of Central and Eastern Europe.

The major challenge is to develop an understanding of the social, economic, and cultural forces that underlie these trends, and to trace out how they have their effects. Can these observations be related to what is known about risk factors, the pathways involved in atherosclerosis, and its thromboembolic complications? If the correlations between social factors and health outcomes reflect causal processes, then there must be biological pathways through which they exert their influence. Whatever the "ultimate cause(s)" of health or disease, there must at some point in the chain be a "proximate biological cause."

In this chapter we start with an account of our current understanding of the pathological basis of CHD. This is then related to the picture that emerges from the historical comparison of trends in different countries and cultures. This leads, in turn, to an analysis of the competing hypotheses about the particular characteristics of populations that seem to trigger or enable the biological responses leading to CHD in individuals.

HISTORICAL PERSPECTIVE ON PATHOGENESIS

Atherosclerosis, which is a thickening of the inner lining of blood vessels ("hardening of the arteries"), is recognized as the underlying process from which coronary heart disease can develop. But at the beginning of this century, atherosclerosis was considered a natural consequence of age and appeared to have little effect on normal life span. Although the relationship between atherosclerosis in the coronary arteries and the clinical complications of coronary heart disease, such as angina pectoris (chest pain), was recognized by Edward Jenner in the late 1700s, it was not until the middle of this century that the increase in the incidence of coronary heart disease led to a major interest in the nature of the disease.

Morris (1951) investigated the pathology records of a London hospital early in the twentieth century, and then reviewed the same data for the middle part of the century. The extent of atherosclerosis in the coronary arteries was similar for individuals dying in each period. He found, however, that there was a major difference in the vessels of those dying in the later period. Although the underlying atherosclerosis was similar, many in the later period had severe localized narrowing, and in many cases complete blockage, of their coronary arteries. Something had happened during the intervening fifty years that led not to more atherosclerosis but to pathological processes building on it, which led in turn to thrombosis (formation of clots), blocking the blood flow to the heart.

Most pathology studies during this century have shown that individuals can have extensive atherosclerosis without clinical manifestations such as angina and heart attacks. Clinical manifestations are associated with focal narrowing of vessels, rupture of the atherosclerotic plaques in the inner lining of the arteries, thrombosis, and occasionally spasm (Davies and Thomas, 1985).

These observations are compatible with at least two processes being involved in coronary artery disease: those causing thickening of the lining of the blood vessels, and those causing focal narrowing with thrombotic occlusion (blockage by clots) of the narrowed vessels. This realization of more than one pathway aids understanding of the epidemiology of coronary heart disease. Features of life-style or of the environment may be related to only one of the pathways.[2]

Seldom-noted early animal experiments set the stage for the explosion of interest, in the middle of this century, in the role of cholesterol in CHD. Ignatowski (1909), a Russian scientist early in the twentieth century, fed rabbits diets rich in saturated fat and cholesterol and found that they developed extensive lipid-rich atherosclerotic lesions—fatty deposits in the arterial linings. Subsequent work showed that these thickenings of the inner lining of major arteries were associated with increased levels of cholesterol in the blood of these animals. Experiments carried out by Ignatowski's colleagues demonstrated that, for rabbits, diets rich in unsaturated fats from vegetable or fish sources produced little or no atherosclerosis and did not raise blood cholesterol levels (Anitschkow, 1915). All the subsequent animal studies (from primates to mice) have shown a clear relationship between diets rich in saturated fat and cholesterol, hypercholesterolemia, and the development of atherosclerosis (Roberts and Straus, 1965).

All of these studies have also found, however, that animals with the same level of cholesterol may develop different degrees of atherosclerosis. This variance, which can be quite marked, has never been satisfactorily explained. Furthermore, with a few exceptions, these researchers did not find the thrombotic complications of atherosclerosis. The exceptions were extremely long term studies in which the animals were also often stressed (Taylor, Cox, Counts, and Yogi, 1959). The animal experiments thus showed that dietary fat influenced the development of atherosclerosis, but did *not* show that this fat-induced atherosclerosis was a key pathway causing focal narrowing and thrombotic occlusion.

The emergence of coronary heart disease as a major cause of death in developed countries led to a number of epidemiological studies to explore what might be causing the "epidemic" (Keys, 1980). The earlier animal experiments, combined with the observation that coronary heart disease appeared to be a disease of the affluent, led to an interest in diet, and particularly the cholesterol content of the diet.

One group of investigators found that individuals living in countries with diets lower in fat, particularly less saturated fat, had lower blood cholesterol levels and a substantially lower incidence of death from coronary artery disease (Keys, 1980). Some of these populations lived in Mediterranean countries in which fish and olive oil are important dietary ingredients. The results from these studies and from very detailed longitudinal studies, such as the U.S. Framingham study, gradually established that elevated blood cholesterol, particularly LDL (low-density lipoprotein) cholesterol, was associated with an increased risk of dying from coronary artery disease (Kannel and Gordon, 1973; Johnson, Epstein, and Kjelsberg, 1965; Tibblin, Wilhelmsen, and Werkö, 1975).

Although the animal and epidemiological evidence concerning saturated fat and cholesterol showed that the fat content of the diet was an important factor in the development of atherosclerosis, there was still the nagging problem that most of the events that produced clinical symptoms were actually thrombotic—depending on the formation of clots in the blood, not merely the thickening of the arterial walls. Some degree of atherosclerosis appears to be a prerequisite for thrombosis but it is likely that high levels of blood cholesterol are not, in themselves, sufficient for thrombosis to occur.

The contribution of thrombosis to atherosclerosis also has its champions (Duguid, 1948; Morgan, 1956; Woolf and Crawford, 1960). The idea that thrombosis might contribute to the development of atherosclerosis is generally credited to Von Rokitansky (1852) in the last century. He suggested that fibrin clots occurring on the surface of blood vessels, in response to injury to the vessel walls, would become incorporated into the inner layer of arteries and produce thickening. In the middle of this century, Duguid (1948) and others (Morgan, 1956; Woolf and Crawford, 1960) demonstrated from human autopsy studies that mural thrombi—

clots on the arterial walls—are in fact incorporated into the walls themselves and thus contribute to atherosclerotic thickening. A number of investigators found that stenotic lesions (narrowing) could be produced by the accretion of material from repeated episodes of mural thrombosis (Duguid, 1948; Woolf and Crawford, 1960; Jørgensen, Rowsell, Hovig, and Mustard, 1967). This is clearly a key pathway in producing advanced stenotic atherosclerotic lesions. Vessel injury and thrombosis is also the key pathway that produces clinical manifestations of coronary artery disease. Repeated injury to the lining of arteries without cholesterol feeding will produce the full spectrum of atherosclerosis. Thus atherosclerosis produced by diet or by repeated vessel injury can be the basis for development of stenotic atherosclerotic lesions that set the stage for thromboembolic events that cause heart attacks.

Until late in the 1970s, thrombosis was not generally recognized by clinical cardiology (in countries such as the United States) as important in the story of coronary heart disease. The emergence of modern imaging techniques, however, and more detailed pathological studies have now established that thrombosis is the primary end stage event causing clinical complications (Fuster, Badimon, Badimon, and Chesebro, 1992). As described earlier in this chapter, a dominant process is rupture of atherosclerotic plaques in stenotic areas with the formation of thrombi at these sites (Davies and Thomas, 1985; Fuster et al., 1992). The process of thrombosis involves platelets adhering to the damaged vessel wall and to each other, and blood coagulation. Plasma lipids and cholesterol have only a slight effect on this process, which is largely influenced by other factors (Taylor et al., 1959; Mustard, Packam, and Kinlough-Rathbone, 1981). In theory, then, factors influencing atherosclerosis and factors influencing arterial thrombosis will both determine the incidence of clinical coronary heart disease.

THE RISE AND FALL OF CORONARY HEART DISEASE

In examining the epidemiology of coronary heart disease, risk factors, and approaches to prevention, our interpretations should take into account the knowledge we have concerning the underlying process and particularly the fact that several processes are involved.

It is instructive to contrast the experiences of Western Europe, North America, Eastern Europe, and Japan, focusing particularly on possible relationships between the incidence of CHD and socioeconomic differences across, and changes in, societies. This is not to deny the potential importance of risk factors such as smoking, diet, exercise, or other "life-style" patterns. These may well be part of the explanation for the broad changes in the rate of occurrence of CHD. In fact, a review of CHD trends suggests three classes of factors at work: nutrition, cigarette smoking, and socioeconomic characteristics of a society that are not as well defined. But the last of these has been by far the least extensively explored.

The rise and fall of CHD, because it is such a major cause of death, is intimately bound up with changes in life expectancy. We begin with a review of these changes.

Western Europe and North America

In regions of the world where CHD rates are high, such as Western Europe or North America, the higher the rate of CHD, the higher the mortality from all causes. This is in part because CHD is such an important contributor to the total death rate. But it is also because there is a correlation between mortality from CHD and mortality from other causes. This is true for areas within a country, such as regions of England and Wales or states of the United States, social classes within a country (OPCS, 1989), and to a lesser extent differences between European countries (Uemura and Pisa, 1988).

On the other hand Preston and Nelson (1974) found an inverse association between CHD and all-cause mortality in a review of data from 165 countries. This is because countries with low CHD mortality are most typically developing countries with high mortality from infectious disease.

This reversal corresponds to what is known as an epidemiological transition (Omran, 1971). As infectious disease mortality declines, it is replaced by a different pattern of chronic diseases: predominantly cardiovascular disease and cancer. This transition or health development is broadly related to the level of economic development. There are examples of developing countries where infectious disease mortality has declined, but has not as yet been replaced by an increasing burden of chronic disease. More typically, in Western countries the rise of CHD occurred with economic development. In mature industrial economies, however, continuing development is associated with a decline in prevalence of CHD.

This epidemiological transition was well under way in Britain in the 1920s. In 1921, CHD and cancer together accounted for approximately the same number of deaths as infectious diseases. By 1931 these chronic diseases had become the major causes of death in both men and women (Davey Smith and Marmot, 1991).

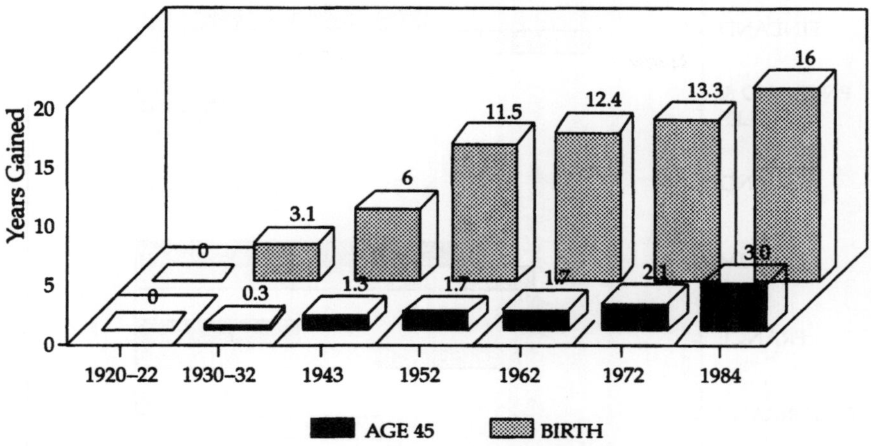

Figure 7.1. Increase in life expectancy for men in England and Wales compared with 1920–1922.

The decline of infectious disease mortality had a considerable impact on life expectancy. Figure 7.1 shows that in England and Wales, from 1922 to 1984, life expectancy at birth for men increased from 55.6 to 71.6 years and for women, from 59.6 to 77.6 years. This rapid improvement is mainly the result of reductions in infant mortality. At age 45, the increase in life expectancy over this 60-year period was only 3.5 years for men, though a more impressive 6.7 years for women. This rather modest improvement at middle age reflects the rise of chronic disease mortality, particularly from CHD and lung cancer, a rise that was more marked for men. In fact, during the early part of this period, in the 1930s, life expectancy for men at age 45 actually fell.

After a long period of virtually no improvement in male life expectancy at middle age, there was an increase of 1.4 years in only 12 years. CHD and lung cancer, although still major causes of death, have passed their peaks and are now on the way down. (Lung cancer deaths among women are still rising rapidly, however, as a direct result of the increase in smoking among females twenty years before.) Figure 7.2 shows the decline in CHD mortality in England and Wales, and other European countries, over the period 1970–1985. Such declines have also occurred in other countries, notably the United States, Canada, Australia, New Zealand, and Japan (see below).

The general picture in Western countries is of sharp increases in CHD mortality in parallel with the rapid increase in prosperity following

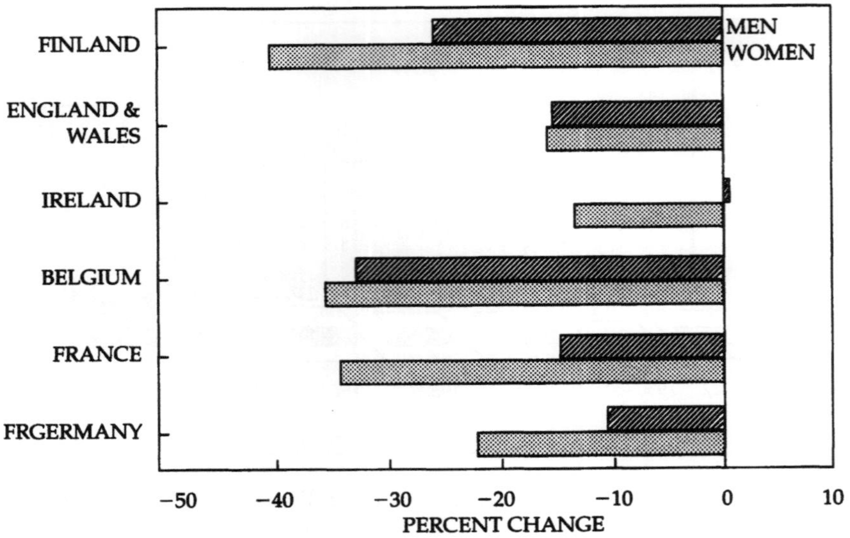

Figure 7.2. Change in heart disease mortality, 1970–1985, age standardised 30–69.

World War II, followed by sharp falls as economic development in the affluent countries has continued.[3]

East versus West Europe

Figure 7.3 shows trends in CHD rates for the European countries of the former socialist block. In all cases, the rates for men increased during 1970–1985. In each of these countries, except the former German Democratic Republic, all-cause mortality increased concurrently. Data from Hungary, for example, show that life expectancy decreased through this period. The picture for CHD is similar to the earlier experience of Western Europe, up until the 1950s and 1960s.

When CHD was rising rapidly in England and Wales, infant mortality was declining. Thus life expectancy at birth continued to rise, although there was little improvement in life expectancy in middle age. In Eastern Europe, by contrast, the increase in CHD was not balanced by a decline in infant mortality, so overall life expectancy has fallen (Hertzman, 1992). One might then speculate that the same causes responsible for the earlier rise and fall of CHD in Western Europe are now operating in

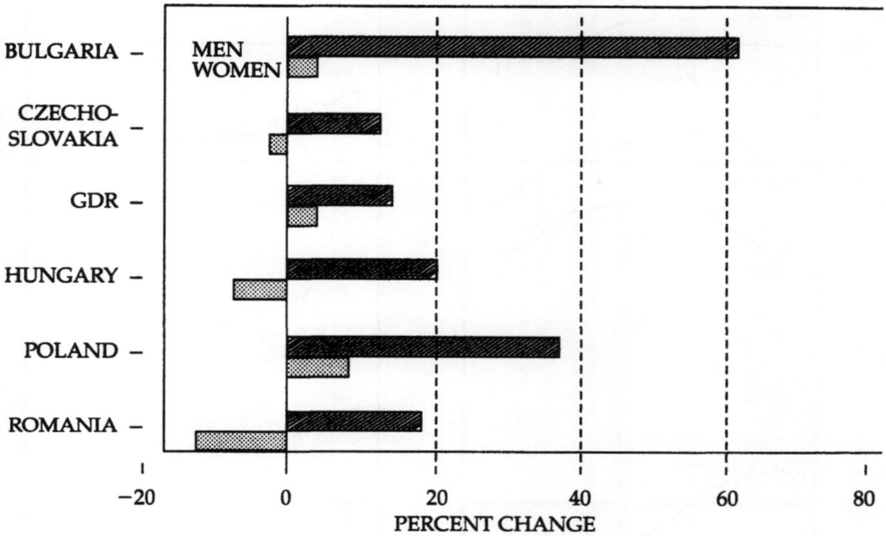

Figure 7.3. Change in heart disease mortality 1970–1985, age-standardised mortality rates 30–69 years.

Eastern Europe, a generation later and with similar effects on life expectancy.

Why should Eastern Europe now be going through an epidemiological transition like that of England and Wales in an earlier period? It is perhaps not fanciful to suggest that this reflects the relative state of economic development. Those countries may be at the point in industrialization and economic development that, in the West, corresponded to the upswing of the CHD epidemic before it reached its peak. A striking feature of recent studies is that the east-west life expectancy gap cannot be accounted for by differences in disease-specific *individual* risk factors (Hertzman, 1992).

Comparison with Japan

A rise in CHD rates is not, however, an inevitable consequence of economic development, industrialization and the decline of infectious disease. Japan's experience makes this clear. Despite dire warnings of the effect of industrialization, and supposed Westernization, Japan escaped the CHD epidemic and has had among the lowest rates of heart disease of any industrialized country (Marmot and Davey Smith, 1989).

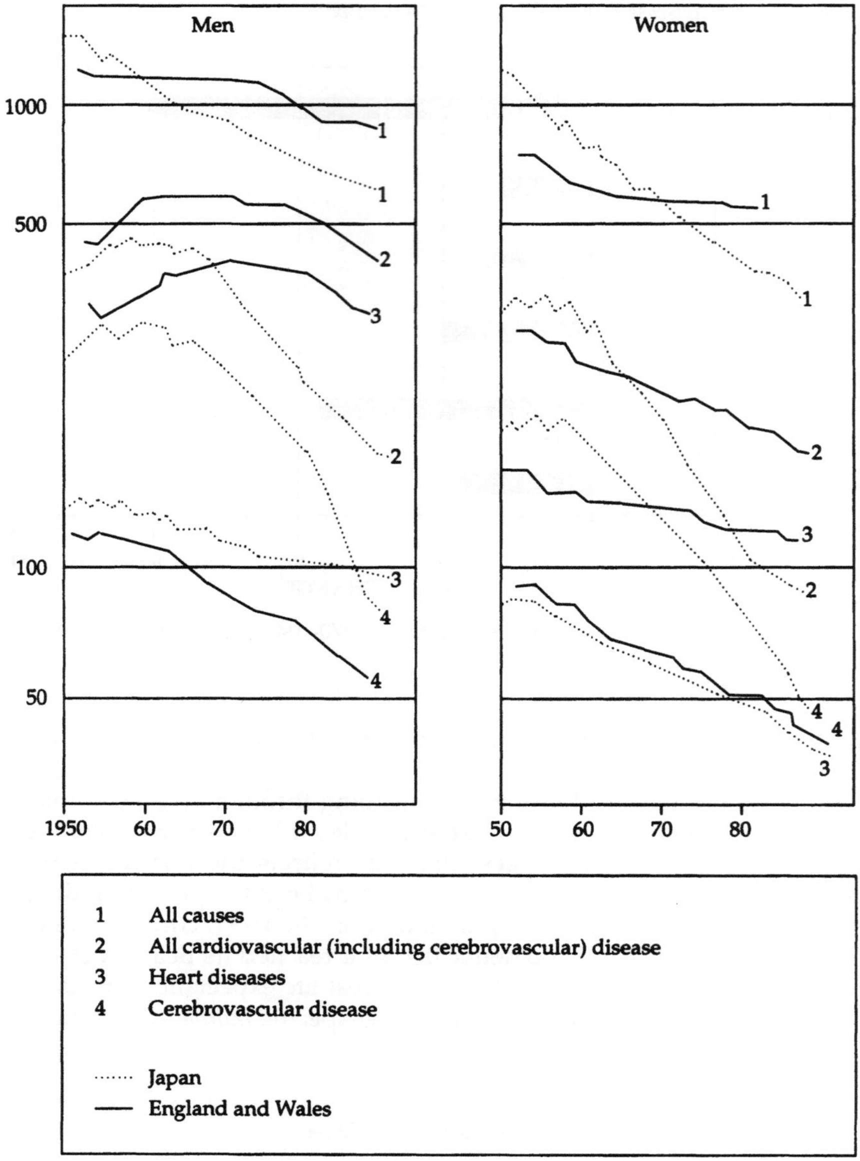

Figure 7.4. Age-adjusted mortality rates in Japan and England and Wales, 1950–1990.
Source: Marmot and Davey Smith, (1989)

Nevertheless, as Figure 7.4 shows, age-adjusted rates of death from CHD have declined steeply in Japan as well, even more so than in England and Wales.

More generally, trends in mortality in Japan have been more favourable than other countries for virtually all causes of death over the last twenty-five years. For example, at one time Japan had the highest mortality rate in the world from stroke, but this has since declined steeply. Figure 7.4 contrasts mortality rates in Japan with those in England and Wales (Marmot and Davey Smith, 1989). Japanese all-cause mortality rates in middle age were higher up to the early 1960s (Uemura and Pisa, 1988). They then began to fall much more steeply, and by now are well below those in England and Wales.

Since the decline in infectious disease mortality in Japan was not offset by increased CHD, there has been a marked increase in life expectancy (Table 7.1). At birth, a Japanese boy could expect to live 75.2 years (assuming today's mortality rates applied) compared to 71.9 years for a boy born in England and Wales. A Japanese girl could expect to live 80.9 years, compared to 77.7 for her English counterpart (Marmot and Davey Smith, 1989).

The speed with which life expectancy has increased is also impressive: 7.5 years for men and 8 years for women in the 21 years from 1965 to 1986. To put this increase in perspective, abolishing all heart disease (and assuming that other causes of death did not increase in age-specific frequency) would add only 4.7 years to life expectancy in England and Wales.[4] The improvement in life expectancy that has occurred in Japan

Table 7.1. Life Expectancy (years) of Japanese and of English and Welsh Populations Since 1955

		Males		*Females*	
		At birth	*At age 65*	*At birth*	*At age 65*
Japan	1955	63.6	11.8	67.8	14.1
	1965	67.7	11.9	72.9	14.6
	1975	71.7	13.7	76.9	16.6
	1980	73.4	14.6	78.8	17.7
	1986	75.2	15.9	80.9	19.3
England and Wales	1955	67.5	11.8	73.0	14.8
	1965	68.5	12.1	74.7	15.8
	1975	69.5	12.4	75.7	16.4
	1980	70.4	12.8	76.6	16.8
	1984–1986	71.9	13.4	77.7	17.3

Source: Marmot and Davey Smith (1989).

in 21 years is equivalent to the abolition of all heart disease and most cancer in England and Wales. This is worthy of some attention.

Life expectancy at birth is, of course, heavily influenced by mortality in the first year of life. But Table 7.1 shows that even at age 65, life expectancy has improved 4 years for men in Japan and 4.7 years for women since 1965, compared to 1.3 and 1.5 years for men and women, respectively, in England and Wales, and these increases were on very comparable (identical for male) "baseline" life expectancies in 1965.

Given the unusually favourable Japanese experience, and its departure from the "typical" European pattern, considerable further exploration would seem to be in order. The lessons learned might well have broader applications. In particular, the determinants of health and illness that are operating so powerfully in Japan may well have parallels to the equally powerful, though still incompletely understood, forces emerging in the data from the U.K. Civil Service studies (Marmot and Davey Smith, 1989; Marmot, 1985; Marmot and Theorell, 1988).

THE DETERMINANTS OF VARIATION IN CHD MORTALITY: ALTERNATIVE CANDIDATES

Migration, Cultures, and Genetics

CHD, like other epidemic diseases, relates closely to social conditions. Its frequency of occurrence has much more to do with the social and cultural features of a society than it does with the genetic makeup of that society's population. The strongest general arguments for this are, first, the rapid changes that have occurred in the rate of occurrence of CHD. In the United States, for example, death rates from CHD declined by 48 percent between 1970 and 1985. In Japan, the reduction was 39 percent in men and 30 percent in women (Uemura and Pisa, 1988). Gene frequencies do not change at that rate.

An equally powerful argument against genetic determination emerges from studies of migrant populations. Migrants tend toward the rate of CHD of their country of adoption (Marmot, Adelstein, and Bulusu, 1984). Men of Japanese ancestry living in Hawaii have higher rates of CHD than Japanese in Japan. Japanese in California have higher rates than those in Hawaii but less than average for the United States (Worth, Rhoads, Kagan, Kato, and Syme, 1975; Marmot et al., 1975). Presumably, they take on the life-style of the host country with its attendant disease consequences. Indeed, there is evidence that in California those

Japanese who adopted American life-styles have higher CHD rates than those who retained more traditional Japanese styles of life (Marmot and Syme, 1976).

This is not to claim that hereditary factors play no part in CHD; clearly they do. But while differences in genetic makeup provide part of the explanation for differences in disease experience among the *individual* members of a particular population, they cannot explain the large observed differences between *populations*. These findings underscore the importance of the definition of "heterogeneities" established in Chapter 3, as systematic differences in aggregate measures of health between population groups, not among individuals.

Health Care

It is natural, of course, to ask whether the improvements in rates of CHD, or health status more generally, are a result of greater consumption of higher quality health care. The contribution of improved medical technique to the decline in CHD mortality is controversial, but it is worth noting that Japan does not spend a high proportion of its national income on health care. In 1965, Japan spent 4.3 percent of its gross domestic product on health care, not very different from the United Kingdom (4.1 percent), and substantially less than Canada (6.0 percent) or the United States (5.9 percent). By 1990 the percentage of GDP spent by Japan and the United Kingdom had increased to 6.5 and 6.1 percent, respectively, while the United States was up to 12.4 percent, and Canada, along with several European countries, was in the 8–9 percent range (Schieber, Poullier, and Greenwald, 1992).[5] These high-expenditure countries all have shorter life expectancy than Japan and a higher incidence of CHD.

It is not, of course, the amount spent that is of crucial importance, but its effect. Charlton and Velez (1986) have examined mortality trends from 1951 to 1980 for a group of conditions that could be prevented or cured by medical intervention. The countries included were Japan, England and Wales, the United States, France, Italy, and Sweden. Japan started with by far the highest rate for these conditions in 1951 (largely due to stroke), and it showed the most dramatic decline of all the countries studied.

However, unlike the other countries, Japan also showed a steep decline in mortality rates from causes not amenable to medical intervention. It started the period with the highest rate of such mortality, but by the late 1960s it had the lowest, and the downward trend has since continued. It is very unlikely that improvements in medical care could explain a decline of this magnitude and rapidity (Hertzman, 1992; Marmot and Davey Smith, 1989).

Nutrition and Smoking

McKeown (1976) attributed much of the decline of infant mortality and infectious disease mortality that occurred with industrialization in England and Wales to improvements in nutrition. Adequate nutrition means largely adequate calories. Internationally, higher calorie consumption is related to lower mortality rates. The maintenance of adequate nutrition may have prevented an adverse effect on infant mortality of the high unemployment and poverty that went with the 1930s in Britain (McKeown, 1976; Winter, 1983).

Poor nutrition may also mean too much as well as too little. There has been controversy as to what has happened to fat intake, for example, in Britain and the United States during the twentieth century. The rise in consumption of polyunsaturates, in the United States since the 1960s and in the United Kingdom since the 1970s, may have played a part in the decline in CHD (Marmot and Theorell, 1988). Data from food consumption surveys in the United States suggest that saturated fat intake has declined since the 1960s (Stephen and Wald, 1990). But it is unclear whether or to what extent saturated fat intakes increased over the first half of the century, before the subsequent decrease.

The role of nutrition in the rise of ischaemic heart disease can, therefore, be questioned. High intake of saturated fat and consequent high mean levels of plasma cholesterol may have played an enabling role, providing the conditions for a high population rate of heart disease. But if these existed throughout the period, some other factor(s) may be directly implicated in the increase in CHD.

An obvious candidate for the missing factor is cigarette smoking. Smoking increased relatively early in England and Wales. During the period of increased CHD, lung cancer was also on the rise. This may well be a key factor in Eastern Europe. Smoking is highly prevalent in Hungary, for example, while it is declining in frequency in many of the countries of Western Europe and North America.

On the other hand, the current rapid rise in lung cancer rates among women in North America is associated with falling rates of CHD. Moreover, two-thirds of Japanese men smoke (Ueshima, Tatara, and Asakura, 1987). This is extremely high by world standards. It is a puzzle as to why they do not, therefore, have high rates of CHD. In the seven-countries study, smoking was a weak coronary risk factor in Japan, somewhat stronger in Southern Europe, and a strong risk factor in the United States (Keys, 1980). It may be that the importance of smoking as a risk factor is related to the background level of risk as determined by diet and level of plasma lipids, or by other factors in the environment in which people live and work.

Dietary fat makes up less that 25 percent of the Japanese diet compared to 42 percent in Britain (Ueshima et al., 1987). The ratio of polyunsaturates to saturates is 1.1 compared to 0.34 in Britain. Fat intake may have increased in Japan, but it is still far below Western (or Eastern European) levels.

It may be that the coronary epidemic in the countries of Eastern Europe is related to high levels of smoking combined with a high intake of saturated fat. In Japan, the high level of smoking takes place against a background of a low level of fat intake. This may help to explain why Japan appears to have carried off the balancing act of a decline in its "own" diseases—stomach cancer and stroke—without taking on the "West's" diseases—CHD and cancer of the lung, colon, and breast.

While the Japanese diet may help to explain why CHD did not increase in Japan in the face of widespread smoking, however, it cannot explain the dramatic 38 percent *fall* in male CHD rates between 1970 and 1985. A decline in salt intake may be playing a role in the decline in stroke and, to a lesser extent, in CHD. But there must be other factors operating as well.

Prosperity and the Social Environment

The rise and fall in CHD in Europe and North America was, as noted above, broadly related to economic development and changes in the environment in which individuals live and work. The most dramatic change in Japan's circumstances in the postwar period has been its rise as an economic superpower. There is a sharp contrast between Japan's economic performance and that of Britain, during the period when Japan's life expectancy raced past Britain's (1965–1986; Marmot and Davey Smith, 1989). Japan maintained low inflation, a high growth rate (4.2 percent per annum, 1965–1987, compared to an OECD average of 2.3 percent), and low unemployment; Britain's performance was worse than the OECD average. Japan's gross national product per capita, lower than that of Britain in the 1970s, was 50 percent higher in 1987 and ranked fourth among the OECD countries (after Switzerland, United States, and Norway). The United Nations Development Programme Human

Development Index (HDI) ranks Japan at the top for the same time period (*Economist* 1990). (The HDI combines life expectancy at birth, adult literacy, and purchasing power.)

Wilkinson (1989) emphasizes the international correlation between income and life expectancy, but the relationship is stronger with measures of income distribution than with per capita gross national product alone. Japan, with the fastest growth rate of any OECD country and now the fourth highest GNP, has the smallest relative differences in income among high and low earners (World Bank, 1988). This may be part of the explanation as to why Japan's life expectancy has surpassed Britain's (Marmot and Davey Smith, 1989).

Work and Social Relations

The creation and distribution of wealth in a society profoundly affects its social environment. Economic development brings wealth, but it also brings a change in the nature of working and social life. The NI-HON-SAN migrant study of men of Japanese ancestry living in Japan, Hawaii, and California showed that the higher rate of CHD among Japanese in California was related to their abandoning a Japanese life-style. Californian Japanese men had a higher fat diet and higher mean serum cholesterol than men in Japan (Marmot et al., 1975; Nichaman et al., 1975; Kato, Tillotson, Nichaman, Hamilton, and Rhoads, 1973). Independent of the level of serum cholesterol, men who were more traditionally Japanese in the sense of retaining ties to a closely knit community had a lower prevalence of CHD than men who were Westernized in their culture and social relations (Marmot and Syme, 1976).

These findings are consistent with Matsumoto's (1970) hypothesis that features of Japanese society mitigate stress. He proposed that work patterns and the collective nature of Japanese society provide social support and psychological security. These in turn may provide protection from diseases such as CHD. There is a larger body of work relating social supports to protection from CHD and premature death (Berkman, 1984); animal experiments also show significant effects of social environment on cholesterol-induced atherosclerosis (Nerem, Levesque, and Cornhill, 1980; Kaplan, Manuck, Clarkson, and Prichard, 1985). Nor is there yet any evidence, despite popular fears, that the distinctive mode of Japanese social life is changing to resemble Western culture. Westernization appears more confined to superficial aspects of life-style.

The influence of psychosocial features of the work environment on CHD risk has been reviewed by Karasek and Theorell (1990). An impressive body of evidence suggests that work characterized by lack of control, little opportunity for personal development, and boring repetitive tasks is associated with increased cardiovascular risk. These characteristics may be less a feature of the Japanese work environment than in many Western countries (Marmot and Davey Smith, 1989).

Yet, again, this cannot be the whole story. Japanese women show the same large and rapid gains in life expectancy as do men. But their participation in the labour force and experience of work have been quite different from that of Japanese men. This argues against the primary importance of "healthy" work environments as the key determinant of long life expectancy in Japan.

In summary, the Japanese experience suggests that to explain the broad trends in CHD, we need to consider at least two classes of factors: Characteristics of the socioeconomic environment and life-style patterns such as nutrition and smoking may both exert their influences in a variety of ways. Moreover, "life-styles" do not emerge in a vacuum; they are powerfully influenced by socioeconomic factors.

SOCIOECONOMIC FACTORS

As noted above, life expectancy appears more closely related to income inequalities than to overall income or wealth levels (Wilkinson, 1989). It is therefore important to consider not only how aggregate economic changes may relate to mortality changes for a whole society, but also how they affect the economic and social environment of sub-groups within the population.

Social Class Differences within a Country

As discussed in Chapter 3, there are in most Western countries differences across social classes in death rates both from CHD and from all causes (Marmot, Kogevinas, and Elston, 1987). These differences are indicative of the influences of socioeconomic factors on health and disease, and of their varying impact on different groups in the overall population.

The analysis of class differences in health status has been subject to both political and methodological controversy. The concept of class itself is an intellectual (or ideological) construct; and there is no "natural" or overwhelmingly compelling single approach to the measurement of class status. Income or years of education are commonly used indicators. In Britain, social class has traditionally been based on occupational prestige—the registrar-general's social classes ranging from I (Professional) to V (Unskilled Manual)—and these are highly correlated with (age-specific) mortality rates. However, other indicators such as access to a car or home ownership (housing tenure) also turn out to "predict," or be correlated with, mortality, independently of social class based on occupation (Fox and Goldblatt, 1982).

The strong (inverse) relationship between social status and mortality that emerges from the registrar-general's data is open to several methodological criticisms. But any suggestion that it is artefactual runs up against the strong confirmation provided by the Whitehall study of British civil servants (Figure 7.5), which does not share these methodological weaknesses. Grade of employment shows a clear inverse relation with mortality: the lower the grade, the higher the risk. The smooth nature of the relationship is striking. It is not only the men at the bottom who are at increased risk; each grade of employment is associated with higher risk than the one above it (Marmot, Shipley, and Rose, 1984). The gradient in mortality is the same for CHD as for other causes of death.

The Whitehall study also found that other measures of status or economic position—whether the individuals had access to cars or owned their own homes—added further "explanatory" power (Davey Smith, Shipley, and Rose, 1990). Position in the civil service hierarchy was a

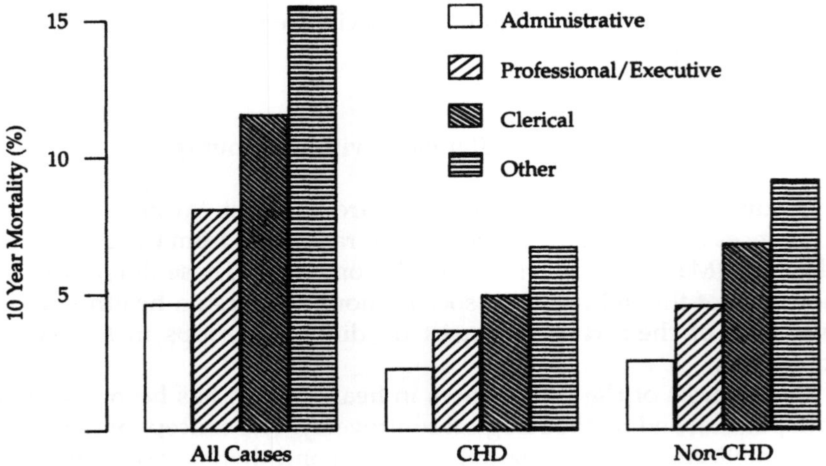

Figure 7.5. Percentage of men dying in ten years from all causes, from CHD, and from non-CHD, by grade in the British civil service (age-adjusted figures). *Source:* Marmot and Theorell, 1988:662

primary indicator of status and correlate of mortality, but not an exclusive one.

An obvious question arises as to the role of smoking, the prevalence of which itself is inversely related to social class. But the social gradient in CHD observed in the Whitehall study was as strong among nonsmokers as it was among smokers. Those few men in the higher grades who smoked were at lower risk *from smoking-related diseases* than were smokers in the lower grades, though at each grade (with the exception of the bottom grade), smokers were at higher risk than nonsmokers. Smoking *does* kill; but it is clearly not the main explanation for the social gradient in mortality.

These British findings recall the Japanese experience of low rates of CHD despite the high prevalence of smoking. Both suggest that to explain the broad trends in CHD, we have to consider other factors. The Japanese population may have a low tendency to arterial thrombosis or, because the Japanese have less atherosclerosis, they may be less susceptible to arterial thrombotic occlusions. If smoking mainly affects the thrombotic pathway, then it would have little effect unless there were extensive atherosclerosis. In animal experiments, smoking was not found to cause or enhance the development of atherosclerosis (Rogers et al., 1988).

Time Trends in Social Class Differences

In contemporary Britain, social class differences in CHD parallel those for mortality from all causes. But it was not always so. Changes in diagnostic fashion create difficulties in interpretation, but it appears that in the 1930s, when CHD was on the rise, it was more common in classes I and II than in semiskilled and unskilled classes IV and V (Marmot, Adelstein, Robinson, and Rose, 1978). The changeover occurred by the early 1960s. The subsequent decline in overall CHD rates has been concentrated among men in nonmanual occupations; there has been no decline at all among men in manual occupations—or their spouses (Marmot and McDowell, 1986).

These changes in the relationship between social class and CHD indicate that it is not economic or hierarchical position per se that correlates with disease, but some underlying factor(s) whose relationship with socioeconomic status can change over time. They thus parallel the observation in Western countries that, as economic development proceeds, CHD appears to increase; but as development proceeds further, it declines. CHD seems to pass through society in a wave, affecting first the more privileged and subsequently the less privileged. It declines first in those better off and, presumably, subsequently in the rest (Marmot and McDowell, 1986). This is similar to the "social history" of peptic ulcer (Susser and Pisa, 1988).

Social Class Differences in Different Cultures

The relationship between social class and disease will therefore depend on other features of a society. This is illustrated by the study of mortality in migrants to England and Wales. Migrants bring their pattern of disease with them, which then changes toward that of the host country as they become integrated into that society. Among migrants to England and Wales, we see three social class patterns of mortality (Marmot, Adelstein, and Bulusu, 1984). Immigrants from Ireland show the same inverse association of illness with class status as in England and Wales. But within each class, the mortality rate for immigrant Irish is higher than the average rate for that class in England and Wales. Immigrants from the Indian subcontinent, by contrast, show little relation between class and mortality. Finally, immigrants from the Caribbean show a reverse pattern, of higher mortality rates in nonmanual classes than in manual.

The varying relation of mortality to class appears to be related to stages of economic development in the societies from which these different cultural groups come. The Afro-Caribbean picture is more like that of England and Wales in the 1930s; the South Asians, like England and Wales in the late 1950s; the Irish, similar to England and Wales at present.

A dynamic and evolving relationship with class status such as that found for CHD can also be seen for an individual risk factor, such as smoking (Figure 7.6; Yach, 1990). In South Africa, the relation of class to smoking is different for different ethnic groups and is dependent on where those groups are in the socioeconomic spectrum. For groups lower in socioeconomic status, smoking is *positively* correlated with (within-group) status; in higher status groups, the relationship flattens out and is then reversed.

Links Between Socioeconomic Position and CHD

The association between social class and mortality was discussed in more detail in Chapter 3. As noted there, the weight of the current evidence seems to indicate that the relationship is real, not artefactual, and that it is not a result of the selection or sorting of unhealthier people

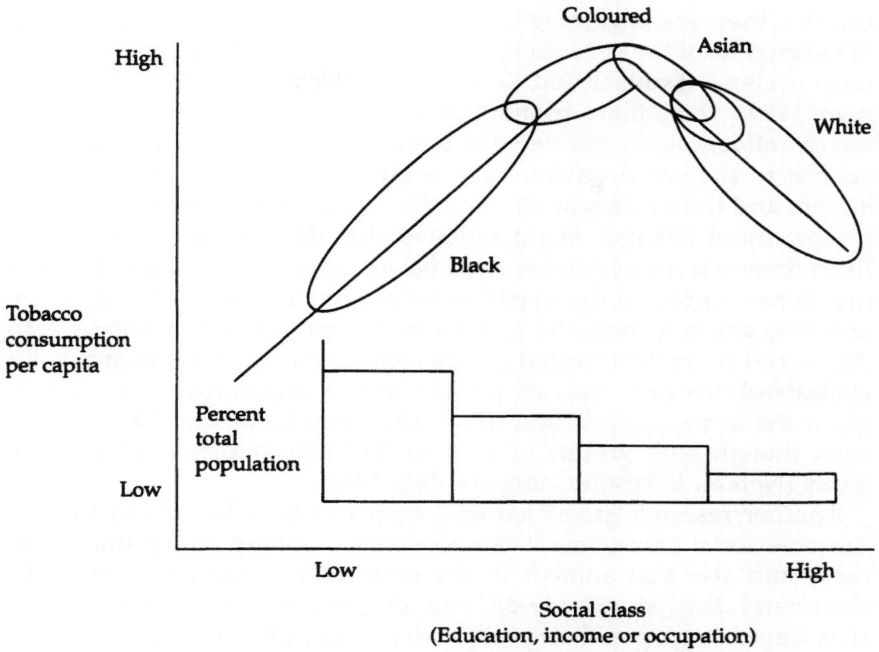

Figure 7.6. Simplified relationship between tobacco consumption, social class, and race in South Africa.
Source: Marmot (1992)

into lower status positions. An extensive review of this evidence in Britain led the authors of the Black report (Black, Morris, Smith, Townsend, and Whitehead, 1988) to favour a materialist explanation—income and wealth provide one with access to superior food, housing, work, transport, and environment in general.[6]

But the Whitehall civil service study shows a smooth *gradient* for most of the major causes of death and sickness, with significant differences even between "top people" and those immediately below them. This seems inconsistent with an explanation in terms of deprivation: People in the professional and executive grades of the U.K. civil service are not in any sense deprived of any of the material conditions of life. These data indicate that some underlying factors related to social environment are at work. One is left with a fundamental puzzle as to the nature of the factor or factors that produce these gradients regardless of the "fashionable causes" of death or sickness.

Evidence is now emerging from studies in cell biology, however, that may have a bearing on this question. As discussed in the previous chapter, these are beginning to show the molecular basis for interaction between cells of the nervous system and cells of the immune and endocrine systems (Dantzer and Kelley, 1989; Zalcman, Richter, and Anisman, 1989). Thus, there are now potential biological pathways through which influences on the nervous system—such as an individual's response to the social environment—could influence the host defence system and the expression of a number of different diseases.

How these linkages might influence the development of coronary heart disease is not at present clear. But at least one set of animal experiments has confirmed the hypothesis that a gentle, friendly, supportive environment influences the process of diet-induced atherosclerosis. In these studies, rabbits treated gently—music played to them and fed a cholesterol-rich diet—had 60 percent less atherosclerosis than rabbits given the same diet and the usual laboratory treatment. This was so even though both groups of animals had similar plasma cholesterol levels (Nerem, Levesque, and Cornhill, 1980).

Another research group working with monkeys has found that an unstable social environment can accelerate coronary artery atherosclerosis, and also that animals in the same colony, fed the same high-cholesterol diets, show very different degrees of coronary artery occlusion, depending upon their position in the status hierarchy of the group (high is better; Kaplan et al., 1985; Kaplan et al., 1991).

These differences in the extent of atherosclerosis, in the presence of equivalent elevated levels of blood cholesterol, are compatible with the variation, referred to above, found in nearly all animal experiments with cholesterol-rich diets. Animals with the same level of cholesterol in the blood develop very different degrees of atherosclerosis (Clarkson, Kaplan, and Adams, 1985).

There is now substantial evidence that pathways linking the nervous system to the immune system can lead to immune responses that damage the lining of arteries (endothelium) and thus contribute to atherosclerosis (Bondjers et al., 1991). Furthermore, injury to the lining of arteries in the presence of hypercholesterolemia leads to more extensive atherosclerosis than injury by itself. Do people with more control of their jobs and better satisfaction at work develop less atherosclerosis than other individuals with the same level of plasma cholesterol?

A further observation in the Whitehall study (Minick and Murphy, 1973) has implications for how one interprets the processes at work. There is a gradient in blood fibrinogen levels, with the lowest levels in the top class of civil servants. A number of investigators have shown that individuals with elevated fibrinogen levels have an increased risk of dying from coronary heart disease. Since fibrinogen is known to be involved in blood clotting and therefore to be a factor in thrombus formation, it has been assumed that elevated fibrinogen levels represent an increased risk for thrombosis. While this may be the case, it is also known that the normal blood levels of fibrinogen and platelets are far in excess of those needed for thrombus formation or the formation of haemostatic plugs. Thus, it is unlikely that the increased risk for CHD seen with increased fibrinogen levels is due to an enhanced probability of thrombus formation.

The known factors that influence arterial thrombus formation are platelet adhesion to the vessel wall, platelet aggregation, the pathways of blood coagulation (particularly the enzymes that catalyze the coagulation reaction such as factors X, IX, VII, and thrombin), the degree of vessel stenosis, rupture of the atherosclerotic plaque, and the extent of disturbed flow at the site of vessel injury (Davey Smith and Marmot, n.d.). Could the gradient in fibrinogen levels be related to something else? Fibrinogen is a reactive protein that takes part in host defence responses and is elevated in circumstances where the host response is stressed (Mustard, Packham, and Kinlough-Rathbone, 1986). Fibrinogen levels rise in most cases of illness, for example, and they are commonly known to be raised after injury and in chronic disorders such as rheumatoid arthritis. It is possible, therefore, that the gradient in fibrinogen levels represents differences in the stress on the body's host defence system and the variations in host response.

CONCLUSIONS

The trends and variations in CHD mortality described in this chapter point to the importance of social and economic forces in determining the rise and fall of coronary heart disease. There is also substantial and increasing understanding of the pathways involved in the development of atherosclerosis and its clinical thromboembolic complications. The results from these studies are compatible with epidemiological findings. It is useful to keep both perspectives in mind when considering socioeconomic differences both between and within countries.

Socioeconomic differences within countries have come to assume such major importance that continued exploration of underlying connections between social position and CHD is likely to be fruitful. Investigation should be focused on the broad categories of factors discussed: material conditions, social environment including work and social life, nutrition, early environment and life-style including smoking and exercise (Marmot et al., 1987; Hardwicke and Squire, 1952). These factors may operate, in part or in whole, through linkages between the nervous system and the body's host defence systems. Attention will have to be given not only to explanations of what "risk factors" might account statistically for socioeconomic differences in CHD within (and between) countries, but to the prospects for changing them.

Examining the problem of CHD from a population base provides a perspective that allows the incorporation of a wide variety of sources and types of knowledge and provides an understanding different from the traditional disease focus. It shows that the occurrence of CHD is intimately bound up with the fundamental nature of the social structures in which we live.

CHD thus provides a detailed and concrete illustration of the theme developed throughout this book. The focus on a particular disease or disease complex shows how observations of populations can be woven together with clinical observations of individual cases, and with evolving biological understanding. This in turn indicates the biological pathways through which the characteristics of social and physical environments have their impact on health. But CHD is only a leading example, chosen because of its importance as a (proximate) cause of illness and death in modern populations. The same sort of molecule/cell-to-person-to-population (and back again) analysis could be carried out for a number of other diseases.

One can also, as shown in Chapter 6, focus on particular biological systems—the immune system or the endocrine system—and trace out the way in which that system responds to environmental characteristics, and thus gives rise to more general responses by the organism that lead to, or are themselves interpreted as, "disease" or "health." And in Chapter 5, we emphasized the significance of the genetic makeup of the individual in interaction with these environmental factors.

This chapter also provides illustrations of the general theme of Chapter 4, the role of social interpretation in determining the nature of "disease." Is atherosclerosis a disease or merely part of the normal aging process? Is an elevated (how high?) level of blood lipids a disease, to be screened for, diagnosed and "cured"? A high cholesterol diet? (A morbidly excessive concern for one's health?) The answer will vary with who one asks, and when; the definition of a disease depends upon both the "scientific" understanding of biological processes and the interpretation and labeling of probabilistic chains of (hypothesized) causation.

Some of these ideas are new; biological science in particular continues to make rapid progress. But others are quite old, and it is remarkable how, even at the bench or experimental science end of the knowledge continuum, findings from decades ago either reemerge or, worse, become ignored and lost as the stream of interpretation takes, or is pushed into, a new channel. Firmly grounded scientific observations that do not fit comfortably within the dominant contemporary structures of social interpretation carry little weight and are fortunate to survive.

Such dominant social interpretations may be incomplete, or wrong, or grossly oversimplified: "Eating fats causes heart disease." "People (especially males) will live longer if they keep down the level of fats in their blood, if necessary by taking drugs." But they also serve important social or political purposes—or they would not be dominant. In the next section of the book we begin to explore why it is that health policy tends to be so resistant to certain kinds of information on the determinants of health, and so exquisitely sensitive to others.

Why is it that in some areas we know without acting, in others we act without knowing? Or more generally, why are the standards of evidence required before observations are accepted as knowledge, or knowledge accepted as a basis for action, so stringent for some and so flimsy for others?

"Health policy" in this context includes clinical policy, the activities of providers of care, the decision rules that guide those actions, and the processes by which those evolve. Chapter 9 focuses particularly on health care interventions, and the growth of knowledge as to their strengths and limitations. Chapter 10 moves upstream to consider the context from which specific policy interventions emerge, and the scope for changing that context (or at least some of the outcomes). Chapter 8 takes a broader view of public policy with respect to health. It explores the historical evolution of health care systems in this century, and the ambiguous role of "health promotion" as either an alternative to or a component of the health care system.

NOTES

1. CHD remains a major cause of death, but at older ages. Since everyone dies, and vital statistics recording conventions require that they die of *something*, a reduction in the absolute number of CHD deaths is not necessarily a sensible objective. The total number of deaths cannot change—one per person—so some other "cause" must increase. The alternative may be cancer. The decline in CHD is thus measured by a *deferral* of death and of the onset of disease.

2. For example, since the main cause of myocardial ischemia (heart attacks) is a thromboembolic event it is difficult to see how changes in cholesterol levels in adult males will dramatically change outcomes since there is no evidence that cholesterol has a major clinical effect on the thromboembolic process. This may be one of the reasons why risk modification by trying to lower cholesterol levels has not had a dramatic effect on the incidence of heart attacks.

3. "Economic development" is used in a loose sense here. During the 1930s the decline in infant mortality in England and Wales was what would be expected with continuing economic development. This was, however, the time of the great economic depression and of great economic hardship for many. Similar hardships presumably resulted from "developments" in Eastern Europe during the 1970s and 1980s. Nevertheless, conditions in "depressed" twentieth-century European economies were likely to have been very different from those characteristic of rural and urban poverty in developing countries, or urban poverty in Britain in the nineteenth century.

4. We are grateful to Dr. Peter Boyle, IARC Lyons, for this calculation.

5. In principle, one might prefer to compare the actual levels of health care used, per capita, in different countries. This would require both expenditure data and data on relative prices of health care services that reflected the different mix of services (e.g., pharmaceuticals, medical, hospital) consumed in each country. Some data of this nature now exist, and suggest that Japanese consumption levels are really quite similar to those in Canada and the United States (Schieber et al., 1992; Gerdtham and Jönsson, 1991). But the mixes of services are quite different in these countries (e.g., very high relative rates of pharmaceutical use and low surgery rates in Japan), and we cannot yet be confident that the price indexes developed for these purposes are up to the task.

6. Barker's studies suggest that it may not only be conditions acting during adult life that are important. Circumstances *in utero* or in infancy may have a persisting effect on mortality rates throughout life (Barker, 1989).

III

8

The Determinants of a Population's Health: What Can Be Done to Improve a Democratic Nation's Health Status?

T. R. MARMOR, M. L. BARER, and R. G. EVANS

I. INTRODUCTION

As we began the 1990s there was in each of the industrial democracies a widely shared sense of apprehension about health care policy (Evans, 1992). Everywhere rancorous, embittering disputes regularly break out, largely but not exclusively about how much more should be spent on curative medicine. These contests center on the familiar world of doctors and nurses, hospitals, and clinics. And they feature regularly the medical world's claim that more must be spent if the people (of Canada, the United States, France, Great Britain, Sweden, etc.) are to rightly enjoy the fruits of modern medical science.

Yet these conflicts show little or no awareness of the issues and evidence raised in the preceding chapters. The debates are carried on in almost complete isolation from the growing understanding that the determinants of health are much broader than the medical care system itself. No one seriously challenges the evidence for this broader viewpoint, yet the medical care debates proceed as if these broader determinants were irrelevant to decisions about how much should be spent for narrowly defined medical services. Indeed, the continuing pressure for expansion of traditional medical care has tended to preclude the development and support of programs addressing other and more significant determinants of health status.

The expansionary dynamics of traditional medical care have been met, not by the competing claims of broader health-related policies, but by charges that the present medical system already costs too much. In the period after the Second World War—from roughly the late 1940s to the late 1960s, the most pressing health policy question for the developed world was how to bring the wonders of modern medical care to all its citizens. For the past two decades, however, there has been a startling shift in policy focus, from expanding access to care to containing its costs. Some see the problem as "insatiable demands" by "consumers with unrealistic expectations"; others put more emphasis on inefficiencies and inadequate management within the medical care systems themselves; still others stress the extensive evidence of inappropriate and ineffective care (Marmor, 1986; Schieber, Poullier, and Greenwald, 1992).

For all these reasons, *controlling* the rate of growth in health care costs had by the mid-1970s assumed center stage throughout most of the industrial democracies (Pfaff, 1990).[1] And although the precise timing varied across countries, by the early 1980s almost all had succeeded in restraining the growth of their health care costs to a roughly constant share of their national incomes. Yet in every country that has managed to achieve some stability, it has been a precarious balance, with escalating political costs. None of the OECD countries is in a position to declare victory over the escalation of medical costs.

In the course of this struggle, and as the public agenda shifted, a new version of public health emerged in a number of countries. Canada's Lalonde report (Canada, 1974)—perhaps the most widely distributed of all the national documents on the role of preventive approaches in national health policy—expressed a widely shared view that the determinants of health go well beyond medical care.[2] If improving the health of a population is the key objective, then, according to these reports, the richer western democracies—all but the United States with universal health insurance—had accomplished much of whatever gains in health status could have been expected through widened access to medical care services. What mattered now, in the "new" view of public health, were the more basic determinants of health: the work and physical environment, the genes one inherits, and the style of life one adopts. These items constituted the appropriate agenda of intervention, the right "fields" for health improvement. If this "new perspective" provided supporting argumentation against the resource demands of medical care providers, so much the better. But the case for improved health outside medical care could be (and often was) made on its own merits.

Despite nearly two decades of repeated intellectual efforts to redirect health policy away from curative medicine to more fundamental interventions, the task remains largely undone. Why?

There are two elements of a plausible answer. First, health policies at any given time reflect the prevailing conceptions of what health is and what factors contribute to its improvement or deterioration. Ergo, any significant policy change requires the modification of a nation's underlying belief system—what intellectual historians would regard as the prevailing health paradigm.

Changes in the state of knowledge within the scientific community alone are clearly inadequate for such paradigmatic shifts. The general knowledge and beliefs shared by the majority of citizens constitute the "prevailing system of beliefs" (Sabatier, 1987; Lomas, 1990b). And there is typically a wide gap between scientific understanding and popular beliefs. Changes in the beliefs of that broader constituency come slowly.

Second, the pace of change varies with the degree to which the prevailing system of beliefs has found expression in the structure and practices of professional organizations whose participants' interests are threatened by change. In the twentieth century, the health paradigm that assigns a central role to medical care in combatting disease became embodied in what has become the largest single industry in the OECD world. This concentration of economic power and (with it) political influence must, and does, resist significant change in the supporting system of beliefs. Little wonder, then, that the "new perspective on health" has to date found so little practical expression.

The twentieth-century evolution of health beliefs, then, has had pervasive effects on modern medical care. The prevailing beliefs, in turn, provide a partial explanation for the present state of health policy. As a consequence, we cannot understand contemporary health policy apart from the history of both health care institutions and the prevailing beliefs about health and its determinants from which those institutions were spawned. What follows, while surely not a complete history of that development, is an evolutionary sketch of health policy in North America from the second to the seventh decade of this century.

II. HEALTH POLICIES AND THEIR HISTORIES: PATTERNS FROM THE PAST

A. 1920–1970: The Sickness Insurance Movement and Later Efforts at Rationalizing the Costs of Medical Care

This half-century marked the dramatic spread of insurance against the costs of illness. While there were considerable efforts before the First

World War to organize sickness insurance for the industrial worker, the 1920s represented (in North America most clearly) the broadening of the sickness insurance movement.[3]

What is central here is that the early effort was not only motivated by egalitarianism (allocate care by medical need, not income). The advocates of sickness insurance also believed that the development of a more scientific medicine would transform the treatment of common diseases, and thus assumed that making medical care more accessible would improve considerably the health of a nation. They took for granted that access to improved pre- and postnatal care for pregnant women and children would reduce the mortality associated with childbirth and they were right. The later emergence of dramatically effective treatments for infectious diseases provided further support for the assumption that the most direct road to health was through better medical care, more widely available.

These optimistic assumptions about the benefits of medicine were reinforced by the experience of the next two decades, which greatly increased the appeal of universal health insurance. The wartime demand for personnel brought into public view, for the second time in three decades, just how unhealthy were some of the young men within these populations. Battlefield medicine not only trained large numbers of young physicians, but extended the scope of their surgical and medical talents. Finally, the very experience of waging a long war against the Axis powers—with all the sacrifice required in this common cause—powerfully reinforced the sense of community on which postwar expansions of the welfare state would rest. After the war, there was a clear presumption that progress lay in widely distributing the benefits of a remarkable medical care world, a mix of science, professionalism, and dedication that would both improve and extend the lives of those it treated.[4]

Others have charted the economic and social details of medical care's expansion after the Second World War. Any time series of national expenditures shows the remarkable year by year, decade by decade growth in financial outlays (Abel-Smith, 1992; Schieber et al., 1992). What is striking to our contemporary sensibilities—themselves so conditioned to complaints about the costs of health care—is the degree to which these expenditures were interpreted as social progress. Budget officials, as always, worried about the consequences of growing expenditures in public programs. The negotiators in European sickness funds and North American health insurance firms were from time to time quite agitated about the required increases in employer/employee contributions and premiums. But none of that was a threat to the widespread optimism about medical care's beneficence. The relevant question seemed to be how one should go about improving the organization and financing of these beneficent services, not to speak of the scientific research that would further extend medicine's reach (Starr and Marmor, 1984).

This, broadly speaking, was the state of health affairs in North America and Western Europe from the late 1940s to the late 1960s. Such a summary picture obviously misses the details (and the contradictory elements) of some places and periods. The pace of growth was faster in Sweden than it was in Britain, France lagged behind West Germany for a time, while Canada and the United States followed each other very closely in the expansion of health insurance coverage and overall health outlays. But expansionary enthusiasm was the common element that changed so radically and widely in the economic turmoil of the 1970s.

B. The Transformation of the 1970s: Medical Care, Health, and the New Skepticism

By the early 1970s, all developed countries but the United States had reached the end of this policy road. And they found there three things: First, it was much harder to turn off the flow of resources into medical care than to turn it on. There is no built-in shutoff valve; medicine can indefinitely absorb large quantities of resources, and if permitted to do so, will. Second, universal access to ever-expanding medical services did not lead to equal access to health. Large inequalities in health status persisted, despite (more or less) equal access to care (Black, Morris, Smith, and Townsend, 1982). And finally, the early and dramatic improvements in health status resulting from medical intervention were not repeated. Diminishing returns had set in, though many major health problems remained.

These observations generated two different responses from those interested in health policy. One group became concerned to place some limit on the flow of resources into medical care, in order to protect other competing social priorities.[5] The other focused on the remaining inequalities and inadequacies in health status. They began to explore the prospects for health improvement, either by refocusing the activities of the medical care system or by developing programs outside that system.

The "cost controllers" found that the expansion that had been supported prior to 1970, far from meeting all the needs, had created stronger constituencies for even greater expansion. On the other hand, the universal public funding systems were new, countervailing constituencies for cost control. Thus the stage was set for the battles over cost control that have been with us ever since (Marmor and Smithey, 1989).[6]

On the other hand, the "health improvers" found that the intense conflict between cost expanders and cost controllers left few resources available for developing health-enhancing programs outside medicine. Nor did the members of the traditional medical world show much enthusiasm for redirecting their efforts into unfamiliar health care channels—unless, of course, those activities brought in more money.

The two groups have from time to time found uneasy common ground in the hope that greater health promotion might lead, through better health, to reduced costs of care. But experience has yet to provide any support for this hope. In any case, the two objectives are logically quite distinct. But it was from this mixture of motives and constituencies that the governments of the industrial democracies came at various times during the 1970s to reject quite publicly the medical care enthusiasm of earlier decades. The breadth of this change should not be underestimated.[7] While acknowledging the central role of cost considerations in this shift, we will in the remainder of this chapter focus on the growth of the health promotion movement, and its impact on contemporary conceptions of health itself.

C. The 1970s and After: The Promotion of Alternative Pathways to Health Improvement, and Resistance to the Rise of Health Care Expenditures

1. *The New Perspective on Health*

As noted above, the Canadian Lalonde report became one of the most widely distributed public health documents. In the United States, a new office devoted to promoting prevention sounded the same themes in the mid-1970s and by the latter part of the decade was regularly producing documents charting the progress or decline in national health status.[8] And the North American examples were typical, not exceptional, as governments across Europe were simultaneously squeezed for revenues and pressured to use additional public funds to counteract the social and economic impact of the oil crisis and stagflation (Klein and O'Higgins, 1988).

The common thread through the various national "perspectives on health" was the claim that much improvement was possible without continually increasing health care budgets.[9] If attention were paid to individual habits (life-styles), to work and the workplace, to the physical environment, and to human biology and genetic inheritance, according to Lalonde, Castonguay, and many others, we could improve health beyond what had already been achieved through the broader distribution of medical services. It was not that progress through medicine was impossible, but that diminishing marginal returns had set in for wealthy societies—epitomized by Canada, Sweden, West Germany—that amply financed medical services for all. The Lalonde report (Canada, 1974)—and, to be fair, most of the comparable official documents—insisted on the need for a *broad* view of the scope of health policy—hence the reference to a "new perspective."

In practice, however, the breadth of policy response did not match the breadth of the "new perspective" rhetoric. The role of "life-styles" was seized upon with a vengeance, for a variety of different reasons, by politicians, health promoters, and the mass media. The public policies that they developed or supported, interpreted life-styles very narrowly, as "chosen" individual behaviours:

> Personal decisions and habits that are bad from a health point of view, create self-imposed risks. When those risks result in illness or death, the victim's lifestyle can be said to have contributed to, or caused, his own illness or death. (Lalonde, 1974:32)

The health promoters thus individualized both the root of the problem and many of the remedies. In this way they avoided challenging either the conventional world of work, income distribution, and control over the environment, or the conventional medical establishment. It was politically much safer to exhort individuals to live better, often implicitly blaming them for their own illnesses.

The best example in Canada was the "Participaction" program, a publicity campaign to urge individuals to engage in more physical activity. Other publicity efforts encouraged them to stop smoking, to drink less, and to eat better. The consistent theme throughout was that self-improvement constituted the key to a longer and healthier life. There was no suggestion, in any of these programs, that individual behaviour arose in and was shaped by a social and economic context, and that there might be some collective responsibility for changing that context.

The campaign against smoking was an interesting exception to this pattern. Antismoking efforts were everywhere started or strengthened within the OECD nations (Goodin, 1989). By the late 1980s, they had become a standard element of public policy. All but the most libertarian defenders of the "nightwatchman" conception of the state now accept rules against smoking in public places, workplaces, airlines, and so on. In addition, taxes have been increased to discourage consumption, and restrictions have been placed on advertising. The presumption of "individual choice" is particularly inappropriate to the consumption of a toxic substance that is also addictive, and to which people typically become addicted during early adolescence (Barer, Evans, Stoddart, Labelle, and Fulton, 1984).

But the regulation of smoking has individualistic roots as well. It is now recognized that one person's smoking affects the health of identified others. Yet even before the harm of passive smoking was clearly demonstrated, nonsmokers claimed control over their own airspace simply because they found smoke and smell offensive. The collective responses arose out of a clash of individual choices.

The combination of individual exhortation and collective regulation of behaviour not only avoided challenging traditional structures of power, but also required no new major public expenditures. It was cheaper (fiscally and politically) to regulate specific forms of individual conduct than to try to modify the circumstances giving rise to them.

2. *Other Pathways: The Environment and the Workplace*

There was at the same time a quite separate development of environmental activism.[10] This movement did not get its inspiration from the Lalonde report or its counterparts, but rather emerged from the cultural revolution of the 1960s. No health minister became the symbol of this movement; the Green parties are the European and Canadian heirs to its initial zeal in the early 1970s. This political movement emerged by 1970 (the year, it happens, of the first Clean Air Act in the United States), went underground in the midst of the economic misery of the late 1970s and early 1980s, and had returned with force by the end of the decade. Not primarily a movement for health improvement, environmentalism is a broad ideological force that encompasses health aims within its more general hostility to unrestrained consumption and its positive embrace of a simpler standard of life (Tesh, 1988).

There was as well pressure to change the workplace, to make it less risky, less conducive to accident, less a source of deadly diseases like black lung, and of contaminants like PCBs and other carcinogens. In the United States, the road taken was federal regulation of the work environment. Actual change was quite restricted by extended court challenges by some employers, and a tendency to invoke idealistic rules that few workplaces could in fact follow.[11] In Canada, there was action in practically every province. But it is important to note that some of the changes redistributed power and rights, not just changed health and safety rules. The creation of committees to oversee health and safety was the obvious manifestation, and the "right to refuse" dangerous work became the symbol of this new order.

On the other hand, practice in the United States ranged from contests over OSHA rules to company programs to promote healthiness. The campaign for a healthier work force (as against workplace) typically included gymnasia (or "health clubs") within the workplace or subsidized outside, cafeterias that advertise how healthy various foods are, and programs for individual casualties within the work force (alcoholism, drug dependency). Policies were selected that emphasized encouraging the individual worker to behave in "healthy" ways—reshaping the worker rather than the workplace (Warner, 1990).

What remained unchallenged was the basic governance of the workplace and the legitimacy of the present distribution of income, power, and status that work largely determines. At best, the new health promotion was, so to speak, managerial paternalism "at work." At worst, it has led to the labeling and exclusion of the "unhealthy" worker.[12]

3. *The Original Pathway, Revisited*

The impact of the "new perspective" on modern medicine was also much less than might have been expected from the initial rhetoric. Since the policies actually implemented avoided challenging established distributions of power, medicine's expansionary dynamic largely persisted. Prevention became not a substitute for cure, but a basis for further expanding the range of services offered by medical care professionals. Physicians, for example, offered and wished to be paid for antismoking counseling; nurses offered counseling for everything. Surgeons offered liposuction and breast implantation to improve the quality of life by correcting "deformities." A wide variety of practitioners, from iridologists to aroma therapists, vied for inclusion under health insurance coverage.

Far from serving as a basis for restraining the expansion of the medical care sector, therefore, the new perspective could be converted into new calls for more medical funding. Any improvements in health that might follow from either preventive medicine or healthier ways of living, were located in the indefinite future and could not be expected to result in cost savings now. The current levels and patterns of activities must therefore be maintained, while prevention expanded alongside them. The new perspective, thus implemented, led to neither structural reform in medicine nor to cost containment. The cost controllers were on their own.

D. Contemporary Preoccupations and Their Immediate Roots

In the 1990s, governments everywhere in the OECD world are still preoccupied with restraining the costs of medical care. The notion that cost restraint could be achieved if only everyone were a health promoter and disease preventer was revealed for what it is—a mirage.[13] And so, the never-ending resource struggle with the professions and the hospital world continues under straitened circumstances and with a more rancorous tone (Culyer, 1991). In every country (with the possible exception of the United States) claims of "underfunding" form a continuing theme from providers of care, regardless of the actual level of expenditure. Payers, government or private, are constantly reacting to new developments in the production of new medical technologies or patterns of care. Gone are the days when physician claims were accepted as gospel by public authorities (Renaud, 1989). The problem of limiting this endless expansion remains a fundamental policy challenge, one addressed in subsequent chapters.

The resistance of payers to the health industry's claims of underfunding is described by the latter as "rationing"—deliberately emotive language intended to convey the impression that patients are suffering in consequence (Blustein and Marmor, 1992; Hadorn, 1991). But these claims appear to arise whenever available resources *increase* less quickly than the expectations of providers and their patients, irrespective of the actual *level* of spending. Even if resources could be increased at a rate to match those expectations, "rationing" would still occur—"needs" are capable of infinite expansion. But the *rhetoric* of rationing will continue to be used as a rejection of the legitimacy of any attempt to constrain the growth of the medical care sector.

The cost controllers have, however, gained an increasing sense of their own legitimacy from another major theme in contemporary debates. Research concerning the effects of medical care on health is generating a growing body of evidence, summarized in the next chapter, that calls into question the relationship between medical care and its promised outcomes. Against the claim that "rationing" results in "unmet needs," the counterclaim that cost restraint will sacrifice (mostly) inappropriate and inefficient care is emerging with growing force of evidence behind it.

Excessive evidence does not yet encumber either claim, but the conflict between them has spawned an entirely new subindustry, variously labeled as quality assessment and assurance, continuous quality improvement, total quality management, managed care, utilization review, and outcomes research, all with roots in either clinical epidemiology or productivity enhancement. It may take some time for the realization to dawn that these activities, like health promotion before them, will not in themselves control costs—though they will certainly create new jobs (Rachlis and Kushner, 1989; Wennberg, 1990a; CIAR, 1991).

The spirit of the "new perspective" was not, however, entirely diverted into modification of individual behaviour and victim blaming, or into justification for the control of medical care costs. The collective emphasis resurfaced as the "healthy public policy" movement. It is being championed by an international organization—the WHO—and by particular policy entrepreneurs there like Ilona Kickbusch. Theirs is a political agenda of reforms from the 1960s—the redistribution of power through wider participation in the decisions that determine the conditions of modern life. But the agenda includes the rearranging of those conditions: more parks, more restrictions on cars, fewer high-rise buildings, less pollution and waste, and, in general, a less frenetic pace of life. (The unexamined assumption appears to be that wider empowerment will necessarily lead to these changes.)

The most dramatic extension of the concept of collective determinants of health has to do with mobilizing whole cities. The WHO advocates envision "healthier cities" not only, or even necessarily, as places with good vital statistics (Tokyo would not qualify whatever its health statistics). Rather they would be more humane sites for human interaction, which bear witness to our capacity to live more wisely in our environment.

At best, "healthy public policy" represents modern utopianism. At worst, it is simply a form of clever propaganda, piggybacking a set of other policy interests onto the powerful and broadly based public support for health (Marmor, 1990). In its extreme forms, this line of argument detaches the concept of "health" from any of its conventional and (potentially) objectively measurable manifestations, and declares that health is whatever the people (which ones?) of a community (how defined?) declare it to be. If the state has a legitimate interest in, and indeed an obligation to promote, "health," then surely it must support these local initiatives.

There is, however, a much more optimistic interpretation of this worldwide movement. Proceeding from the undeniable fact that socioeconomic factors shape the health profiles of modern populations, the advocates of change seize on one or another important causal factor—early childhood experiences, the degree to which one can control one's working environment, the direct threats from pollution and accidents, and so on—and press for change on health as well as other grounds. This is a reasonable interpretation of what has taken place within Ontario in recent years (Mendelson and Sullivan, 1990).

This strategy of highlighting the health implications of a wide range of desired policies has the possibility of either great effect or great disappointment. Health is after all a matter of enormous concern, for some an obsession. There is a health component to almost all public policies if one looks hard enough. It may be that this will be used with force in fashioning policies that improve our health on the way to equal or more compelling visions (of fairness, environmental balance, etc.). But the strategy may backfire if the health effects of reforms turn out to be less than promised, or simply unmeasurable.

Governmental consideration of this vast array of other "potentially health enhancing" public policies will also be affected by a final "contemporary preoccupation"—a growing array of extraordinarily difficult ethical decisions regarding traditional medical services. Should the medical care provided to the aged who have lived out their "natural" life span be limited to the relief of suffering? Should certain types of services (e.g., coronary bypass surgery, kidney dialysis, or organ transplants) be withheld from the very elderly? Should research into diseases that typically affect this group not be funded? Should governments allow for active euthanasia, in addition to the now relatively common practice of passive euthanasia? Should procedures involving the use of fetal tissue be supported by public funding? Should decisions as to the funding of particular medical treatments be made in the public arena, or should they be left to doctors and their patients?

These ethical concerns confuse several different issues. There is, for example, a major distinction between the purely ethical questions surrounding euthanasia, or the use of fetal tissue to treat Parkinson's disease, and those which are entangled with economics, such as decisions not to treat people above a certain age, or whose probability of benefiting from the intervention is below a certain level, or who will indeed benefit but at a cost that is vastly out of proportion to that benefit (however measured).

In the first case the cost/benefit ratio is irrelevant; the question is simply whether the intervention is right or wrong. In the second case the argument is over whether the anticipated benefits are large enough to justify the costs. And this in turn leads, or *should* lead, into a consideration of the costs and health effects of these medical interventions relative to the broader range of potentially health enhancing public policies. This comparison must include a careful and ongoing examination of the benefits of particular medical care interventions. Thus a number of the "ethical" issues blend into those of evaluation, and cannot be resolved or even seriously addressed in isolation from them.

But the task of evaluating competing uses of resources both within and beyond the traditional boundaries of medical intervention is as yet relatively uncharted territory (Drummond and Stoddart, 1992). There is thus a very real danger that decisions on matters only partially ethical (if at all) will come to be taken on supposedly "ethical" grounds alone, simply because the pace of progress rarely waits for the definitive evaluation. And what one person asserts as an "ethical imperative" can to others look very much like pursuit of an interest.

Pressures to expand the scope and intensity of medical care will not disappear. The past successes of medicine in alleviating pain and suffering and in curing certain diseases have created so many expectations that public support for medical care services will remain extremely strong. Yet the immense increases in health care capacity—people, facilities, and know-how—in all Western industrialized nations over the last four decades also present some of the key health policy problems for the coming decades. With this capacity comes a set of personal expectations held by those who derive from it their incomes and professional sustenance. For them, the system becomes an end in itself, creating ever new "needs" by nurturing ever greater public expectations.

As the following chapter suggests, there are growing concerns that a significant component of the care provided by modern health care systems is inappropriate. This suggests, in turn, that we may have overinvested in health care capital. Unfortunately the capital—both physical and human—will be with us for a long time. Chapter 10 offers some suggestions on how it can be more effectively and productively harnessed to work toward better health for all.

NOTES

1. Control, of course, is not equivalent to restraint (Evans, 1990a). Some seek to exercise control over costs in order to increase them.
2. See, for example, the discussions of this period in Breslow (1990) and Omenn (1990).
3. For the United States, see Starr (1982); for the United States and Britain, see Fox (1986) and Hollingsworth (1986); for Canada, see Naylor (1986).
4. For this development in the United States, see Starr (1982, especially, pp. 280–86 and pp. 333–51; for an extended account of the origins and enactment of Canadian national health insurance, see Taylor (1978); for Britain and the United States, see Fox (1986), Hollingsworth (1986), and Marmor and Smithey (1989); for a fascinating account of the impact of the British wartime experience on the support for the postwar National Health Service, see Titmuss (1950). For more on the actual origins of the NHS, see Klein (1989). For an account of the development in a particular area of medical care (mental illness), see Grob (1983). There is, of course, a detailed bibliography of the postwar expansion of government and nongovernment health insurance across Europe and North America, but we will not review it here.
5. Additional dollars spent on medical care have an opportunity cost. These funds cannot be used to address other social needs that might actually have a greater marginal effect on a nation's health status (e.g., highway maintenance,

education, police protection, environmental cleanup). In a single-payer system (like Canada's) the provincial governments have control of an overall budget of which medical care is one of many items. Cost control is achieved, in part, by different departments competing for a share of a fixed level of financial resources.

6. While the struggle to contain costs is universal, the capacity to do so depends on the organization and strength of the countervailing constituency. In the one country in which such a constituency is fragmented—the United States—the cost control battle has thus far been unambiguously lost. See *Consumer Reports* (1992).

7. In Canada there is considerable evidence of the rhetoric of health promotion by nonmedical means, but relatively weak reorientation of public policy. See the commentary in Mendelson and Sullivan (1990).

8. For details on the Office of Disease Prevention and Health Promotion within the United States Department of Health and Human Services, and what has been claimed for its successes, see Mason (1990). What is striking is the dominance of individualistic forms of health promotion in the appraisals published by this office.

9. There are actually two phases distinguishable during this period. The earlier phase, roughly 1970–1975, was typified by concern about medical inflation, about increases in the *prices* of services. In the second phase, following the oil crisis of 1974, there was great pressure to reduce the rate of increase in health care expenditures, whether price or volume driven.

10. See Ackerman and Hassler (1981) for one story of American environmental activism. For a spirited history of the movement, see Scheffer (1991).

11. For the story of the fight over the Occupational Safety and Health Administration in the United States, see Bardach and Kagan (1982).

12. See the recent work of Stone (1990a,b,c, 1987) on the use of health screening to select out from the potential work force those with unhealthy habits or unfortunate genes. This development, of course, is a special preoccupation in the United States, arising from the employment-related character of private health insurance.

13. See Warner (1990) on the exaggerated benefits attributed to corporate wellness campaigns and the subsequent more sober assessment of the financial consequences of trying to shape up workers.

9

Small Area Variations, Practice Style, and Quality of Care

N. P. ROOS and L. L. ROOS

INTRODUCTION

The first section of this book set out a framework for understanding the health of populations. In the second section that framework was used to explicate the role of particular factors such as genetics, social class, and culture. In the present chapter we bring together evidence of a different type. Not only is it true that non–health-care factors play a powerful role in shaping the health status of modern societies, but questions are increasingly being asked about the effect on a population's health of large segments of conventional health care.

Medicine has traditionally been oriented toward care for the individual patient. Using their knowledge, physicians intervene to cure or ameliorate the diagnosed illness. Given a choice of treatments, they select what seems most suitable for the patient. This logical model of medical practice implies a tight link between needs, interventions, and outcomes. Yet, such a link is radically inconsistent with the results of extensive research on patterns of medical care utilization in North America and Western Europe. The conventional model presumes a degree of

Reprinted with permission from "Assessing Quality Health Care: Perspectives for Clinicians," R. P. Wenzel, ed., pp. 223–238. Copyright © 1992 by Williams and Wilkins. Reprinted with slight authorial and editorial revision.

precision in both diagnosis and therapy—and a knowledge of patient needs and of effective responses—which is currently beyond the capabilities of most individual practitioners and of the health professions collectively. The blunt reality is that there is little hard evidence available to evaluate the effectiveness of many medical acts and procedures, within or outside the acute care sector. Furthermore this lack of evidence is pervasive. It includes everything from commonplace procedures to high-tech interventions.

In the absence of such evidence, opinions within the medical profession differ widely as to how conditions should be both diagnosed and treated. Patterns of practice vary widely. This implies that patients of particular physicians (or in particular regions) might sometimes not receive helpful treatment, while others might receive unnecessarily costly or otherwise inappropriate services. There is no empirical basis for the general claim that "more is better" when patterns of intervention vary so markedly from region to region, hospital to hospital, physician to physician, and when reliable evidence of benefit is so often lacking. Physicians' decision-making is influenced by many things other than biomedical science, including the psychological dynamics of and the uncertainty about the short- and long-term consequences of alternative treatments.

UNCERTAINTY AND VARIATION

Uncertainty Permeates Medical Practice

The variation in patterns of medical practice may be largely caused by uncertainty (Eddy, 1984). The relevant uncertainty may be about the choice or the meaning of diagnostic test results, or about the effectiveness of alternative courses of treatment. To the extent such uncertainty is reduced or eliminated, the forces producing practice variation will greatly diminish.[1] Eddy (1984) has described both the uncertainties surrounding how conditions are diagnosed in the first place and how they are treated once diagnosed. For example, in the diagnosis of disease, the line between normal and abnormal findings is often unclear. Many signs and symptoms are common, and knowing which ones will require treatment is difficult to determine. When two (or three) physicians see the same signs, symptoms, X-rays, or other test results, they are likely to interpret them differently (Koran, 1975a,b).

Similar problems surround the decision on how to treat diseases once they are diagnosed. For any given patient, a wide variety of procedures "can be ordered in any order and at any time"; the list of procedures that might be included in a workup of a patient presenting with chest pain or hypertension could easily take more than a page (Eddy, 1984). Even choices between major treatments are by no means obvious. Kassirer and Pauker (1981), for example, found that a significant number of clinical problems referred to their division of clinical decision-making at Tufts–New England Medical Center for consultation were essentially "toss-ups." The differences in expected result among the alternative treatments were so small as to be clinically irrelevant.

This uncertainty in medical practice affects established as well as new and relatively untested areas of medicine. Vayda et al. (1982) developed a series of hypothetical cases describing patients who would be candidates for five common procedures (including cholecystectomy, inguinal herniorrhaphy, hysterectomy, cesarean section, tonsillectomy and adenoidectomy, and colectomy). These case histories were mailed to Ontario physicians who were asked to recommend treatment for each patient. Recommendations made for every case showed substantial disagreement. For example, 65 percent of the physicians recommended cesarean section in one case whereas 35 percent said they would not perform a cesarean.

Physician consensus panels have also drawn on experts to define the "state of the art" in medical practice. The lack of agreement over appropriate medical treatment in the most common of situations is striking. For example, in a panel examining the appropriateness of various indications for bypass surgery, initial levels of agreement among the nine physician panel members ranged from 12.2 to 22.2 percent, depending upon how stringent the criteria for agreement were. After two days of panel discussion, the agreement levels improved somewhat. But even using the least strict definition of consensus, panel members failed to agree on more than half of the indications for bypass surgery (58.8 percent) (Park et al., 1986).

Not surprisingly, physicians fail to agree on indications for specific procedures because of the substantial uncertainties about the effectiveness of these procedures. Eddy (1984) has described a meeting of experts in colorectal cancer detection, all of whom were very familiar with the diagnostic occult fecal blood test and most of whom had participated in two prior meetings on cancer detection. Physicians were asked, What is the overall reduction in colorectal cancer incidence and mortality that could be expected if men and women over the age of fifty were tested with fecal occult blood tests and 60-cm flexible sigmoidoscopy every year? The answer to this question is obviously central to estimating the value of fecal occult blood testing. Physician judgments of the value of this test combination ranged from useless to a capacity to wipe out the disease. When these results were communicated to those attending the conference, the physicians "had no idea that they had such differences of opinion" (Eddy, 1984). This uncertainty about the value of a particular diagnostic test is also reflected in the fact that a recent economic evaluation of colorectal cancer screening was faced with the prospect of having to evaluate over twenty different combinations of diagnostic workups then found in clinical practice (Brown and Burrows, n.d.).

There is considerable scientific uncertainty about the results of even the most common of procedures. When patients are observed over long periods of time after treatment, they typically experience more adverse outcomes than the literature suggests. Thus, although expert opinion suggested that the frequency of additional surgery after transurethral prostatectomy was very low (Grayhack and Sadowski, 1975), the cumulative probability at eight years of having a second operation was found to be 20.2 percent (Wennberg, Roos, Sola, Schori, and Jaffe, 1987). When treatments diffuse outside large hospitals (the site of most evaluations but not where most care is delivered), the outcomes are usually worse (Wennberg et al., 1987; Roos, Nicol, and Cageorge, 1987; Steinbrook, 1988).

Variations and Practice Style

Population-based estimates of health care use have been widely developed. There are comparisons of utilization across countries (Bunker, 1970; McPherson, Wennberg, Hovind, and Clifford, 1982), across states (Chassin et al., 1986; Mindell, Vayda, and Cardillo, 1982), and across smaller hospital service areas (Dyck et al., 1977; Knickman, 1982; Gormley, Barer, Melia, and Helston, 1990). These variations occur across all age groups, from children (Perrin et al., 1989), through middle aged (Wennberg, 1984), to the elderly (Chassin et al., 1986). Their implications are substantial, as several analysts have emphasized. Using surgical rates to calculate lifetime probabilities of organ loss, Gittelsohn and Wennberg (1976) estimated that in the early 1970s the chances of a Vermont child reaching age twenty with tonsils in place ranged from 40 to 90 percent, depending on community of residence. If the United States' expenditures on seven common surgical procedures (hysterectomy, tonsillectomy, etc.) were based on the rates of low-hospital-service areas of Vermont and Maine, the costs were estimated to be \$2.4 billion, while the outlays based on the high-use areas of these two states would have been \$6.6 billion in 1975 dollars (Wennberg, Bunker, and Barnes, 1980).

A number of factors surely influence these practice patterns (McPherson, 1990). Yet, most of the variation is explicable not by underlying health differences in the populations of these different areas but rather by the practice style of the physicians (Roos, Henteleff, and Roos, 1977; Roos and Roos, 1982; Roos, 1983; Wennberg, 1987a,b; Wennberg and Fowler, 1977). Some of the most persuasive evidence of the impact of practice style comes from the work on "surgical signatures." Wennberg and Gittelsohn (1982) have demonstrated marked differences in rates of surgery for five common procedures across several areas in Maine. Rates of hemorrhoidectomy in the areas studied stayed much below the state average over each of the five years, whereas prostatectomy rates remained quite high. Left undisturbed by review, feedback, or the migration of physicians in and out of the area, the surgical signature of a community remained relatively constant from year to year. Although consistent variation in rates across small areas points strongly to the influence of physician practice style (since several physicians typically practice in these areas), the evidence is somewhat indirect. However, in Manitoba the surgical workloads of other area physicians remained stable over time when a surgically active physician moved into an area, while population utilization was increased by the new surgeon's activity (Roos, 1983).

Marked differences in the practice patterns of individual physicians seem to have produced the variation in rates. For example, the rate of primary cesarean section across eleven physicians treating low-risk women in a Detroit suburb was found to range from 9.6 to 31.8 percent. Close examination of the data yielded "no obvious explanation for variations in cesarean section rates across physicians" (Goyert, Bottoms, Treadwell, and Nehra, 1989). Devitt and Ironside (1975) observed several years ago that 85 percent of one surgeon's patients at the Ottawa Civic Hospital undergoing cholecystectomy had operative cholangiography,[2] whereas none of the patients operated upon by another surgeon had this procedure.

Manitoba elderly patients reporting good or excellent health were found to have very different probabilities of being hospitalized in the two years after their interview, depending upon the practice style of their physician. Thirty-three percent of the patients of those physicians scoring high on an index of physician hospital practice style (PHPS) were hospitalized in the two years following the interview, compared with 20 percent of the patients of physicians who scored low on the index. After adjustment for such patient characteristics as age, education, self-reported health status, proximity to death, and nursing home entry, and for such system characteristics as supply of hospital beds and occupancy rates, a patient of a physician who scored high on the index was *twice* as likely to be hospitalized as a patient of a physician scoring low on the index (Roos, 1989).

IS MORE BETTER?

Rates and Results, Benefits and Costs

The health care ethos in most Western industrial nations is that "more is better." Expenditures rise every year and yet media headlines constantly decry underfunding. Does this suggest that areas delivering the most care also have the best quality of care? Are, for example, areas with the highest hysterectomy rates delivering the best gynecological care to area residents? Examining the hospital records of diabetic cases treated in high-, medium-, and low-rate counties, Connell, Blide, and Hanken (1984) reported that the patients admitted by physicians in high-rate counties were tested substantially less thoroughly than those admitted in low-rate counties. Intravenous insulin treatment for severe metabolic emergencies was also less appropriately used in high-rate counties.

Some practice patterns are not only costly, but almost surely unhealthy. Both a well-publicized clinical trial in Pittsburgh and extensive Manitoba analyses of administrative data (Paradise et al., 1984; Roos et al., 1977) emphasized the desirability of conservative standards for tonsillectomy. Nonetheless, considerable differences across areas remain. Canadian children in Lethbridge, Alberta, for instance, are much more likely to have their tonsils removed than are children in the city of Edmonton (Halliday and LeRiche, 1987).

Assuming that high rates must be better also overlooks the fact that hospitals can be dangerous places. In Steel, Gertman, Crescenzi, and Anderson's (1981) study of patients admitted to a medical service of a university hospital, 36 percent of the patients were found to have acquired an iatrogenic illness (one caused by treatment). For 9 percent, the event was considered major (something life-threatening or producing considerable disability). Compared with research done over a decade earlier, the risks associated with hospitalization have, if anything, become worse over time. This has happened despite enormous increases in hospital funding over the period, much of which was justified as necessary to improve the quality of hospital care.

How could this be possible? Orkin (1989) has suggested that even relatively innocuous-sounding improvements in care should not be approved without clear demonstrations that the benefits exceed the risks.

His editorial focused on monitoring standards forwarded by the American Society of Anesthesiologists to improve the quality of care for patients undergoing anesthesia. Since the benefits from new monitoring equipment are so few (deaths associated with anesthesia are estimated to occur at a rate of less than one per hundred thousand anesthetics), the risks and financial costs need to be carefully considered. The information gained from monitors such as pulse oximetry and capnography, although beneficial in specific situations, are neither riskless nor costless:

> At the least, these new monitors engender complacency with regard to direct observation of the patient: less attention is directed to the patient and we are lulled into believing that all is well if the monitors do not alarm. However, their alarms sound all too often, spuriously; a recent prospective study in a pediatric hospital noted that alarms (principally pulse oximeters) sounded an average of 10 times per case, every 4.5 minutes. Seventy-five percent of the alarms were false while only 3 percent indicated possible patient risk! (Orkin, 1989, p. 570)

Anesthesia is not, however, an isolated case. It has been suggested, for example, that all those thirty-five years of age or older planning to take up jogging should be assessed by their physicians and should consider exercise stress testing. Aside from the two-billion-dollar cost of performing twenty million stress tests (a 1980 estimate of the number of American joggers; Graboys, 1979), what could be wrong with finding out whether one is fit enough to undertake strenuous physical activity? Unfortunately, the benefits of using a stress test to screen the average person about to begin an exercise program are unknown. Whether the stress test can screen for sudden cardiac death from exertion is not clear. However, undergoing a stress test, which in itself carries few risks, is known to produce side effects. It results in the identification of certain conditions (sometimes falsely, sometimes correctly) that will lead some physicians to further investigations that carry known risks, and potentially to further treatments, again with certain risks.

Graboys (1979) estimated that the stress-testing program described above would result in two million individuals undergoing coronary angiography (approximately 10 percent of asymptomatic persons undergoing stress tests have positive results), and approximately five hundred thousand people going on to bypass surgery (approximately 25 percent of such asymptomatic individuals will show some degree of multivessel coronary disease worthy of invasive intervention according to some cardiologists and surgeons). The risks and costs of these subsequent treatments are reasonably clear. Given the 1 percent mortality rate associated with angiography, two million procedures would result in two thousand deaths. Graboys' estimates suggested at least a 2 percent mortality rate from bypass surgery, as well as an 8 percent risk of a perioperative myocardial infarction. At least ten thousand deaths and forty thousand myocardial infarctions might be expected following five hundred thousand bypass procedures.

The Case of Bypass Surgery

The continuing growth of coronary artery bypass surgery (along with continuing concerns about the population to which this technology is applied) illustrates the dangers associated with the "more is better" philosophy. Although Canadian rates are still much lower than American, they are more than twice those in Britain. No one knows if this is good or bad (Anderson, Newhouse, and Roos, 1989; Detsky, O'Rourke, Naylor, Stacey, and Kitchens, 1990). Nonetheless, controversies about falling behind American rates have surfaced repeatedly in Canada over the last several years. Provincial governments have made special allocations to increase the availability of bypass surgery for their residents (Detsky et al., 1990).

Differences within Canada are also large—more than a twofold variation in rates of bypass surgery among twelve metropolitan areas (Statistics Canada, 1990). The population served by one referral centre in Ontario, for example, has undergone bypass surgery at a rate almost twice that of a population served by a second referral centre (the two areas show rates of bypass surgery of 77.8 versus 42.8 per 100,000 population, respectively; Anderson and Lomas, 1989). Physicians in one region of Manitoba have referred their ischemic heart disease patients to Winnipeg at a much lower rate than those in the other regions (Roos and Sharp, 1989).

As described below, appropriateness studies have shown that, even in areas with relatively low rates of coronary artery bypass surgery, some patients with equivocal or inappropriate indications may well be having surgery. As Canadian cardiovascular surgeons complain about waiting lists and the need to expand surgical programs, some patients with triple-vessel disease (those with quite high probabilities of benefiting) may wait for surgery, while others for whom the benefits of surgery are more doubtful are receiving the operation, simply because of their particular region or surgeon.

Certain technologies are so important and contentious that population-based programs both to monitor and manage waiting lists and to evaluate outcomes almost certainly should be instituted (Naylor, 1991). In Canada, such programs for coronary artery bypass surgery have been initiated in Toronto and are planned in Manitoba. By collecting information at several points from entry onto the waiting list for coronary angiography to coronary artery bypass surgery the characteristics of patients who do and do not receive these procedures can be studied in a timely manner. Among those who do receive angiography or bypass surgery, patient characteristics can be compared according to their length of time on a waiting list. Although expert panels do disagree among themselves, consensus standards based on expert panels can be applied to the data immediately (Naylor, Baigrie, Goldman, and Basinski, 1990), while information can also be accumulated for outcome studies.

TYPES OF EVIDENCE

Appropriateness and Discretion

Since definitive evidence is lacking, expert opinion informed by such evidence as does exist has been used to specify what is and what is not appropriate care. Analyses based on such expertise reveal high levels of inappropriate and equivocal medical decision-making (Leape, 1989). North American studies found, for example, that only 35 percent of carotid endarterectomies (Chassin et al., 1987), 14 percent of tonsillectomies (Roos et al., 1977), and 80 percent of pacemaker insertions (Greenspan et al., 1988) were responses to appropriate indications. High rates of inappropriate utilization are found in more general reviews of hospital use. Rates of inappropriate admissions ranged from 6 to 19 percent and rates of inappropriate days of care ranged from 20 to 39 percent in the studies reviewed by Payne (1987).

Some evidence suggests that high rates identify discretionary decisions about the delivery of health care and indicate overuse, possibly unnecessary use, of the health care system (Wennberg, Freeman, Shelton, and Bubolz, 1989; Roos, Roos, Mossey, and Havens, 1988; Paul-Shaheen, Clark, and Williams, 1987). Dyck et al. (1977) found that a larger proportion (52 percent) of hysterectomies were inappropriate in the Saskatchewan city with the higher rate than in the city with the lower rate (17 percent). In a study of twenty-three adjacent counties in one state, Leape et al. (1990) found that 28 percent of the variation in coronary angiography was explained by the level of inappropriateness. For the other two procedures studied (carotid endarterectomy and upper gastrointestinal tract endoscopy), however, there was no relationship between the overall surgical rate and the rate of appropriately selecting individuals for surgery.

Not only can particular treatments be studied, but hospitalization as a whole can be analyzed in terms of its discretionary or nondiscretionary nature (Roos, 1992). In Manitoba, the relationship between a physician's practice style and the type of patient hospitalized was examined to determine if physicians more likely to admit patients to hospitals did so for more discretionary indications and for patients who were less ill. We used the index of physician hospital practice style (PHPS) noted previously; a physician's score on this index was strongly related to the probability of his or her patient being hospitalized after controlling for factors related to patient health status, access to care, etc. (Roos, 1989; Roos, Flowerdew, Wajda, and Tate, 1986).

A 197 percent difference in hospital admission rates was found between those physicians most and least prone to hospitalize their patients (Roos, 1992). Physicians scoring highest on this index were 6 percent more likely to admit patients with a condition for which the hospitalization rate varies markedly across areas. But they were 34 percent more likely to admit patients with a diagnosis judged to be discretionary. Patients of physicians least prone to hospitalize were also somewhat more likely to show a higher illness level: They were 32 percent more likely to be admitted with a high-risk diagnosis.

We perhaps should not be surprised at these differences between rates of hospitalization and rates of discretionary or inappropriate use. After all, Wennberg (1987a) has suggested that "precisely because so many accepted theories concerning the treatment of common illnesses have not been adequately assessed, the number of potential patients who can be appropriately treated by medical or surgical alternatives is very large indeed." Similarly, Brook (1990) persuasively contends that the bias inherent in our processes of judging appropriateness "may mean that elimination of inappropriate or equivocal uses would improve a population's health, but that increasing appropriate use may only increase health care expenditures."

Considerations of Cost and Effectiveness

Funding choices among alternative medical treatments are continuously made in all health care systems. Decision analysts have attempted—using data of various kinds—to answer the most critical questions that face responsible decision-makers:

1. Are there treatments providing some benefit to the patient (regardless of cost) that could be expanded?
2. Which treatments are likely to be more cost-effective compared with other uses of the funds?

Summarizing information on the comparative cost-effectiveness of a number of programs is difficult. Data from various sources, using different methodologies, must be forced into a common framework. Table 9.1 summarizes some of Detsky's (1989) work on the comparative cost-effectiveness of a number of programs. Choices within groups are ex-

Table 9.1. Hypothesized Cost-Effectiveness Ratios[a]

Program	*Approximate cost/QALY gained*[b,c]
Phenylketonuria screening	Money is saved
Coronary artery bypass surgery for left main coronary artery disease Neonatal intensive care, birth weight of 1,000–1,499 grams Thyroxine (thyroid) screening Treatment of severe hypertension (diastolic blood pressure >105 mm Hg)	Relatively inexpensive programs (approximately $5,000–12,000/QALY gained)
Treatment of mild hypertension (diastolic blood pressure 95–104 mm Hg) in men aged 40 years New radiocontrast media, provision to 30% of the population at highest risk Estrogen therapy for postmenopausal symptoms in women without a prior hysterectomy Neonatal intensive care, birth weight of 500–999 grams Coronary bypass surgery for single-vessel disease with moderately severe angina School tuberculin testing program Continuous ambulatory peritoneal dialysis Hospital hemodialysis	Moderately expensive programs (approximately $20,000–70,000/QALY gained)
New radiocontrast media, provision to low-risk patients Liver transplant	Very expensive programs (approximately $200,000 /QALY gained)

[a] Adapted from Detsky (1989).
[b] QALY indicates quality-adjusted life year.
[c] Reported values were adjusted to U.S. dollars using the U.S. Consumer Price Index for medical care for all urban consumers.

tremely difficult to make. Choices between program groups may well be appropriate. On reexamination, several of the treatments within the moderate and highly expensive groups could turn out not to bring any benefit to the patient. Indeed, the calculated cost-effectiveness of some interventions is probably unduly optimistic for a number of reasons.

First, the analyses are most likely based on efficacy data. Efficacy is concerned with whether a particular treatment works under ideal conditions, typically on patients selected using a strict protocol in a teaching hospital. Effectiveness studies deal with whether or not a specific treatment works in practice, when the treatment is widely diffused. For example, hospitals where relatively few surgical procedures of a particular type are performed often have poorer outcomes than do those performing larger numbers of the procedure (Luft, Bunker, and Enthoven, 1979). Bypass surgery in particular shows a very wide range of risk-adjusted mortality among hospitals (Steinbrook, 1988).

Second, most decision analyses are unclear about the role of comorbidity and age. For example, the selection criteria used in the major randomized clinical trial of bypass surgery (the CASS study) were applicable to less than 10 percent of the patients receiving bypass surgery in CASS participating centers and other hospitals (CASS Principal Investigators and Their Associates [CASS], 1981; Hlatky et al., 1988). The remainder of the patients were either older or sicker than the CASS group (CASS, 1981). Although the CASS researchers developed a registry to follow individuals who were not randomized, most clinical trials do not follow the patients whose characteristics may exclude them from randomization (Davis, 1990).

Surgical interventions are in general less beneficial for older patients and those with more comorbidity. The risks of surgery are greater, whereas the benefits are available over a shorter life span. Decision analysts need to take this into account, as Barry, Mulley, Fowler, and Wennberg (1988) have done for prostatectomy.

Third, the baseline population mortality will vary markedly among areas, even across such large areas as U.S. states (U.S. Bureau of the Census, 1990). The baseline mortality affects the benefits and risks calculated for particular interventions (Roos et al., 1990). Calculations of quality-adjusted life years (QALYs) are in particular likely to change when done for different populations. All else equal, the higher the baseline mortality rate in a given area, the lower will be the QALY gain from the intervention.

Fourth, the quality of the information used in decision analyses is often poor. Although Detsky's summary used some meta-analyses and randomized trials, this is not always the case with published decision analyses. Population-based, nonrandomized research is scarce. Weak research designs are typically biased toward showing improved outcomes from a new treatment (Chalmers, Reitman, Hewett, and Sacks, 1989; Colditz, Miller, and Mosteller, 1989; Miller, Colditz, and Mosteller, 1989). Such biases are important because sensitivity testing with small changes in the data may well reveal a wide range of plausible cost/QALY values.

Additional uncertainties arise from the "dating" of research. Because of the time gap between data collection and publication, proponents of a particular new treatment often claim that the innovation should have a better cost-effectiveness ratio than the literature suggests. Although improved results and reduced costs often do result from experience (Yeaton and Wortman, 1985; Cromwell, Mitchell, and Stason, 1990), this need not be the case (Orkin, 1989). Manitoba data on several common surgical procedures show that increasing expenditures over time do not necessarily translate into significant declines in postoperative mortality or in the rate of related hospital readmissions (Roos, Roos, and Sharp, 1987). In fact, an equally plausible scenario is that as an innovation diffuses, new programs typically start up and new teams have to work up the learning curve.

Desirable results are usually not well specified for different types of patients. Although Table 9.1 suggests the very different benefits of coronary artery bypass surgery for two types of patients (those with left main disease and those with single-vessel disease and moderately severe angina), benefits need to be estimated for the other types of patients likely to receive bypass surgery. Often, as has been demonstrated for tonsillectomy, just a small portion of the patients receiving the procedure can be shown to benefit from the surgery (Roos et al., 1977; Paradise et al., 1984; Roos, 1979).

Finally, cost-effectiveness ratios are likely to differ "at the margin" as fewer or more patients receive a procedure. Cross-sectional data (from Manitoba and New England) show no clear relationship between surgical rates and population risk factors (Roos et al., 1990). As rates increase, a given treatment may bring in older, sicker patients (as appears to have happened with coronary artery bypass surgery) or younger, less ill patients (Anderson, Newhouse, and Roos, 1989). As rates fall, patient risk may increase (cholecystectomy) or decrease (hysterectomy) (Roos et al., 1987).

Patient Preferences

The shared responsibility "among clinicians, patients and policymakers who act as societal agents" increases the complexity of clinical decision-making (Mulley, 1990). The expected benefits of any intervention vary with patient preferences. Some evidence suggests that risk-averse patients would have lower rates of surgery. Specifically, patients seem likely to avoid "a choice that has a high expected utility because it includes a possibility of the worst outcome." Moreover, "when offered a choice, patients often choose differently than their physicians" (Wennberg, 1987a).

McNeil, Weichselbaum, and Pauker (1978) found that, when confronted with choices of treatment for lung cancer, the sufferers preferred radiation therapy, which had higher probabilities of immediate- and one-year survival, over surgery, which had a higher probability of five-year survival. Although the physicians in this study seemed less risk-averse than the patients, physicians as patients might behave differently. A study investigating how physicians would want to be managed if they had non-small-cell lung cancer found that only between 3 and 16 percent of Canadian oncologists would have wanted to be treated with chemotherapy (as recommended in the standard textbooks; McKillop, O'Sullivan, and Ward, 1987).

New educational technology developed for prostatectomy provides additional evidence (Wennberg, 1990b). After receiving information on treatment alternatives and the probabilities of different results, patients were more likely to make conservative choices. Preliminary data suggest that, after watching the video explaining the treatment choices, many patients adopt a "watchful waiting" strategy, postponing prostate surgery as long as the symptoms are tolerable.

PHYSICIAN BEHAVIOR

Improving the information physicians have about appropriate treatment or the results associated with different treatments may or may not change their behavior. Part of the problem may be clinician overconfidence. Baumann, Deber, and Thompson (1990) noted such overconfidence in two different situations: the treatment of breast cancer by physicians and the management of intensive care patients by nurses. In both, clinicians were highly confident they had made the right decision ("micro-certainty"). But there was no consensus about precisely what the optimal treatment in fact would be ("macro-uncertainty").

Although high rates of care are not consistently associated with high rates of inappropriate use, rates sometimes fall when aggressive physicians are fed back information on their practice style. When practitioners learned their rates of surgery were substantially above state averages, there was, for example, a 50 percent decrease in the rate of hysterectomy. Similar changes in practice, following feedback, occurred in Maine and Vermont for tonsillectomy and in Norway for lens extractions (Wennberg, 1984). Physicians in these high-rate areas apparently concluded that some of their previous surgery had been unnecessary.

On the other hand, some physicians can be very hesitant to change established practice patterns, even where improved quality of care is directly involved. Research on the behavior of cardiovascular surgeons participating in the CASS study, a major clinical trial that helped develop criteria for coronary artery bypass graft surgery, produced rather discouraging findings (Maynard et al., 1986). Despite their surgeons' cooperation with this high-profile clinical trial, the participating hospitals differed markedly in the extent to which the CASS practice guidelines were followed. Among the fifteen hospitals, the number of bypass procedures that took place ranged from 75 to 124 percent of those expected from CASS guidelines, given the patients' clinical and angiographic characteristics.

Whether physicians left to their own devices reduce only inappropriate and equivocal care is not at all clear. The Rand Health Insurance Study provided relevant, but disappointing evidence (Siu et al., 1986). Although cost sharing reduced the rate of admissions to hospital, it did not disproportionately reduce the rate of inappropriate admissions. Moreover, identifying "good practice" and then disseminating such information apparently is not enough to change practice patterns. For example, a widely disseminated and nationally endorsed practice guideline for cesarean surgery had almost no impact on the pattern of obstetrical practice in Ontario, Canada (Lomas et al., 1989). Similarly, the consensus conferences of the National Institutes of Health have not in general been able to change practice style in the United States (Kosecoff et al., 1987). In both of these examples, the guidelines were communicated and physicians were generally aware of what they should be doing. They just were not doing it.

Physicians resist the monitoring of their practice, particularly if they interpret such monitoring as "cookbook medicine." This ideological stance is very widespread, but has its severe critics within medicine. For example, Hampton (1983) claims "clinical freedom is dead" and argues that "no one need regret its passing." According to Hampton, "the doctor's opinion was all that there was . . . in the days when investigation was nonexistent and treatment as harmless as it was ineffective." But now, for critics like Hampton, the "opinion" of doctors alone "is not good enough." How medicine copes with this tension between autonomy and clinical accountability will be an increasingly important area of health care policy in the coming decades.

WHAT HAVE WE LEARNED?

The evidence summarized above supports the following propositions:

1. Patterns of medical practice differ substantially from one physician to another.
2. A significant amount of care is inappropriate and the rate of inappropriate care is often as high in low-rate areas as in high-rate areas.
3. The lack of evidence of clear benefit from certain procedures suggests that some existing rates are too high.
4. Clinical uncertainty explains some practice variation.
5. Reducing uncertainty does not guarantee appropriate care.
6. Informed patients tend to prefer conservative treatment (at least where there are risks involved).
7. Both expert panels and cost-effectiveness studies tend to overestimate the benefits of treatment.
8. Applying practice guidelines may lower surgical rates in certain areas, but this is not guaranteed.

The politics driving expansion of acute care is well documented (see, e.g., Detsky et al., 1990; Evans and Barer, 1989), and is taken up in more detail in subsequent chapters. Continued pressure on health care budgets is inevitable in all Western industrialized societies, particularly pressure for more, and more sophisticated, diagnostic and surgical procedures. Where the risks are very low, patients and physicians are likely to want what they believe to be "better" diagnoses, even if the worth of the diagnostic procedures has not been demonstrated. On the other hand, there is evidence that better-informed patients are less willing to undergo invasive procedures.

The uncertainties of medical practice and the large variations in hospitalization rates should focus attention on the link between health care and the health of populations. The health status (of both individuals and populations) and the effectiveness of medical interventions are related, but "experts" differ widely in their judgments as to the nature and strength of the relationship. This diversity of opinion highlights both the potential for saving resources through eliminating inappropriate care and the difficulty of getting agreement to do so.

POLICY SUGGESTIONS

Reduce Utilization in High-Rate Areas

The lack of evidence on the effectiveness of many treatment strategies suggests that policies to contain costs could, at one extreme, focus on bringing utilization rates down toward the lower end of their range. A more moderate approach would target only regions with above-average use rates; utilization in these areas might safely be reduced toward mean levels. This conservative strategy may have considerable appeal to those who pay for care.

This strategy implicitly assumes that inappropriate care is more common in high-use areas. Yet, surprisingly, high rates of inappropriate care have been found in both low- and high-rate areas. Moreover, various biases in the process of evaluation have led to overestimates of appropriateness of care. Even RAND's expert panels have been shown to be generous in their assessments. When viewing the same research and patient histories *and told to ignore resource constraints,* British physicians were much more conservative in their assessments than were their American counterparts (Brook et al., 1988)! For example, they judged 35 percent of bypass surgery procedures to be inappropriate; the American physicians, viewing the same set of patients, considered only 13 percent to be inappropriate. These findings suggest that the "true" rates of inappropriate care are higher than those reported in the North American literature; they do not, however, explain the similarity of those rates in both high- and low-use areas.

What, then, is the basis for thinking that efforts at reducing utilization in high-rate areas will not adversely affect health? Perhaps the relative rates of use reflect differences in underlying need. In fact, however, researchers have not found these variations in use rates to be correlated with indicators of need.

Socioeconomic factors, for example, do affect both rates of utilization and the associated expenses for hospital care (McLaughlin, Normolle, Wolfe, McMahon, and Griffith, 1989; Epstein, Stern, and Weissman, 1990). But in both New England and Manitoba, it has been shown that the regions with low incomes are not those with the highest hospital use rates. Conversely, dramatic differences in utilization between Boston and New Haven occur despite demographically similar populations receiving most of their care in university hospitals. Most of the higher utilization in Boston "is devoted to the hospital admission of adults with common acute but often minor illnesses or with chronic diseases. . . . These findings indicate that academic standards of care are compatible with widely varying patterns of practice" (Wennberg et al., 1987). More generally, regions with high utilization have not been shown to differ systematically from regions with low utilization in terms of access to care, health status, or mortality (Roos and Roos, 1982; Wennberg and Fowler, 1977; Roos and Sharp, 1989; Wennberg, Freeman, Shelton, and Bubolz, 1989).

Which utilization should be reduced? Targeting both areas with high overall use and areas with high rates of particular treatments is a place to start (Phelps and Parente, 1990). Such targeting must be supported by both information and expertise to ensure that reductions occur primarily among the inappropriate and highly discretionary services.

Some American observers believe that "as provincial plans restrain the use of technology, [Canadian] physicians [will] increasingly face the difficult choice of providing care on the basis of medical need rather than rendering it to all who could benefit" (Iglehart, 1990). Yet, as we have clearly seen, this misdiagnoses the nature of the problem in what is, in fact, the second most expensive health care system in the world. If a significant proportion of the care delivered is inappropriate or of unknown benefit, then there is no necessary connection between restraining use and denying services to those who could benefit. Expansion of resources for procedures of proven effectiveness can in principle be achieved through better management and restraint of inappropriate use.

Evaluate Treatments

Too few procedures have been proven effective. We need better information about what does and does not work, and for whom. The value of clinical trials is well recognized; Detsky (1989) has suggested that the trials themselves are (potentially) highly cost-effective as ways to identify inappropriate care. Well-designed studies using disease registries or population-based cohorts may have similar benefits.

New and expensive technologies pose special problems, both for cost containment and for rigorous evaluation. Their advocates argue that traditional methods of evaluation or technology assessment have been outstripped by the dramatic benefits promised by new technologies. They claim, on the basis of clinical impressions rather than rigorous evaluation, to help at least some patients. If subsequent evidence fails to uphold the promise, the argument is always available that the most recent (and as yet unevaluated) version is better. This could be true. For example, Luepker (1988) has summarized care of the coronary heart disease patient as: "rapidly evolving, driven by new knowledge and technological innovations. . . . Old methods of clinical trials and epidemiologic surveillance are not rapid or sensitive enough to characterize or justify many of these new approaches. Thus, new methods of testing and surveillance seem essential to better understand [*sic*] and evaluate the population effects of new therapies." The need for practice guidelines is not removed by the absence of concurrent evidence.

Such guidelines are most important for controversial interventions that significantly affect patient outcomes or system costs (Leape et al., 1989). Procedures showing high variation across service areas indicate professional disagreement. Phelps and Parente (1990) have developed an index of expected gain from technology assessment that combines measures of resource use, the coefficient of variation in rates across regions, and the estimated rate at which the incremental value of a medical intervention changes as its rate of use changes. The index provides an estimate of the cost implicit in observed variations, which can be used for setting priorities for assessment. Coronary artery bypass surgery had the highest index score, but most of the high-index interventions were nonsurgical (including hospitalizations for psychosis, cardiac catheterization, chronic obstructive lung disease, and angina pectoris; Phelps and Parente, 1990).

The nature and importance of the treatment problem should influence the approach to evaluation. Thorough assessment of the appropriateness of coronary artery bypass surgery, for example, requires detailed data on the patient's condition. Such research is costly but, if the data are collected concurrently, they can also be used to guide treatment. On the other hand, administrative data appear suitable for better understanding the differences among hospitals in outcomes after hip fracture (Roos, Sharp, and Cohen, 1991).

Quality of Care Assessment Must Include Judgments of Appropriateness

Some recent efforts to monitor quality of care have focused on comparing mortality rates of patients treated at different hospitals (Brinkley, 1986). In-hospital reviews often focus on deaths, although progress has recently been made in targeted reviews of performance of particular procedures. Such reviews using administrative data offer the possibility of identifying quality problems in a cost-effective way. Hannan, O'Donnell, Kilburn, Bernard, and Yazici (1989) have reported the success of a targeted study (testing eleven explicit criteria) of uniform hospital discharge data. Cases identified using the discharge abstracts were more likely to have quality of care problems (as validated by record review) than were those chosen at random.

Questions such as, Was the admission appropriate in the first place? Should the surgery have been done? or Should the MRI have been performed? are typically not regarded as pertinent to reviews of quality of care, although they might be asked as part of utilization review. Quality assurance focuses on doing things right; utilization review on doing the right things. Yet, economics aside, modern medical treatment has significant potential to do harm and to produce pain and suffering. Given the enormous variations in physician practice patterns, quality of care assessments should encompass utilization review.

Develop Explicit Guidelines Drawing on External Sources

If practice guidelines are developed by local practitioners without reference to clinical trial evidence and work done elsewhere, they may well generate idiosyncratic guidelines. Local input is critical to local acceptance of guidelines. But it is equally important that physicians come to realize the marked variation that occurs among well-meaning practitioners, and the extent to which the practices in particular communities of physicians can depart from appropriate norms.

Leape et al. (1989) have reviewed practice guidelines developed in several contexts by specialty societies: the Clinical Efficacy Assessment Project, the Joint Commission on Accreditation of Healthcare Organizations, etc. These guidelines proved to be useless for assessing the appropriateness of particular procedures because they lacked specificity. They were so general as to leave everything up to the judgment of the individual practitioner or review body.

This problem was underscored by recent experience with reviewing indications for cesarean section (Jessee, Nickerson, and Grant, 1982). The use of subjective criteria such as "failure to progress in labor" and "fetal distress" led to the identification of 98.9 percent of the procedures as justified. In contrast, admission rates fell and mortality was reduced after guidelines for management of head-injured adults, developed by a national group of neurosurgeons, were adopted (Jennett, 1988).

Worthwhile Activities

Significant funds will be needed to develop practice guidelines, to do outcome assessments, and to monitor practice. The evidence reviewed above indicates that there is no reason to add new monies for these purposes. Redirection of current funding from some of the ineffective care that we now provide should be sufficient not only to finance these activities, but to support expansion of services found to be effective. But initial funding will be needed, because capturing the savings will be dependent on identifying areas of inappropriate or unnecessary care.

A good deal more information will also be needed, about both providers and patients. Careful thought must be given to the type and quality of data collected (see Chapter 11). Analysis of administrative data can often provide a cost-effective first cut, yielding answers to some questions, and more precisely focusing more detailed analyses. Interregional comparisons of such data may suggest evaluations of particular importance in a given region. A comparison of postsurgical mortality between Manitoba and New England, for example, showed generally better results in Manitoba, an advantage that became more pronounced by three years after surgery (Roos, Fisher, Brazauskas, Sharp, and Shapiro, 1992). Repair of hip fracture, an exception with relatively poor survival in Manitoba, has now been targeted for special attention in that province. Finally, the "natural experiments" that would take place if use rates in high-use areas are reduced would, if organized suitably, provide administrative data for both cost containment studies and the assessment of particular treatments.

The greatest challenge may be finding the political will to manage health care in a cost-effective fashion. In the next chapter we turn our attention to that challenge. The evidence reviewed here, regarding variations in patterns of medical practice, their suggested "determinants," and the difficulty of encouraging the uptake of guidelines, focuses our attention on provider practice styles or "signatures." The next chapter considers some possible approaches, through both public and self-regulatory policies, to modifying these practice styles, reducing the provision of inappropriate care, and releasing resources for other activities contributing to population health.

ACKNOWLEDGMENTS

The authors gratefully acknowledge the help of the Manitoba Health Services Commission. This research was supported by National Health Research and Development Project No. 6607-1197-44, by Career Scientist Awards No. 6607-1314-48 and No. 6607-1001-48, and by the Canadian Institute for Advanced Research. Interpretations and viewpoints contained in this paper are the authors' own and do not necessarily represent the opinion of either the Manitoba Health Services Commission or Health and Welfare Canada. The authors also wish to thank Kerry Meagher and Phyllis Jivan for the preparation of the manuscript.

NOTES

1. Uncertainty in medical practice has two quite distinct meanings, which are often confused. An individual practitioner may be uncertain, in a particular case or class of cases, about diagnosis or treatment. A community of uncertain practitioners (who are not in close communication) may be expected to show a high degree of variation in their behaviour. This is the situation hypothesized in this section. Better information will, if accepted as authoritative, lead to reduced uncertainty and convergence of practice patterns.

Alternatively, however, each individual practitioner may be quite certain about both diagnosis and treatment, but his or her opinions may differ from those of his or her colleagues. Such a divergence of certainties, across the community of practitioners, will also produce practice variations. We may if we wish say that the *community* of such practitioners is uncertain, although each individual enjoys perfect certainty. In the absence of close communication, they may never become aware of their disagreements, let alone resolve them.

There is evidence for both forms of uncertainty as sources of observed practice variations. But the considerable difficulty of changing practice patterns is suggestive of diverging, strongly held opinions—or else a very selective view of what constitutes relevant evidence.

2. Radiologic examination of the bile ducts after ingestion of a radiopaque substance.

10

Regulating Limits to Medicine: Towards Harmony in Public- and Self-Regulation

J. LOMAS and A.-P. CONTANDRIOPOULOS

The previous chapter has emphasized that the contribution of medical care to health, though substantial, is nonetheless limited.[1] Furthermore, a significant proportion of the medical care now provided has unevaluated or questionable effects on the health of its recipients. Earlier chapters have reviewed some of the extensive evidence that many important determinants of health lie outside the health care system.

These observations present three problems for societies wishing to maximize the impact of their investments in their population's health:

1. how to reduce or at least stabilize the total expenditures on medical care in line with our understanding of its relative value as but one contributor to a population's health;
2. how to maximize the effectiveness of health care resources within the domain of medical care organizations and practitioners;
3. how to generate among the public and policymakers a more balanced understanding of, and support for, both social and health care investments in health.

Success in dealing with these problems may lead, in the future, to a more effective allocation of resources among the alternative pathways to health.

In this chapter we address each of these issues in turn, although for the last we offer little more than an analysis of its intractable nature.

Historically these three problem areas have usually been addressed independently within different and often unconnected policy domains. The budgetary allocation power of governments and other payors is the avenue used to control total expenditures on medical care. The "self-regulation" power vested in the medical profession is the tool of choice for improving the precision with which medical care inputs are used to produce health outputs.[2] Information campaigns and other tools of public education have been used in attempts to broaden public understanding of the factors that contribute to health.

Our thesis, developed in the following section, is that a greater degree of coordination across these policy domains, particularly between medical self-regulation and government regulation, may create synergies that would speed our progress toward solutions in each of these areas. In subsequent sections we analyze the implications of this thesis for the design of medical self-regulation, government or "third-party" regulation, and public and policymaker education.

I. THE INTERDEPENDENCE OF GOVERNMENT HEALTH POLICY, THE SELF-REGULATION OF MEDICINE, AND PUBLIC PERCEPTIONS OF HEALTH

Medical care dominates public perceptions of how societies invest in their populations' health, for reasons that have been described from a variety of disciplinary perspectives: sociology (Friedson, 1970; Starr, 1982), political science (Alford, 1975; Marmor, 1983; Klein, 1989), economics (Fuchs, 1974; Evans, 1984), geography (Eyles, 1987), and medicine itself (Naylor, 1986; Caper, 1988). Starting with the local community doctor dedicated to doing what he or she could, an entire set of institutions, aspirations, and commitments has grown that equate "medical care" with "health." The institutions thus created—pharmaceutical manufacturers, the medical device industry, hospitals, organized medicine, indeed all who draw their income from the provision and support of medical care—reinforce this public perception. Health is achieved and maintained by the application of medical care to eliminate or alleviate disease. Presenting itself as a "science," medicine has been able to claim open-ended budgets on the strength of the alleged scientific link between "needs" and services provided. Presenting itself as a "profession," medicine has been able to deflect any external examination of this relationship, retaining in the hands of the medical practitioners themselves responsibility for ensuring the linkage between medical care and health.

With the changing understanding of the determinants of health and a growing realization of the questionable scientific basis for a good deal of medical practice has come a willingness both to question open-ended budgets and to scrutinize self-regulation. This willingness, however, is as yet largely restricted to the policymaking elites. Translation into policy is slow, because in all industrialized societies medical care continues to dominate public understanding of the production of health, and to be the first port of call for individuals suffering anxiety about deviations from "good health."

Consequently, revenue shortages have been used as a justification for the resource caps and expenditure limits introduced by governments in Canada and western Europe, and under discussion in the United States (McLachlin and Maynard, 1982; Evans et al. 1989; Abel-Smith, 1992). Left largely unexploited are rationales based on the limited value of additional resources committed to medical care rather than other determinants of health. Furthermore, such budgetary limitations have tended to be blunt instruments—overall supply constraints or tightened expenditure envelopes—with no accompanying incentives for practitioners and their organizations to address concerns about inappropriate or wasteful provision of care. Physicians' considerable economic freedoms and their influence over the total allocation of resources *have* been affected—hence the claims of "underfunding." These measures, however, do not challenge the dominance of physicians over the institutions, approaches, and values of the health care system. Nor do they promote (directly) improvements in the precision of medical practice.

Similarly, quality assurance measures and competence assessment initiatives within medicine, whatever their motivations, have not been justified by the profession on resource constraint grounds. Indeed, "cost containment" is considered, by both the profession and the public, as a tainted justification for the measures taken by the medical profession under the rubric of self-regulation. Insofar as initiatives such as technology assessments or practice guidelines may free up resources by improving the precision of medical care, these are expected to be redeployed elsewhere in medical care. The redirection of such resources to alternative (nonmedical) pathways to better population health is not contemplated, and in the absence of coordination with public regulation will not occur. Medical care will continue to dominate the production of health, at least financially.

There are thus two distinct reasons for reexamining the resources used for medical care: to ensure that we are "doing the right things" (for the maintenance and promotion of health), and "doing things right" (within the context of medical care itself). While these have different policy implications, they can be mutually compatible and complementary. In the one case policies are applied to release resources from medical care, while also justifying such release in ways that encourage awareness of a broader set of alternative paths to health. In the other case, the relationship of medical care inputs to health outputs is improved, thus increasing the likelihood that if resources shrink the degree of health improvement does not shrink in parallel. On its own the latter may improve the quality of care, but it will leave unexploited other possibilities for improving health because it will not automatically release resources from the grasp of medical care. The former on its own may release some resources from medical care that could be used to promote health in alternative ways, but will not realize the full potential of those remaining.

Policy coordination and compatibility have not been encouraged either by public understanding about the relationship between medical care and health or by the way in which government or professional regulatory tools have been used. Two solitudes exist for "regulating" medical care, each actively avoiding consideration of key objectives of the other. Governments avoid sharing responsibility for the activities of medical care, not wishing to be seen as encroaching on clinical decision-making. Instead they focus on the balance between limiting the resources available and satisfying the electorate. For their part the medical profession avoids sharing responsibility for the resource allocation activities of government. The self-regulation process in medicine has focused on the individual practitioner-patient encounter, a framework that both discourages resource consideration in making judgments of "good care" and makes it difficult to ascertain overall impacts on population health.

What can be done with public regulation to facilitate the goal of precision, and to reorient self-regulation to resource allocation as well as medical concerns? What can be done with self-regulation to support the public objective of reduced resources to medical care for equivalent impacts on population health? Both types of regulation require broadening and the two must be brought closer together. The common ground is (or at least should be) improving health. The battle grounds are physicians' claims to autonomy and control over the content of medical care (in the interests of their patients), and governments' responsibility to allocate resources to those areas most likely to improve health (in the interests of their public). One of the key instruments in this battle is, and will continue to be, public opinion.

In the next two sections we analyze in more detail both medical self-regulation and public regulation. We reject at the outset such panaceas as "free-market" solutions or technocratic state regulation. The latter is incomplete; the former is simply wrong. So-called "free market" approaches have been discredited often enough as a mechanism for the allocation of resources in medical care that the arguments for their rejection need not be revisited here (Evans, 1984; Rochaix, 1985; Reinhardt, 1987; Pouvoirville, 1990).

In the state regulation approach we recognize some potential, especially in establishing the framework of expectations from the state and acting as a precipitating factor for change. Ultimately, however, we believe it is incomplete because its standardization and inflexibility are unable to handle many of the areas of discretion and uncertainty that are inherent to the practice of medicine. New attitudes, beliefs, and values cannot be legislated, either within the profession of medicine or across the broader public. Technocratic state regulation may be *part* of the solution but it will not *be* the solution.

Underlying our proposals is the vision of a "third way" in which redesigned institutions and incentives, catalyzed by regulatory change, produce a new ethos among policymakers, the medical profession, and the public. This will replace the current dominant belief system that equates ever-expanding medical care provision with ever-improving population health. The goal is a "public investment" model in which limited societal resources flow by design and desire to the best bets for improved population health. The final section addresses this issue of developing a new dominant belief system.

II. THE MEDICAL PROFESSION AND SELF-REGULATION

The Origins and Responsibilities of Self-Regulatory Power

The self-regulatory power of the medical profession has all too often been used as a way of perpetuating and capitalizing on the monopoly held by physicians over medical care (Slayton and Trebilcock, 1978). This, of course, is almost the opposite of the intent of self-regulation—or at least of the justification offered to the rest of the community.

If their activities are to be consistent with society's goals and expectations, monopolies must be accountable and under some external control. Because of the technical and expert knowledge required to adjudicate upon actions of their members, professional monopolies are granted self-regulatory responsibility. This makes the profession accountable to itself, yet it does not remove a broader social accountability. The rules of self-accountability imposed upon members of the professional group and its institutions are based on professional codes of ethics that reflect that broader set of expectations.

The self-regulating profession thus has responsibility for divining society's goals and expectations, and for developing accountability mechanisms that translate them into the actual behaviour of its organizations and members. These goals and expectations of society are of at least two types.

First, held by both the public and government, is the expectation that each physician will treat each patient ethically and with the most appropriate therapy given the particular presenting symptoms. The professional responses are licensure and disciplinary bodies, which, once established and operating, historically have represented for most citizens the entirety of medicine's self-regulatory responsibility. The focus of such bodies is on establishing (at a point in time) the competence and technical ability of individual physicians—the *potential* for each member of the profession to improve health. (They have also attempted to respond to situations involving clinical malfeasance.) But such bodies have not generally considered the extent to which this potential was realized. Assessment and action based on the individual physician's ability to use medical care selectively in ways that clearly *do* improve health has been neglected. The origin of this approach can be traced to the automatic identification of the provision of medical care with the production of health. Improvements in this aspect of accountability are aimed at increasing the precision with which medical care is used to produce health.

More significantly, there has been no assessment of, or action based on, the relative impact of the profession as a group on society's health. The second and less recognized type of societal expectation, held largely by those who pay for care, is that both individual physicians and the profession as a whole will attempt to maximize their impact on the population's health *within the constraint of the resources that the rest of society chooses to commit to medical care.*

This expectation has been brought into much sharper relief in most western nations by the virtually universal public funding of medical care services, establishing a relationship that some have called the "social contract" (Evans, 1973). The profession is expected to ensure that its members are, individually and in aggregate, providing cost-effective services, i.e., those most likely to maximize the health of the population within the given resource pool. As yet the profession in most countries has no institutional mechanisms for economic accountability in the way that licensing and disciplinary bodies correspond to accountability for the quality of care delivered by individual physicians.

In meeting these expectations the profession (and society) must contend with the inherent uncertainty surrounding the effects of a particular intervention on a particular patient. Whether prostatectomy for benign prostatic hypertrophy is to be offered cautiously or recommended strongly is within the discretion of a physician; whether the outcome is likely to be better with or without the prostatectomy depends upon the strength and applicability of the evidence on prostatectomy for the particular patient (Wennberg, 1992). The way in which medical discretion is managed, and what physicians use as a guide in the exercise of their discretion, is at the root of how well the self-regulatory process in medicine is working.

In some countries, such as the United Kingdom, resource constraints are accepted as part of individual medical decision-making; they act as one of the guides for physicians' exercise of medical discretion. This can be seen in the higher thresholds for intervention used by U.K., compared to U.S., physicians when faced with the same clinical scenarios (Hartley, Epstein, Harris, and McNeil, 1987; Brook et al. 1988; Bernstein, Kosecoff, Gray, Hampton, and Brook, 1993). Unlike the physicians of most other industrialized countries, U.K. practitioners have operated under fixed rather than open-ended budgets throughout the postwar era (Aaron and Schwartz, 1984).

Reform of the way in which medicine regulates itself requires, as a minimum, recognition of resource constraints. It also requires that each physician has in hand, and is likely to use, the best available information on the cost-effectiveness of the various clinical alternatives. Furthermore, the management of medical discretion requires not only information about the acceptable boundaries within which it *should* be exercised, but also ways of identifying areas of practice and types of practitioners outside acceptable boundaries.

Thus the conduct of self-regulation is mostly a matter of determining acceptable boundaries to the exercise of discretion, generating a sense of responsibility and a willingness to operate within these boundaries, and then monitoring and assuring that the activities of both the profession and the individual practitioner do, in fact, remain within them. Finding ways to manage physician discretion effectively is the new challenge for medical self-regulation, and finding ways to support medical self-regulation in this role is one of the challenges facing public regulation of medicine. The profession must become accountable for both the quality of care (the precision of medicine) and the resources used to provide such care (the cost-effectiveness of medicine). These two forms of accountability are addressed below.

Accountability for Producing Health

It will be no small matter to move from assessment of individual practitioners' technical competence to assurance of the profession's actual contribution to the population's health. Measuring this contribution requires data systems that focus on the population as well as on the individual practitioner—one component of the system of health statistics described in Chapter 11. It also requires comparative information on the relative worth of different interventions for producing health—what has become known as clinical epidemiology and disseminated as practice guidelines. Finally, professional self-regulation must include mechanisms to bring about the individual and professionwide changes indicated by the results of monitoring and assessment—the actual process of improving precision in the link between medical care and health.

One may hope that such changes will further encourage the growth of constructive scepticism among the medical profession about the general worth of what they do in everyday practice—in Osler's (1909) terms the replacement of "placid faith" by "the fighting faith of the aggressive doubter."

The technologies required to support such changes are available, and for the most part have been available for some time. Their use, however, is not presently encouraged by the focus on the individual rather than the profession, and on the process rather than the outcomes of medical care. For example, the administrative data sets generated by the processes of hospital oversight and physician payment, described in Chapter 11, can be used as demonstrated in Chapter 9 to identify areas of questionable medical practice. Yet they have rarely been turned to the uses envisioned here. The literature on small-area variations dates back to the 1960s, but with few exceptions (Keller, Chapin, and Soule, 1990) has not been used by the medical profession to generate changes in practice, or even to encourage more detailed investigation of high-variation interventions (Evans, 1990b).

Even more rare is the use within self-regulatory processes of administrative data on physician performance in comparison with the population-based practice patterns expected on the basis of clinical epidemiology. Dyck et al. (1977) did use such a comparison to alert colleagues in Saskatchewan to the overuse of hysterectomy, with the result that rates of such surgery fell sharply. But in the succeeding fifteen years few emulated this example.

Indeed, professionwide initiatives such as practice guidelines, intended to limit the boundaries within which discretion may be exercised, are tolerated only so long as they do not impinge on a physician's clinical autonomy. Commenting on the U.K. situation, the Royal College of Radiologists recently stated that "pressures to consider only the guidelines and their further refinements, and to ignore monitoring and peer review, continue to be enormous. The problem of how to assure compliance with an agreed standard of practice needs to be resolved" (Royal College of Radiologists Working Party, 1992:743). This is despite the fact that the literature evaluating physician behaviour change has uncovered, again more than ten years ago, a number of approaches that consistently appear able to improve the precision with which medical care produces health (Eisenberg, 1986).

Whether through the formal regulatory authorities of medicine, or through new roles for medical schools, specialty societies, or other medical organizations, improved accountability for producing health will require greater exploitation of:

- population-based measurement of medical care activity and its health outcomes,
- syntheses of formal evaluations of medical care interventions such as those conducted by clinical epidemiologists (Pauker, 1986; Chalmers, 1991), and
- strategies known to bring about changes in physician behaviour.

These activities will enable action to be taken when discretion is clearly identified as being exercised outside defined parameters.

Although the responsibility for such activities may lie largely with the medical profession (at least until such time as they clearly demonstrate an unwillingness to take it on), public regulation can both encourage and facilitate this process. Perhaps of most import is a clear and explicit expectation from public regulators that the responsibilities of the profession include assurance of the contribution of the profession at large to the population's health. The legislation assigning self-regulatory responsibility continues in most countries to address only individual practitioner competence.

Such a change in responsibilities obviously has to be complemented by changes in the resources and infrastructure supporting medical self-regulation. The administrative data sets that currently reside mostly within the government or payor domain have to be not only made available, but modified and presented in ways that facilitate their use by the medical profession. The governance structures for the data sets should reflect the fact that access to and quality of the data are equally important to both government *and* medical self-regulators (Ellwood, 1988). Clearinghouse functions for technology assessment, quality assurance, and practice guideline initiatives can be shared between government and the profession. An often-quoted model for this is the National Initiative for Quality in the Netherlands, where the medical specialty societies have joined forces under one umbrella to promulgate guidelines for medical practice, to facilitate their use to change hospital-based practices, and to monitor and evaluate progress (Reerink, 1990).

Such central activities are, however, only predisposing factors for improving the precision of medical care. Improved precision in medical care ultimately depends upon the incorporation of new information, such as guidelines, into the practice of individual physicians at the local level (Greer, 1988; Lomas, 1990a). The identification of problem areas of medical practice (i.e., areas that appear to be imprecisely linked to health outcomes) and ongoing monitoring of improved performance are most efficiently done centrally. However, changes in the approaches and behaviour of individual physicians—the development of that new ethos based on greater scepticism and cautious acceptance of the worth of particular medical interventions that Osler called for nearly a century ago—must occur within local medical communities.

Exploiting the influence of local opinion leaders and local lines of communication (Wenrich, Mann, Morris, and Reilly, 1971; Lomas et al., 1991) can be facilitated by establishing a more formal presence for medical self-regulation in each community. Public funding for such activity and decentralization of significant behaviour change initiatives to local bodies accountable for medical regulation would be steps in this direction. Indeed, this could be formalized through appointing physician "geographic scholars" responsible for the quality of care of one hundred to five hundred local physicians, affiliated with a medical school but resident in the community, employed by the local self-regulatory body but paid by government, and trained in the requisite quality assurance skills. These geographic scholars would not only be the conduit for relevant findings from central monitoring, but would also be the principal agents of change through their influence and pressure on local colleagues.

Finally, this major change in the perspective and responsibility of medical self-regulation may be complemented by a more formal and public monitoring of the accountability function. Through public regulation the medical profession could be required to report annually on its current estimated contributions to the population's health, its targets for improvement in the next year, and its major achievements and improvements in the preceding year. This might be analogous to an "auditor general's" annual report on government performance—with just the same degree of public and media interest.[3] Obviously, such reporting would focus on *demonstrable* improvements in health outcomes attributable to the entire profession and not, as tends to be the case at the moment, on processes and procedures undertaken and directed at individual practitioners.

Accountability for Cost-Effective Production of Health

The collective funding of medical care, public or private, has been associated with a dramatic expansion in the quantity, range, and sophistication of services used, and increasing concerns as to the necessity or appropriateness of all this activity. It is often alleged that patients are "abusing" the system because their out-of-pocket costs are reduced, although the claim is more strongly based in rhetoric than in evidence (Barer, Evans, and Stoddart, 1979; Woodward and Stoddart, 1990; Rachlis and Kushner, 1992). Less commonly noted, however, is that *physicians* practising in such environments do not have to consider the financial repercussions of their clinical recommendations.[4]

Cassel, writing about U.S. Medicare and Medicaid, points out that this consideration acted as a significant brake on the treatment decisions made by practitioners prior to the establishment of those programs. The removal of accountability for cost, *increases* the freedom of physicians to deliver any care they may wish: "It [Medicare] was a freedom, in its most positive sense, from the question of how far to go with the poor and the elderly. . . . The implicit cost-benefit analysis no longer had to be made" (at least for those covered by these programs; Cassel, 1985:551).

All developed societies other than the United States have established health care systems that provide universal coverage for their populations. Combined with generous and (until the last decade) open-ended funding for medical care (Abel-Smith, 1992), this has accustomed a generation of physicians to an environment of (from the perspective of the individual practitioner) "costless care." Studies of physicians' knowledge about the costs of the drugs or laboratory tests that they order as part of their everyday activity demonstrate a significant ignorance. Even when physicians are made aware of such costs they are resistant to incorporating such knowledge into the treatment decisions they make (Wones, 1987) or actively oppose the concept of such cost considerations on what they believe to be "ethical" grounds: "A physician who changes his or her way of practising medicine because of cost rather than purely medical considerations has indeed embarked on the "slippery slope" of compromised ethics and waffled priorities" (Loewy, 1980:697; but see Williams, n.d.).

Should a schoolteacher, holding the public responsibility to educate our children, take this attitude we would presumably have particle accelerators purchased for every science class, professional theatre companies hired to act every English literature play, and chronically expanding deficits in education funding.

Accordingly, physicians have not until recently really considered judicious management of the resources under their control as part of their job. Triage expertise and the skilled managerial ability to trade off competing priorities for limited beds, operating rooms, diagnostic equipment, and so on are not usually part of the current training of a physician. The only incentives to practice efficient medicine are the frustrations that physicians feel from repeatedly encountering the limits on total resources available, but they receive no guidance as to how to respond. Any resource constraints are thus perceived by physicians and their organizations as a barrier to be removed (at someone else's expense)—"the system is underfunded"—rather than as a challenge requiring the acquisition of managerial skills to complement their technical and clinical abilities.

The privilege of self-regulation should include a responsibility for contributing to public objectives by incorporating the concept of cost-effectiveness into the definition of "good medical practice." The profession should be accountable not only for the quality of care, but also for the efficiency with which resources are used to achieve that quality. Even if the activities described in the previous section—to improve the precision of medical care—were all successfully implemented, resources would likely still be used wastefully.

Various policies that signal and underline the finite nature of resources for medical care—capped budgets, priority-setting mechanisms, limited capital capacity—are outlined in more detail in the next section on potential government initiatives. Introducing these policies in isolation, however, assumes that medical practitioners are both able and willing to make the allocation decisions that will maximize the health impact of the finite resources.

At present, however, economic considerations are largely excluded from the mandate and expectations of medical self-regulation. Nor is the individual physician rewarded for managerial ability in clinical practice. Practitioners perceive that their responsibilities have been discharged by their taking account of their individual patients' needs and desires, and by answering when necessary to the existing accountability mechanisms of disciplinary or licensing bodies. Consequently medicine has few formal mechanisms to make the physician accountable for the cost-effectiveness of what he or she does, or the profession accountable for its share of public resources.

Recent initiatives in Oregon would incorporate more formally into decision-making the fact of resource constraints. Oregon has instituted mechanisms for attaching explicit priorities to the various claims on limited Medicaid funding. For example, low-cost, high-payoff care for children, such as vaccination, is favoured over organ transplants (Office of Technology Assessment, U.S. Congress 1992). There is much wrong with the Oregon proposal: its applicability only to those dependent on Medicaid, or its organization around defined disease-treatment pairs, which reinforces the perception that there should be no discretion in the application of particular treatments for particular patients in particular circumstances. Nevertheless, the design of a process that forces physicians to confront the resource constraints under which they operate is commendable. Less draconian and more defensible alternatives can also be found.

Experiments in the United Kingdom demonstrate that providing "clinical budgets" to physician-led hospital departments generates increased appreciation for the relative costs and effects of different interventions (Coles and Wickings, 1976). These have led more recently to the development of clinical budgets for general practice "gatekeepers" (Glennerster, Matsaganis, and Owens, 1992). In Canada some medical organizations have, with partial success, recommended cautious use of expensive but not demonstrably superior therapies, such as the drug t-Pa (versus streptokinase) for heart attack patients (Linton and Naylor, 1990). Recommendations for explicit triage criteria to improve the efficiency of waiting lists are another managerial example of the same concept (Naylor, 1991). Without more fundamental institutional reform, however, widespread appreciation of the importance of cost-effectiveness and incorporation of the concept into the daily practice of medicine is unlikely to occur.

Self-regulatory reform might include encouraging the incorporation of concepts of cost-effectiveness into the medical education process by imposing licensure and competence requirements that include appreciation of the balance between risk, benefit, *and* cost, or defining cost-effective practice as a major criterion for the granting of hospital privileges. Changes in public regulation might include requiring explicit consideration of information on both costs and benefits in proposed new technology acquisitions; including not only the safety and efficacy but also the cost-utility of new drugs as part of the government approval process; establishing remuneration schemes that penalize practitioners who fail to take account of the relationship between cost and outcome; or devolving budgetary authority to decision-making units that make trade-offs more visible.

Many of these changes in public regulation have already begun or are well under way. What is not so clear is the willingness of the medical profession and its members to respond to these increasing pressures to be "cost and outcome conscious." This will require them to acquire new skills, and make everyday decisions with cost-effectiveness in mind (Hunter, 1991). If self-regulation does not embrace accountability for cost-effectiveness, then both the entrepreneurial and the clinical content of medical care are likely to become increasingly subject to external regulation. The protracted resistance of the medical profession in the

United States appears already to have resulted in such third-party encroachment, much to the chagrin of the practitioners in that country (Grumbach and Bodenheimer, 1990).

Insofar as public regulation reflects the values and expectations of the population, it is incumbent on medical care regulators and educators to bring about greater harmony in the objectives under which the two forms of regulation operate. The competing interests of funding agent (government/third party) and funded agent (provider/physician) lead to an inherent tension. It was for this reason, however, that separate professional institutions were established to represent the interests of physicians (medical associations or unions) and of the public (colleges, boards of regents, medical schools). From these latter publicly created and accountable institutions, one can reasonably demand change and expect progress toward a more participatory role in ensuring that the resources devoted to medical care are used efficiently in the pursuit of health.

III. GOVERNMENTS AND PUBLIC REGULATION

In addition to those changes in public regulation already proposed or in process to assist and improve the conduct of medical self-regulation, two new forms of public regulation are emerging: global expenditure limits or caps, and improvements in intersectoral linkages. They are intended to address, respectively, the more precise and cost-effective practice of medicine, and the (re)allocation of an increasing share of public resources to alternative paths to health.

Global expenditure controls or caps establish "a global boundary that surrounds the medical commons, setting clear limits on the amount of money budgeted for the health system [with a] focus on the collective behavior of large groups of doctors and patients, rather than on individual physician/patient encounters" (Grumbach and Bodenheimer, 1990:124). Such caps on total expenditures for medical or other forms of health care provide incentives for medical self-regulation: "[I]f the physician community finds that certain members of the herd are growing fat by consuming too much greenery at the expense of others, it becomes the responsibility of the profession to discipline such greedy members" (p. 125). Changes in budgetary and expenditure mechanisms underline the existence of resource constraints by building a fence around the "medical commons" (Hardin, 1968).

Improved intersectoral linkages require organizational or managerial changes to establish better coordination among the public agencies whose activities may potentially contribute to health. These include such traditional ministries as health care, social services, environment, housing, industrial development, labour, and education. The intent is to ensure that all the different pathways are taken into account in attempting to improve the population's health. Coordination is expected to improve the probability that resources freed from one aspect of medical care do not merely return to another medical care use, if health outcome payoffs from a nontraditional health policy are believed to be greater.

Such coordination is still so early in its conception that it is not clear whether it is better done centrally, locally, or in both places. Nor is it clear whether it should include the medical profession to improve their appreciation of the "broader picture," or exclude them to prevent domination and capture by traditional power structures. Also of concern is whether the evidence to support the social investments arising from intersectoral coordination is available, or strong enough to withstand challenges from medical proponents armed with increasingly available evaluative studies of medical effectiveness (Wennberg, 1992).

Although the following discussion of public regulation possibilities draws heavily on the Canadian experience, many of the same trends can be observed in other industrialized countries, and variations on the specific policy proposals are ubiquitous.

Global Expenditure Limits

Stringent expenditure limits, firmly maintained, may encourage the medical profession to set up its own regulatory processes to improve the outcomes and narrow the discretionary boundaries of medical practice. But it is not enough simply to announce that there will be global expenditure controls. Their precise nature and mode of application will determine whether their potential is realized.

Where Do You Put the Cap?

Is it enough to allow the political processes of a country (or its large subdivisions holding responsibility for health care provision such as provinces in Canada or counties in Sweden) to settle on a finite and inviolable cap on medical care expenditure? Such political processes, aided by changes discussed later in this chapter, can presumably achieve the task of freeing resources from medical care for other competing national or regional priorities. We think, however, that with the exception of those jurisdictions where the physician population is so small that interphysician trade-offs become transparent, these regional or national processes will do little to encourage physicians locally to use their finite resources more wisely. This is of particular concern in the context of fee-for-service remuneration (Evans, 1988).

There are major advantages in these circumstances to applying an additional cap at the local level for physicians' (and potentially other) services (Evans, 1988; Lomas et al., 1989; Rice and Bernstein, 1990). If there is a limit at the level of a large jurisdiction on the total pool of funds available for physicians' services, but no limit on the quantity of services billable by each physician, then the "free rider" who merely adjusts by increasing personal fee claims is left unpenalized (Kirkmann-Liff, 1990). The "responsible" physician who carefully adjusts practice patterns in response to the overall cap will suffer some income loss from reduced claims in the current year, in addition to income loss in subsequent years if there is downward fee adjustment to recoup utilization increases generated by less responsible colleagues.

If caps on medical care funds are applied to individual communities, however, local physicians may constitute a small enough peer group to enable them to bring pressure to bear on free-riders, with or without the assistance of formal self-regulatory structures. Moreover, imposing the cap on local funds may lead not only to control over the level of utilization (expenditure), but also, when combined with the kinds of changes outlined in the previous section, to professionally initiated improvements in the precision and cost-effectiveness of local practice patterns.

How Do You Determine the Size of the Local Cap?

The second consideration after establishing the geographic or other unit(s) at which the expenditure cap(s) will be imposed is the method used to establish their size. In the case of the overall national or regional cap, the political processes are presumed to result in a negotiated or imposed sum that reflects the extant belief systems about the value of medical care relative to competing vehicles for improving the population's health.

Within this overall constraint, the principal determinant of any local caps (i.e., the share of the centrally determined funding pool) should be the size and structure of the population covered. Funds should follow citizens and not, as is presently the case in most countries, the providers and institutions. This would avoid freezing in place existing local allocations of expenditure, with whatever inequitable and inappropriate patterns of provision these represent (Glennerster et al., 1992). Each local area would be "weighted" according to variables that reflect the population's size, age, and gender and, in addition, any other variables deemed important in improving the match between resources committed to an area and its actual need for medical care. Such weights could then be used to allocate the local community's particular share of the larger pot of medical care funds available for the country or region.

The methods for supplementing the determination of local weights, over and above the size and age-sex structure of the population, fall into two general classes: first, methods that make rough assessments of the precision of medical care and thereby reward areas having greater precision with larger shares of the overall expenditure envelope; second, methods that relate the health status of the area to the local share of total medical care expenditure—the less healthy the population being served, the larger is the available budget.

The first class of supplementation methods—rough estimates of the precision between medical resource inputs and health outcomes—can be based either on administrative data or on more subjective judgments left under the control of the medical profession. The use of administrative data is illustrated in Chapter 8: The rates of intervention in an area are used to indicate whether medical discretion is being exercised within acceptable boundaries. Areas with intervention rates that are consistently well above average would be subject to reductions in resources, compared to their current allocation, under the assumption that these higher intervention rates are because of higher rates of inappropriate or imprecise medical care. But there is evidence for (Roos, Henteleff, and Roos, 1977; Leape et al., 1990) and against (Chassin et al., 1987; Leape et al., 1990) this latter assumption. Advantages of the proposal are that it can be applied equally to hospitals and/or physicians, and that it is immediately implementable in countries such as Canada, which already have administrative data on medical care activity at the local level.

The alternative subjective method for estimating the precision of local medical care reinforces the responsibility of the medical profession for monitoring and evaluating its contributions to health. Medicine's self-regulatory responsibility can include the ranking of communities according to how appropriately the area's practitioners are exercising their medical discretion. The approach taken to this "quality of care" assessment might be tracer conditions (Kessner, Kalk, and Singer, 1973; Sibley et al., 1975), appropriateness assessments (Brook et al., 1986), variations data (Keller et al., 1990), or any other method agreeable to the medical profession and incorporating a reasonable service-oriented proxy for health outcomes. Obviously these assessments must be done using geographic boundaries that correspond to the unit of the local expenditure cap. The relative scores can, when combined with information on the size and age-sex structure of the populations, be translated into relative shares for all communities in the overall expenditure envelope.

The alternative to these rough estimation methods for assessing the precision of medical care is an approach that adjusts local expenditure caps for estimated differences in health status. This circumvents the problems of including existing levels of (appropriate and inappropriate) provision in the calculation, and the potential biases of using administrative data or professional subjective judgments to proxy optimal health outcomes. Needs-based approaches (Birch and Eyles, 1990) are defined directly by the relative health of the populations in different areas. Larger weights are applied to the areas with higher levels of population-based ill health. This approach has the significant advantage of focusing attention on the relationship between medical care funding and the health of the population.

But this approach requires a suitable measure of, or proxy for, the level of ill health in the population that is amenable to medical care intervention.[5] Standardized mortality ratios, aggregated across cause-specific categories and calculated for each local area, may be a solution—but only if mortality correlates well with ameliorable ill health. These ratios have long been in use in the United Kingdom, as part of a methodology developed by the Resource Allocation Working Parties (the RAWP process) for the allocation of funds from central government to the various regions of the country (Mays and Bevan, 1987), and have been proposed recently for Canada (Eyles, Birch, Chambers, Hurley, and Hutchison, 1991).

Relating medical care funding to health status in each community may be powerful as both a symbolic restatement of societal expectations of medical care and an economic spur for medical self-regulation to be conducted more in harmony with public regulation. Stringent and unyielding local caps on medical care expenditure, tied to population health status, might encourage action by the medical profession not only on the quality of care, but also on the growing per capita supply of physicians in most industrialized countries (Barer and Stoddart, 1991).

Organizational Changes to Encourage Intersectoral Linkage

A more decentralized organizational structure for health care delivery is implied by the dual objectives of resource allocation outlined in the previous section. Making resource allocation decisions more sensitive to local population health status and personalizing the impact of capped expenditure to encourage self-generated changes in physician behaviour may both be more effectively achieved with a decentralized organizational structure. In addition, there is a convergent trend toward decentralization that arises from the need for greater integration and coordination of all services (medical care and other) that may potentially contribute to health (Mills, Vaughan, Smith, and Tabibzadeh, 1990).

These are, however, two separate motivations for decentralization. One is to limit medical care expenditures, while at the same time encouraging better precision by the medical profession in its circumscribed role as provider of medical care. This is largely a financial and clinical motivation. The second intent is to broaden the portfolio of planning possibilities so as to treat medical care, however precisely practised, as only one of the possible pathways to health. The further hope is that such decentralization will increase the opportunity for the local community to influence the choices made from that portfolio. This is largely a planning and governance motivation.

Because these two separate motivations are not always distinguished, decentralization is often taken to imply the reallocation of resources within a unified budget for both health care and the social determinants of health. This does not have to be the case. It is possible to restructure governance and planning across both medical care and its poorer cousins (social services, housing, environmental protection, and so on), while maintaining separate expenditure envelopes. This consideration is important because we do not know whether a combined pool of resources, controlled by a community with current information and subject to medical persuasion as at present, would result in greater or lesser allocations going to medical care. It might be that rather than Robin Hood stealing from the sheriff of Nottingham, the sheriff would simply expropriate Sherwood Forest along with all of Robin's stores. It might be preferable to protect the resources currently available for nonmedical alternatives, and add to them as and when resources are freed from the medical care envelope.

The potential advantage of local decision-making authority is the greater opportunity for input from local community members. Although many claim a pure ideological justification for this, local community members are also more likely than central bureaucracies to be able to divine and represent the values and desires of their communities.[6] It is, however, an empirical question as to whether these values and desires, when translated into service and program delivery decisions, will result in new patterns of resource allocation, or merely mirror or strengthen the old patterns. A true test of the outcomes of locally empowered decision-making must address such questions as the adequacy of current information at the local level, the extent of expertise that can be expected from local community planners in interpreting the information (Keeney, Von Winterfeldt, and Eppel, 1990), and the feasibility of exploiting new information technologies such as interactive videodiscs (Wennberg, 1990c).

Whatever governance structures emerge at the local level, there are arguments for broader interdepartmental decision-making responsibilities at the central level of government. Government departments tend to become imprisoned by their constituencies and besieged by a variety of interest groups to such a degree that their ability to see the forest (production of health) for the trees (service delivery) is severely compromised (Ontario Health Review Panel, 1987; Quebec Government, 1987). A superstructure spanning departments and interests may promote an appreciation of the broader picture, and encourage justification of intradepartmental activity with reference to this broader picture.

Similar "educational" and "sensitizing" arguments can be used to support the inclusion of representatives of various interest groups on such umbrella organizations, in advisory or executive capacities. This is one way in which government can educate and encourage the medical profession to bring its self-regulatory activities more in line with broader social objectives.

Such attempts at central coordination have a checkered history. The Ontario provincial government in Canada abandoned its superministries after only a few years of largely powerless operation (MacDonald, 1980), and in the United Kingdom much energy was put into attempted coordination with little to show (Challis et al., 1988). These attempts, however, either focused on vertical integration of central and local authorities or failed to create a coordinating structure with sufficient status to direct policy change. The recently established Ontario Premier's Council and similar proposed bodies in a number of other Canadian provinces are intended to focus on a broad range of health determinants. The Ontario council is high profile, being chaired by the Premier, and is intended to play a primary role in horizontal coordination through the development of partnerships *across* central government departments. Perhaps the biggest issue still to be clarified for this type of central umbrella structure is how it can best increase awareness of and redistribute funding to health-related public policies other than medical care. They could provide a setting in which the various interest groups representing (the winners and losers associated with) alternative pathways to health "fight it out." In this scenario, research and evidence will tend to be devalued currencies, but the barriers to reform of the power structures will be made explicit and will have to be confronted.

Alternatively, such organizations could bring together "experts" to assemble and synthesize the accumulating evidence on the determinants of health, calling attention to its implications for public policy. They would include support staffs to disseminate these findings. This model relies heavily on the persuasive power of information to alter power structures. Whether both models can be melded into a functioning hybrid or, for that matter, whether either can change the current distribution of power and resources will become evident over the next few years as experience with such umbrella structures accumulates. But they are unlikely, by themselves, to change in any fundamental way the perceptions of either the public or the professions as to the dominant role of medical care in producing health.

IV. THE PUBLIC AND BELIEF SYSTEMS

The Roots of the Medical Care–Health Identity

The previous two sections presuppose a limited role for health care systems and for the physicians around whom they revolve. The proposals there assume that physicians will generally continue to treat individuals who present themselves with disease, with the intent of removing the cause of the disease or ameliorating its effects. This function is in turn based on an understanding of diseases as observable and quantifiable disturbances in the biological, psychological, or physical functioning of individuals. This understanding is, we believe, consistent with the view held by most medical practitioners themselves that medicine is properly concerned with identifying disturbances within the functions of the living organism, discovering their causes, and acting on them to restore normal functioning (De Vries, 1981). It also corresponds to the use of the term *disease* in Chapter 2, as a set of professionally developed concepts and categories.

In that conceptual framework, *illness* was used to refer to conditions as perceived by the patient or those around him/her. While not equivalent to professional concepts, the patient's "illness" is generally closely associated with the presence of the clinician's "disease." And since the cure and care of illness is self-evidently a contribution to health, physicians and health care systems responding to disease are and must remain a significant component of any society's responses to the problems of ill-health in its population.

As observed in preceding chapters, however, the determinants of health even in the narrow sense of absence of illness go far beyond the activities of health care systems. The evidence requires that one take a broad view of these determinants, however restrictive or encompassing one's conception of health itself.[7] A recognition of the importance of these nonmedical factors is quite sufficient to justify the redesign of public programs for health, even if one's objective is merely to reduce the burden of illness and infirmity.

Redesigning public programs requires, however, more than good ideas. Policy change more often reflects than it leads public opinion. In functioning democracies, good ideas can only change budgetary allocations and institutions if they resonate with how the public and/or the relevant elites view the world. On the other hand, how the public views the world is heavily influenced, deliberately and by default, by the current allocations and institutions: "Without a change in our way of thinking . . . there can be no impact on the environment. But without a change in the material and social environment, there can be no change in our way of thinking" (Guattari, 1992:26).

Of course, taken literally, such a view implies that change can come about only through some externally caused change in our material and social environment. A better idea can never achieve sufficient penetration, against the reality of "things as they are" and as they are correspondingly perceived and understood, to change them. We cannot lift ourselves by our own intellectual bootstraps, however hard (some of us) may think about it. But the material and social environment is changing all the time. As noted in Chapter 8, for example, the decline in rates of economic growth in the developed world has resulted in a marked increase in pressure for "new thinking" in health and health care, which may provide an opportunity for change, *even* in the United States. But the interdependence of social power structures and of ideas, the observation that whatever is actual must correspond to generally prevailing views of what is rational, is a caution against overoptimism and impatience.

It follows, therefore, that the kind of pervasive reform outlined in earlier sections will require a long and tedious process in which changes in our ways of thinking about health and medical care stimulate or support structural changes in the health care system, which in turn reinforce social changes that promote further structural reform, and so on. The barriers to reform are not only that it threatens the privileges and interests of currently dominant groups, but also that it is not supported by current ways of thinking about the relationship between medical care and health.

The dominant belief system equates medical care with health. Concretely this affects the way in which physicians are viewed, and so the circumstances in which their assistance is sought. Many people have come to see the physician as the "fixer" in society, and in this capacity they are drawn to use his or her services when they have amorphously defined and self-perceived deviations from health. Such a tendency is greatly reinforced when, as described in Chapter 4, various forms of social dysfunction or personal inadequacy become legitimized, in one's own eyes or others', when redefined as illness. (There is nothing really wrong with me, or my family, or my job, or my community; I am just temporarily "sick," and the doctor can "cure" me.) At the same time, the individual is bombarded with messages promoting health, most of which contain somewhere the advice "and see your doctor"—before beginning an exercise program, or a diet, or if symptoms persist (or if going bald).

The physician is thus faced with hopes and expectations going far beyond the restricted role of medicine outlined earlier—the alleviation of identifiable and observable "diseases." This is flattering, and in his or her interest to reinforce. But it is also frustrating since the armamentarium of medicine and the physician's training provide a much more circumscribed capability. Alternative ways of addressing the broader (nondisease) problems that may bring people into the physician's office, whether or not these are characterized as "health" problems in the WHO sense of the word, lie outside his or her control. Pointing out and encouraging these alternative approaches, even assuming that the physicians knew what they were, would make the limits of medical care explicit and thus lessen the influence and power of medicine. For some physicians, it might also seem like an admission of failure—"There is nothing I can do for you."[8]

It is also, of course, in the economic interest of the physician to reinforce the belief that medical care is the appropriate response to "whatever ails you." In a fee-for-service environment, the physician's income depends on the number of people seeking care, and the quantity of services he or she offers. And if, through processes over which most physicians have little control, the supply of physicians is being increased relative to the population, then on average each person in the population must receive more services, not less, if each physician's workload is not to fall. Public policies in all developed societies have, for most of a generation, supported a rapid increase in physician supply while trying to place limits on their fees—an exact prescription for stimulating physicians to expand their scope of activity. Nor is this pressure exclusive to fee-for-service systems. Even if physicians are reimbursed through some form of budgetary allocation, an increase in budgets to absorb increased supply must be justified in terms of "increasing per capita needs."

And behind the physician stands the drug company, and the medical equipment manufacturer, and even the biomedical researcher, all of whom depend for their incomes on expanding the scope of medical intervention. For every problem there must be a diagnosis—arrived at or confirmed through the use of ever more sophisticated and expensive equipment—and a therapy (involving, preferably, a pill, or several).[9] Thus powerful commercial interests, unconstrained by the professional ethics that may influence the physician's behaviour, place heavy and continuing pressure on physician and patient alike, to find and treat a medical problem, but also to interpret "health" in as broad terms as possible—in effect, the WHO definition. Any perceived inadequacy or unhappiness is a "health deficit," which should be treated through medical intervention, since the absence of health is obviously illness. The commodities necessary for such treatment are heavily promoted to physicians and increasingly to patients as well.

There is thus a powerful collection of interrelated economic interests encouraging both the citizen and the policymaker to continue to equate health with medical care. But there are still further obstacles to change. The alternative way of thinking, upon which a broader portfolio of societal investments in health must be built, faces problems of acceptance because it requires a focus on populations not individuals (McKinlay, 1992), on extended time frames not immediate effects (Frank and Evans, 1990), and on inter- rather than intrasectoral initiatives. In short, it is abstract, and difficult. We will discuss each of these features in turn.

The effects of environmental and social factors on health can often be observed and assessed only at the population level; for the individual they are "invisible." Public investment in a job creation programme, for example, is not seen by the previously unemployed beneficiary as a specific service tailored to meet his or her particular needs. Only a small proportion of the whole population will be employed in the program; many more may benefit through "multiplier" effects, but few of these will realize that they too are beneficiaries. They are, in any event, highly unlikely to be aware of any resulting improvements in their or their families' health (which may be long-term and nonspecific), let alone to attribute them to the public investment in job creation.

Contrast this with public investment in medical care, allowing a recipient to obtain a service tailored to personal needs and assessed for its impact on the basis of the individual benefit received. All citizens will see themselves as potential users of such tailored and tangible services. Moreover, since much illness is in fact self-limiting, a substantial proportion of encounters with the health care system will be followed by health improvement, which is likely to be attributed to the encounter. For most people, medical care is tangibly linked to health while job creation is neither provided specifically for them nor seen as affecting their health. For quite understandable reasons, the average person is led to overestimate the effects of medical care on health, and to underestimate the effects of more general social interventions. The latter can be observed at the population level; the former often cannot. But individuals observe their own experience and that of other individuals; they do not see populations.

Moreover, environmental and social factors are often slow to affect the health of a population. Enriching the circumstances of early childhood appears to pay off in health benefit many years later. Medical care, by contrast, is seen to reduce illness-related pain and anxiety in the here and now. Individuals inevitably build their models of cause and effect based on close rather than distant temporal relations (Fishbein, 1967).[10] The time frames for impact again reinforce the average citizen's view of medical care as the principal determinant of his or her health.

Finally, interventions that might have a powerful influence on health through their impact on the physical or social environment are often outside the immediate health sector, and are not designed with health effects as the primary (or even a recognized) objective. Publicly supported day care is a "women's" or an "education" issue; but it is not seen by feminists or educators as also a health issue. Bureaucracies and advocates who initiate, implement, and support such programmes will rarely use their considerable social influence to emphasize and enhance their programme's link with health. The political and governance structures in industrialized democracies lead to the formation of advocacy coalitions that are specific to particular sectors; this makes it difficult to comprehend, let alone to act upon, cause-effect linkages that extend across sectoral boundaries (Sabatier, 1987).

For example, one of the most successful health policies in the postwar era in the United States was, in fact, an energy policy. The sharp reduction in speed limits on interstate freeways following the oil crisis of the early 1970s led to a marked reduction in deaths from traffic accidents. The American people, however, continue to believe that emergency room physicians are more effective than the U.S. Energy Department in dealing with motor vehicle trauma (Tesh, 1988).

These considerations suggest why the assumption of a close causal link between medical care and health continues to dominate public understanding, and why it is so difficult to generate a new belief system that would support a broader range of social investments in population health. They also illustrate the mutually reinforcing nature of the dominant belief system, and existing institutions and patterns of resource allocation; each protects the other against threats from the continual increase in evidence that is consistent with neither. The reforms outlined in earlier sections offer a start toward changing the existing allocations and institutions so as to break out of this mutually reinforcing cycle. We conclude with some suggestions as to how to initiate parallel changes in the dominant belief system.

Information and Education

Information, and the context in which it is presented, are the nutrient upon which belief systems feed. Current information production and promulgation embody and promote the assumptions that medical care will inevitably expand, and that this is as it should be, adding to the sum total of human happiness. This is reinforced through the media, in news stories, and increasingly through commercial advertisements, with more attention given to medical advances and new technologies than to poorly nourished children or lonely elderly persons. Virtually no attention is paid to the fact that medical technologies, particularly as applied in practice, often do not live up to their promises. And yet this is a commonplace among those who specialize in technology assessment.

The public generally seem to believe that the leading causes of premature death are cancer and heart disease, and that these could be beaten if only more funding could be found for medical research and medical care services. This is, after all, the message of the experts, clinicians, and research scientists, and of the commercial organizations that market the associated commodities. And yet, on the evidence presented in earlier chapters, a more accurate message might be that the leading causes of premature death are lack of social support, poor education, and stagnant economies, and that these must be attacked by initiatives that have little or nothing to do with medical care.

This is reflected in a major imbalance in research funding in most countries, with far greater support given to research that generates information expanding the scope of medical care (i.e., the development of new therapies, drugs, and techniques) than to research into the operations and effects of the health care services themselves (i.e., the assessment of the appropriateness, organization, and even ethics of existing and new therapies). Even less support goes to exploring the nonmedical influences on health, although this is methodologically the most challenging, as well as potentially the most significant of all.

In Canada, for instance, the Medical Research Council received $221 million from the federal government in 1990/1991, a 9.7% increase over the previous year. By contrast the designated agency for funding health services research—the National Health Research and Development Programme—received one tenth that sum at $28 million, and this was a 3.2% *decrease* over the previous year. It is hardly surprising that with almost ten times the rate of production there is at least ten times as much media coverage for, and public attention to, information that reinforces the assumption of a close link between medical care and health.

And even the limited health services research that is possible with this funding "assumes that regulating expenditures for health [care] services and assessing their results are more important than achieving collective welfare or resolving conflicts between social classes" (Fox, 1990:481). What Fox calls the economizing model of research on health affairs predominates, and gives little attention to the broader determinants of health and their policy implications. Addressing the dominant belief system therefore requires changing the nature of the "health" information that is produced, with both a massive shift in funding priorities and a broader view of what constitutes policy-relevant health research.

The concern is not the complete absence of a broader "health message" flowing to the public, but rather the lack of a population focus for that health message. The calls to jog, to eat better, to stop smoking are everywhere. Nevertheless, the motivation for providing this information is the marketing and promotion of products presented as the "cure" for (or the prevention of) any number of medically defined diseases. Such marketing involves, indeed demands, the individualization and medicalization of the target problem. Individual responsibility is emphasized, the victim is blamed, and guilt can be assuaged by purchasing the health club membership or the fat-free meat. Always, however, the message is detached from its social context (Tesh, 1988; see also Chapter 9). To alleviate society's concerns about heart disease we research and market "cholesterol-free" potato chips, provide a safety net for those who can't resist anyway (with a cholesterol-reducing pill), but cheerfully leave unaddressed the stress of the workplace hierarchy or the lack of companionship and support for the widowed elderly. The "life-styles approach" comes to dominate our view of how to improve the population's health, but the "commodification" of life-styles does little to achieve this objective, producing more eager but not more discriminating consumers of an ever-expanding panoply of "medical" products.

To counteract, or at least circumvent, these seductive messages will require equally powerful vehicles that communicate the limits of professional and commercial medical care, and the scope for improved population health through broad social initiatives. At the most aggressive end of the spectrum are proposals for "subvertisements" (e.g., Mackintosh, 1993) that turn the power of marketing to noncommercial ends that might easily include breaking down the medical care—health identity. More restrained approaches involve sponsored mass media campaigns, like that used in a Swiss canton to moderate the overuse of hysterectomy by the local surgeons (Domenighetti et al., 1988), or the U.S. experience with reducing the contraindicated use of aspirin in children (Soumerai, Ross-Degnan, and Kahn, 1992). Community dialogue campaigns have become popular in Canada, under the sponsorship of such bodies as the provincial Premier's Councils on Health (Lundy, 1992). Such campaigns focus first on outlining the general determinants of the community's health and second on identifying what the community can do *in the aggregate* to improve the status of those determinants for their community. Finally, and as yet in a somewhat unplanned way, television and radio soap operas have been used as a vehicle in the United Kingdom to educate the public about broader health rather than medical care messages (Stocking, 1993).

Most physicians share the public conviction that medical care is central to human health;[11] these professional belief systems must also be addressed. This must involve the communication of two quite separate sets of ideas. The first process, focusing on the precision of medical care itself, has already begun. The growing recognition among clinicians of the importance of clinical epidemiology, which provides information on the effectiveness (or lack of it) of various medical services, is particularly significant (Berwick, 1989). Indeed, the elites within medicine are already embracing and/or accepting the power of this body of research through a commitment to practice guidelines (Brook, 1989) and "evidence-based medicine" (Evidence-based Medicine Working Group, 1992). Significant resources are being provided to medicine for the acquisition of the skills and knowledge flowing from clinical epidemiology, although such resources are still dwarfed by the more traditional expenditures on bench science and biomedical research to generate the latest cures and diagnostics.

But the improved precision of medical care itself leaves largely intact the underlying professional belief in the centrality of medical care to human health. It may be that increased professional scepticism about the effectiveness of specific clinical interventions will "spill over" into a more general concern for the relative importance of medical care as a determinant of health in populations; but it is by no means a necessary outcome of that process. Indeed, the more daunting challenge by far will be to instill in a profession that depends for its livelihood on the provision of medical care an understanding of the role of that activity in the broader context of the determinants of health.

This latter would imply a shrinking role for physicians—with obvious economic implications. Accordingly, there are concerns that medicine might use its growing understanding of clinical epidemiology not only to improve the precision of medical care, but also to medicalize other health-promoting activities and services provided by other professionals. Indeed, the tools of clinical epidemiology, and the "monopoly" within the health professions, over the clinical evaluative skills, that physicians appear to be developing, may in fact aid and abet that effort. "If you can't fight them from without, infiltrate and then swamp them from within." Few of the interventions that might influence the broader determinants of health identified above can be evaluated using the dominant methods of the clinical epidemiologist. An insistence that only the "randomized controlled trial" is a valid source of evidence will ensure that the potential of other nonmedical investments will remain suppressed.

This, of course, is no reason to oppose the incorporation of clinical evaluative skills into medicine. But it *is* a reason to ensure that opportunities to acquire and use evaluative skills appropriate to the task at hand (see, e.g., Chapter 4) are available to all programme areas that have the potential to improve the population's health. Only half the task is achieved if critical information on the effectiveness of medical care is produced but comparable information on a broad range of social and environmental interventions does not emerge.

Over the longer term, the key to changing the dominant belief systems in medicine lies in the medical school. Indeed, the present trend in medical education is to do just that by giving greater emphasis to public and community health and other population-based views in the medical curriculum (G.P.E.P. Report, 1984). And if people view the physician as the "health fixer," broadening the perspective of the physician during training may well lead to broadening the perspective of the public. Because it exploits the current pattern of health-seeking behaviour this might also have potential as part of an effective public education strategy. However, it also presents the dangers both of filtering the public's education through a continued emphasis on medical care and of widening the scope (and resource claim) of medical practice well beyond its disease alleviation role.

Medical schools will face other challenges from the significant evaluative role envisaged in the new model of medical self-regulation. This role implies a much greater responsibility for physicians to monitor and assess their own activities, and those of their colleagues and of their profession. The responsibility for providing both the skills in evaluation, and the necessary base of evidence, logically rests with the faculties of health sciences. But they are unlikely to accept these new roles with any enthusiasm, or perform them effectively, under existing modes of medical school funding. Modes of funding will have to be introduced that are more compatible with these training, evaluation, and educational roles (Barer and Stoddart, 1991).

In the more distant future, medical schools also may be pressured to take on some of the responsibility for dealing with any physician surplus that may result from a more circumscribed role for medicine. "Retooling" of existing physicians might be one function that medical schools could perform, simultaneously taking some of the surplus stock temporarily out of practice, finding a substitute activity for the reduction in undergraduate training, and improving the match between the medical care needs of the public and the physician's skills (Barer and Stoddart, 1991; Wennberg, 1992). Furthermore, the medical school is a potentially powerful and credible source of information for the public. Education of the public about the determinants of health, and the place of medical care in the broader context, would be an appropriate function for one of the principal institutions through which the profession should be accountable to the rest of society (Evans, 1973).

Government policy, public regulation, and, given the correct incentives, medical self-regulation can only proceed under assumptions and beliefs that roughly match those of the public. Effectively presenting the public with the evidence we now have on the limits to medicine and the potential of other investments in health may be the most important element in any strategy to uncouple the medical care–health identity. McGuire (1990) has commented that the objectives of our public investments in health care "are bound to change, to reflect the dynamic elements contained in [public] attitudes and expectations" (p. 97). Perhaps the most effective way to harmonise the objectives of both the medical profession and governments would be to have them both struggling to respond to a public understanding that health is more than medical care.

ACKNOWLEDGMENTS

We are indebted to our colleagues in the Population Health Programme of the Canadian Institute for Advanced Research, as well as to those in the Polinomics Research Group of the Centre for Health Economics and Policy Analysis, for comments on an earlier draft. Support to the first author is provided by the Ontario Ministry of Health through a career scientist award.

NOTES

1. While this and the previous chapter focus primarily on the role of medical care as provided by physicians, the observation about limits to the potential of medical care to improve health applies more generally to other types of health care. For example, concerns similar to those reviewed in Chapter 9 have been raised about pharmaceutical use, services provided by other health care practitioners, and long-term institutionalization.

2. *Precision* is used here to underline the need to relate inputs (medical care resources) to the desired output (health). Improved precision means a more direct and demonstrable link between medical care activity and improved health outcomes.

3. Of course, this analogy is imperfect because the auditor general is professionally independent of those (s)he reviews. The challenge, then, will be for a profession to review its performance in a manner consistent with the intent of an independent external audit. This has never been done before (which does not mean that it cannot be done).

4. In mixed public/private systems, costly procedures impose a heavy burden on the uninsured patients who can pay; for those who cannot, the bills become the uncollectible accounts so familiar to physicians and hospitals of the preinsurance era. In those days the physician often faced the unenviable choice of imposing severe financial hardship on his or her patient, or working in effect

for free (and perhaps committing his or her hospital and colleagues to the same charitable sacrifice), or simply not recommending expensive procedures to those without the means.

5. Illness without known remedy may be a misfortune, but is not a need for care.

6. It is often assumed that greater sensitivity to local values is a good thing in and of itself. This is not necessarily so. A small community may well have shared values that are in conflict with those of the wider society of which the community is a part. The capture of hospital boards by antiabortion groups, in the face of provincial legislation guaranteeing access, is a clear case in point. This is quite separate from the issue of majority rule; a majority of the members of a small community may be anti-abortionists. But rights and entitlements assigned by the wider community must not be withdrawn by one's next-door neighbours.

7. For example, one may, in response to the World Health Organization definitions or through personal introspection, wish to embrace the idea that health is more than the absence of illness. One may then extend the term to include any number of aspects of the well-lived life, although as indicated earlier (especially Chapters 2 and 8) we believe that the advantages of doing so are questionable.

8. For that matter, there may not be anything *anyone* can do. Insofar as the patient's "diseases" may be expressions of problems in the social or physical environment, perhaps at some time in the past, there may be no "alternative ways" to health now available. And even if there are, they may not be available to the individual patient, or the physician. How do these two "change the social environment"? And can one develop "coping skills" in mid- or late life? Recall the concept of biological windows in the life of the individual, discussed in Chapter 3. For the population as a whole, it may make sense to consider alternative pathways to health; but for this distressed person in the physician's office, and this physician facing him or her, the only option may be medical care—even if it does not work.

9. Or there will be soon, if only sufficient funding is found for the necessary research.

10. This psychological tendency to retain and be influenced by inferred causes and effects occurring in short temporal cycles is paralleled and reinforced by the pressures of political cycles—"a week is a long time in politics," and policies with costs in the present and benefits beyond the next election may benefit only the opposition.

11. There has, however, always been a tradition of healthy scepticism within the profession itself. Indeed, some of the most articulate and thoughtful commentaries on the limits of medical care have come from physicians (e.g., Thomas McKeown, William Osler, Lewis Thomas, Fraser Mustard, John Wennberg).

IV

11

Social Proprioception:[1] *Measurement, Data, and Information from a Population Health Perspective*

M. C. WOLFSON

I. WHY THINK ABOUT HEALTH INFORMATION?

Preceding chapters have emphasized the power and importance both of information and of its absence. Reliable and valid data are essential to a better understanding of the basic determinants of health.[2] They are also important in understanding how institutions and individuals operate in the health domain, and they are crucial to the effective management of these institutions. As the WHO puts it, "The road leading to health for all by the year 2000 passes through information."

The fundamental importance of data is well accepted in domains as diverse as the physical sciences, economics, demography, and business. Consider the following examples:

• research proposals that are devoted simply to observation and measurement are well funded in the physical sciences (e.g., astro- and high-energy physics);

• the monthly and quarterly movements in major economic indicators like unemployment, inflation, and GDP are regular headline news;

• organized and regular collection of data on population size, growth, composition, and geographic dispersion is by now a universal activity in developed societies; and

- very sophisticated inventory control and financial management information systems are essential to the operation of modern businesses, while the marketplace has evolved comprehensive and generally standardized financial information.

By comparison, data and information on health and health care are more often unreliable, fragmentary, imbalanced, and incoherent. And information of poor quality has costs. The public is bombarded with allegedly health-related information, but much of it is confusing, disturbing, and often misleading or flatly false. Examples include dietary nostrums, the latest cancer risks and cures, news of strikes by health professionals, and waiting lists for surgery or other treatments. In response, much of health policy appears to be in a "crisis management" mode. Citizens, health professionals, the media, and governments are all distracted from recognizing and addressing more fundamental concerns.

Many improvements are needed in health information systems. In this chapter, we single out three strands of development as of particular importance, aiming at the following widely accepted goals:

- to know the levels, trends, and distributions of health (in its many aspects) in human populations;
- to understand the determinants of these different aspects of health; and
- to allocate resources effectively for improving health.

There is a fundamental imbalance between the availability and comprehensiveness of data describing the resources used by health care systems, and the minimal and scattered data on the state of health of the populations they serve. Redressing this imbalance requires the development of a spectrum of reliable measures of health status and health outcomes, including summary measures that will be meaningful to the general public. Only with such information can resources be effectively and efficiently allocated to maintaining and improving health.[3]

Second, there is a serious gap between two "data solitudes." On the one hand, large and growing administrative databases on individuals' utilization of health care services provide a "doctor's- or provider's-eye view" of diagnoses and treatments. On the other hand, there is increasing recognition of the validity and importance of individuals' self-reported information on their health-related problems, and the relation of those problems to their socioeconomic and cultural situation. Such individual-level data have rarely been collected, and still more rarely linked with the former, though this is changing in Canada with the recent development of national and provincial population health surveys. As pointed out in Chapter 4, however, quantitative data even at the individual level cannot be interpreted in isolation from more descriptive information on their cultural context.

Finally, the diversity and complexity of information pertinent to health cries out for a coherent and intuitively plausible organizing structure. A "system of health statistics" might both capture the current state of theory in the health domain and provide a framework for health information. Such a "health information template" can serve as a pedagogical device, a comprehensive classification system, and a means to highlight gaps in our current range of data and collection systems. Such a system of health statistics, and its associated template, could become for health information what the System of National Accounts is for economic information.

Of course, there are many other needed improvements to health information, as well as important impediments to the realization of the three strands of development just singled out. Some of these other topics will be mentioned, though we shall argue in this chapter that these three strands are strategically most important.

Health care statistics in Canada are as well-developed as anywhere in the world. Yet they illustrate very clearly the shortcomings just identified. We will use the Canadian situation as an exemplar in what follows, recognizing in doing so that the problems are common to all developed countries.

We begin with a brief critical overview of the current state of Canadian health-related information from the perspectives of its major users and uses. This is followed by a sketch of the three strategic approaches for improving Canada's health information system. Health information presupposes, of course, systems of measurement, sources of data, and organizations of analysts. While the ultimate need is for appropriate health information, the other items are prerequisites.

II. MAJOR USERS AND USES OF HEALTH INFORMATION

A. In Relation to Health Goals

The importance of health information is illustrated in the recent official statements of health goals in a number of jurisdictions. *Orientations—Improving Health and Well-Being in Quebec* (Quebec Government, 1989), for example, stated the primary goals (p. 19) as:

add years to life by reducing mortality from disease and injury;
add health to life by reducing disabilities and acting on various health factors;

> *add well-being to life* by promoting the optimal use of functional capacity, whether total or partial, and by decreasing the impact of problems that compromise the stability, self-fulfillment and autonomy of individuals.

The Quebec document goes on to express these goals in a number of more specific quantitative and subordinate objectives, and then sets out specific policy and program initiatives whose implementation would be expected to attain them. Data and information are clearly fundamental to this exercise. The subordinate objectives must be stated in measurable terms; otherwise one cannot observe the degree of progress or retrogression. Furthermore, the policy choices require as well at least some knowledge of the causal pathways that connect a given intervention with its health effects.[4]

B. Audiences for Health Information

A commitment to explicit health goals is one source of pressure for better health information, but there are others. Consider the wide range of audiences for or users of such information, and the specific kinds of health information they require. While obviously not exhaustive, the list below indicates both the diversity of information required, and the range of relevant actors.

Provincial Ministers and Deputy Ministers of Health

In Canada, this group, along with their senior officials, has the largest stake in health information. They have formal responsibility for the massive health care industry, and at the same time at least nominal responsibility for health. (Nominal, because an overwhelming proportion of health ministry budgets is devoted to financing and managing health care. Canada's health policy primarily supports a "sickness care system," whose activities are assumed to result in health, notwithstanding the substantial evidence that the determinants of health go far beyond health care.)

Ideally, ministers and their deputies would begin with measures of population health status. This is the proper basis for evaluating all their activities. Yet such measures are almost completely absent from the Canadian health information landscape.[5] Population health status could be measured by regular surveys and summarized in one overall index like the GDP or the CPI. This index would be measured consistently over time and could be broken down by region or population group. Indeed, consistent health status measures could in principle be available all the way down to the level of the populations served by individual hospitals. These would form part of the continuing "outcomes management" process (Ellwood, 1988).

We appreciate that such an index would inevitably require simplifications of concept and measurement. But the impact it could have in refocusing the attention of decision-makers as well as providers and the general public to more appropriate objectives more than outweighs, we believe, any such concerns. After all, economic statistics are far from perfect for their designed purposes, and much less so for their actual uses in the public arena. Yet no one suggests that we would be better off without them. The best should not be the enemy of the good.

In view of the very large share of GDP and provincial budgets devoted to health care, health ministries could also be expected to have detailed management information on the resources being consumed. These systems could provide not only conventional accounting data, which they do moderately well at present, but could also provide the basis for continuous monitoring of quality and effectiveness, information almost totally absent now. Given the range of institutions delivering health care—from private offices and community health clinics to teaching hospitals—this information should use concepts and definitions common across delivery modes, institutions, and provinces. The diffusion of new medical practices and technologies requires particular attention to ensure consistent treatment.

Other Line Government Agencies

Many government policies and activities outside ministries of health nonetheless have health effects. Motor vehicle safety regulation, food policy, workers' compensation boards, environmental regulations, and social services come quickly to mind. They would all be included in a comprehensive system of health information, in a way that highlights their importance for health, relative to health care as conventionally defined. Such information is, unfortunately, extremely limited at present.

General Public

Life-styles clearly affect health. Telling people that smoking is bad for them may not directly cause them to quit. But knowing that smoking is unhealthy is a prerequisite for the many efforts to induce smokers to stop, or at least to restrict their activities. Similarly, there is a very wide range of health information that the public might sensibly use. This includes avoidable risk factors (e.g., dietary elements, household radon, motor vehicle safety features), assurances of product quality (e.g., implantable medical devices, drugs, food safety), and the scope of appropriate self-care.

Such information is now available to the public to a limited extent, but there are two main problems. First, much important information remains highly speculative or unknown. This is perhaps most apparent in the rapid swings among dietary fads and the difficulties governments have in developing consensus guidelines (e.g., cholesterol). The second is that relatively small efforts are put into disseminating the available unbiased information—as compared, for example, to the volume of promotional advertising by food, drug, and other manufacturers.

Managers of Health Care Delivery Institutions

The major examples here are hospital managers. Like provincial ministries of health, they require basic accounting information, though at a much finer level of detail. In addition, automated information systems can assist in the process of patient management and tracking, and are being adopted gradually. Finally, there is a clear need for information for outcomes management, quality assurance, and utilization review. At the institutional level, as in the wider system, we have at present far more data on the resources used in care than on the health benefits produced.

Physicians

Physicians are at the centre of many of the information flows pertinent to health. Many of the services they provide are primarily informational —diagnosing, advising, and prescribing. In the process they draw on a large volume of their own information, most of it acquired in medical school and stored in their human memories. This situation raises two major concerns. First, virtually all the informational transactions are individual to individual. As a result, experience is accumulated at best anecdotally and piecemeal, with all the attendant risks of incomplete and biased impressions. Second, the total available volume of medical information is growing at an extraordinary rate; even with specialization, the human brain simply cannot retain more than a small fraction of it.

These two factors clearly limit the range, accuracy, and currency of the information that any physician can bring to bear on the health problems of a given patient. But there are many impediments to improving this situation, not least the difficulty of altering physicians' attitudes toward their roles. It is hard to reconcile the role of "healer" with all its deeply rooted, almost magical connotations, with that of the skilled retriever and scientific analyst of data. But physicians are coming to see the benefits of automated patient charts, including histories, referrals, and prescriptions. They could also benefit from the broader statistical and epidemiological analysis that is possible with the routine collection and consolidation of data on physicians' diagnoses and services. The willing cooperation of individual clinicians is obviously essential to this process.

Community Agencies

Local agencies other than hospitals are typically not powerful players in the health arena. However, almost every province has a recent major report or study that recommends an increased role for local communities in shaping health policies and programs. The assumptions that underlie these recommendations are in line with many of the arguments made in earlier chapters about the broader determinants of health. But they include a further assumption, that decisions made at local levels will reflect better trade-offs among a wider range of policy instruments, for example inpatient care versus social services for the elderly. Unfortunately, data and information on which to base these trade-offs are virtually nonexistent. (Nor do we, or the authors of these reports, know whether local decision-makers will in fact make these trade-offs differently.)

A great deal of research and analysis is required to support the information needs listed above, and this should be made explicit. These tasks range from developing the foundations for an overall index of population health, to explicating the relevant factors in the causal pathways shown in Figure 2.5. They clearly require far more health information than we have at present, or probably will ever have. But even to begin developing the appropriate information requires basic reorientations in our approaches to data collection. In particular, "longitudinal multivariate microdata" (i.e., data that record the characteristics or experiences of individuals, followed over time, that can then be linked together) are essential. They are generally not available. The incremental costs of producing such data, especially given the likely evolution of health care administrative data systems, need not be great—if these developments are anticipated and planned.

There are clearly many other actors in the health area, and many other health information needs. But any health information system that can respond to the needs outlined to this point will in the process be able to meet many other health information needs. Our sketch has highlighted major gaps in information, which give rise to major social costs. We are at present unable to assess realistically the health impact of our health care system. Nor have we the information base for allocating health resources more effectively.

III. THREE STRATEGIC DEVELOPMENTS

An exhaustive discussion of the vast range of improvements needed in health information is beyond the scope of this chapter. We have chosen instead to identify and describe three particular directions for advance in health information:

- developing an overall measure of population health status as part of a family of health status and outcome measures,
- extending and merging administrative and self-report data systems, and
- creating a template and system for health information.

These developments are very important in their own right. But we believe that creating the data collection systems and information infrastructures that they require will also have major spin-offs: they will provide many of the ingredients to meet health information needs that would appear in any comprehensive listing.

A. Overall Measures of Health Status

Taken in total, the health information now available is as we noted above seriously imbalanced. Statistical compendia are dominated by measures of health care activities and the resources they use (financial outlays, bed-days, pounds of laundry, physician visits). The most common measures of Canadians' "health status" are actually their death status—infant mortality and life expectancy—and these are the only measures available over time. There is very little information on how we feel or function while we are alive.

This imbalance is pervasive. The lack of health status data at the level of individual patient stays in hospitals, for example, means that we cannot identify the effects of various surgical procedures, let alone whether they are being performed appropriately (see Chapter 8).[6] At the other end of the spectrum, the absence of health status data at the national level means that we do not have a solid statistical basis for judging whether the health of the Canadian population is generally improving,[7] let alone for setting the relative priorities for allocating resources to acute care, chronic care, social services, or early childhood interventions.

The need for reliable and systematic measures of health outcomes at the level of individual patient contacts with the health care system is increasingly recognized (e.g., Ellwood, 1988). "Quality assurance" and "outcomes management" are common phrases to describe the processes appropriate to the management of health care. Both are premised on the ability to measure health outcomes.

It is essential, we believe, that outcome measures also be extended to cover large population groups. We noted above that those responsible for the management of our overall health care system—and the public to whom they are accountable—could begin to measure their effectiveness through an overall aggregate index of population health. This kind of index might at first be simply an interesting and novel social indicator, published each year and reported in the popular media in the same way as are such summary economic indicators as the growth rate of GDP, the rate of inflation in the CPI, and the unemployment rate.

Such a summary population health index could also become the object of policy interest. Politicians would support initiatives that they could plausibly claim would increase it. Vested interests would defend their current budget claims and programs on the grounds that they contribute importantly to the increase over time in the population health index. Such uses of the index might well be self-serving, but would in fact be desirable to the extent the index measured what it purported to measure. In any case, the index would tend to focus attention more on health than on health care.[8]

But is it presently feasible to generate such an overall population health status index, satisfying basic requirements of plausibility and reliability? We believe that the answer is clearly "yes"; and to make the argument we will sketch out the way in which such an index might be constructed.

At the outset, of course, it is necessary to recognize that such an index (and a fortiori our preliminary sketch) will not be methodologically ideal. But without wishing to denigrate other statistical efforts, we would simply ask that no higher standards be demanded of a proposed new population health status measure than are met by statistical indicators that are widely accepted at present. Consider, for example, such indicators as GDP, the inflation rate, the TSE 300, municipal air pollution indices, average family incomes, the profits of the Fortune 500, or the probability of precipitation in the weather forecast. All these measures are useful—and used—despite their flaws. By these methodological standards, an acceptable overall measure of population health is certainly feasible.

The construction of an aggregate population health index begins with the level of health of an individual, defined at an instant or preferably averaged over a period of time such as a year. There are, of course, many definitions of health, but the most popularly used concept is the absence of health problems (Blaxter, 1988). Many efforts have been made to structure health problems in a clear and popularly accessible way (Rosser and Kind, 1978; Sintonen, 1982; Torrance, 1987); and a reasonable approach has been adopted for the 1990 Ontario Health Survey, and the 1991 General Social Survey for Canada.

These two surveys both include a set of eight questions on distinct dimensions of health status: mobility, dexterity, hearing, seeing, speech, cognition, emotion, and pain. For each dimension, the respondent's status is determined at one of several levels, in most cases six. This set of dimensions and levels, drawing on work by Torrance (1987), spans most of people's health problems, albeit in a manner more vernacular than clinical. A mapping for the full range of possible responses into an index number between zero and one (more technically, a multiattribute utility function) is currently being developed.[9] Based on these surveys and the forthcoming value scales, we should soon have available a sophisticated summary index of an individual's health status at a point in time, aggregated from a broad range of dimensions of health, and with baseline values measured for a representative sample of the population.

The simplest health status index for the whole population would then be an average of the individual indices for everyone in the survey. This would be comparable, for example, to "average family income"—the most often quoted statistic from household income surveys. This simple average is not, however, the best measure for monitoring trends over time. Since most people's health status deteriorates with age, an increasing average age in the population will tend to reduce the aggregate measure of population health status over time. The measure might be accurate—an older population will indeed be less healthy on average—but could be misleading if in fact the average health status at each age were constant or even improving modestly. An age-standardized average would thus be more informative for a broad determination of whether or not the population's health status was improving (though less so for service planning).[10]

Such survey data permit one to pose and answer "what if" questions with powerful implications. For example, statistics on the distribution of average family incomes have made it possible to measure the redistributive impact of present income taxes and government transfer programs. One simply compares the actual distribution of disposable income to what it would have been without the taxes and transfers. A more detailed exercise serves to evaluate the expected impact of changes to tax and transfer structures.

We can imagine asking similar questions about the way in which overall population health status would change if one could eliminate certain specific problems suffered by the elderly, or a specific dimension of health status like problems of physical mobility. This information is being calculated from the data that are anticipated from the Ontario Health Survey, and the Canadian General Social Survey.[11]

For example, a hypothetical study based on the forthcoming Canadian National Population Health Survey might result in a mid-1990s publication with the following highlights: "Average health status of Canadians was 82.7 percent [where 100 percent would indicate that all residents were in full health on each of the eight major dimensions noted above]. This is 0.3 percent higher than reported in 1990 in the last survey. For those over age sixty-five, average health status was 68.3 percent. . . . If the elderly had not suffered at all from mobility impairments, their health status would have averaged 79.1 percent. . . . Over two-thirds of these mobility impairments were associated with arthritis and other musculoskeletal diseases." These kinds of results are straightforward given the survey data described, and easy to explain. The time trends may, however, be influenced by changing age structure and differential mortality, as noted above.

An alternative way to present this information on average health status and its distribution would be in terms of life expectancies. One could imagine the hypothetical health survey report continuing as follows: "Life expectancy for women is currently 82.2 years. However, adjusting for average observed deviations from full health at each age reduces this to 74.4 years of *healthy* life expectancy. Most of the 7.8 year difference occurs after age 65. . . . A more detailed analysis reveals that limb and joint disorders have three times as great an impact on this healthy life expectancy as all cancers combined."[12]

This hypothetical report could also break the results down by geographic region. The data might support statements along the following lines: "This national average health-status-adjusted life expectancy masks substantial geographic variations. Average health-status-adjusted life expectancy in the healthiest communities was on average 5.7 years higher than in the least healthy.[13] Notably, there was no significant correlation between the average health-status-adjusted life expectancy for a community, and selected health care service utilization measures such as coronary artery bypass graft surgery. However, the healthier communities tended to have a smaller proportion of divorced individuals, higher average family incomes, and lower unemployment rates."

This hypothetical conclusion is deliberately provocative. It might turn out that health-status-adjusted life expectancies did correlate with health care use.[14] The point is that with these kinds of data and analyses, we could answer such crucial questions. Regular publication of results such as these might have a salutary impact on the character of public debate about health care and health policy.

Population health status expressed in terms of health-status-adjusted life expectancy has some of the same characteristics as an ordinary average of individual health values. Both approaches permit one to disaggregate the overall figure by age and sex group, such that the components average or add up to the value for the whole population. And given sufficiently rich underlying data on the correlates of less-than-full health, variations in either measure can be allocated across major "causes" or sources of ill-health (e.g., musculoskeletal disease) in an arithmetically consistent manner.

But the life expectancy form has in addition at least three key advantages over the usual survey averages. First, it implicitly abstracts from changes in age structure, so age standardization is not required. Second, it immediately places morbidity or health status in the same framework as mortality. This allows direct comparisons of life-prolonging and life-improving interventions. The goals of "adding years to life" and "adding life to years" (to paraphrase the Quebec Orientations report cited above) can be encompassed in the same measure.

Finally, the life expectancy concept can encompass a longitudinal perspective, although the average values currently in use are essentially cross-sectional measures.[15] There is overwhelming evidence that a person's health status today is importantly correlated with a very broad range of factors in an individual's history, perhaps decades earlier. Conventional risk factors such as smoking have long been known to operate over many years; more recently discovered associations such as the influence in later adult life of early childhood environment have been noted in earlier chapters. It is clearly desirable to build health status measures that can absorb and reflect back such longitudinal dynamics.

These benefits of summary measures of population health status, expressed as life expectancies, currently come at the cost of some methodological restrictions and challenges. At present, health-status-adjusted generalizations of life expectancy—such as "disability-free life expectancy" (e.g., Robine, 1986)—are computed using conventional life table methods. But these methods generally cannot take account of information on multivariate and/or lagged relationships between risk factors and diseases, such as those just noted.

Popular life table-based measures such as PYLL (potential years of life lost) and cause-deleted life expectancy have been used to indicate the relative importance of various causes of death, such as cancer and cardiovascular disease (e.g., Nagnur and Nagrodski, 1987). However, in their current incarnations, these measures embody mechanical and unrealistic assumptions about disease progression. For example, the increment in life expectancy that results from simply deleting lung cancer as a cause of death is completely oblivious to the fact that the large majority of lung cancers are attributable to smoking. Hence, in a more realistic scenario, these lung cancer deaths would only disappear with the disappearance of smoking. But this in turn would result in a large diminution of coronary heart disease deaths.

Fortunately, there is a generalization of the life table methodology that does not suffer from these limitations. Microsimulation methods can easily incorporate multivariate lagged relationships, as well as quite detailed descriptions of risk factor, disease, and functional health status dynamics. POHEM (for *po*pulation *he*alth *m*odel; Wolfson, 1992a) is an application of this method, permitting the computation of an overall measure of health-status-adjusted life expectancy for national or regional populations.

In a life table, the smallest unit of analysis is a group of people, for example everyone who is female and age seventy-eight. This implicitly imposes a strong assumption of homogeneity—everyone in each age-sex group is exactly the same, for example, being exposed to exactly the same mortality rates. In contrast, microsimulation takes individuals as the basic unit. In POHEM, for example, each individual is followed from birth to death. Individuals are permitted to vary in a number of respects—some may smoke, drink too much, and/or be overweight—according to patterns observed in population surveys or hypothetical policy simulations. This in turn will influence their risks of contracting lung cancer (typically with at least a ten-year lag) and coronary heart disease (depending on a combination of other risk factors like hypertension). POHEM generates a representative sample (say one hundred thousand) of such complete life paths, including information not only on risk factors and diseases, but also on health status along the lines discussed above. Health-status-adjusted life expectancies for each individual are then aggregated by POHEM to produce population health expectancy, or PHE.

PHE is not only an aggregate index; it is a coherent family of indices. Just as the all-items CPI (consumer price index) can be broken down into a CPI for food and another for shelter, PHE can be disaggregated by age, sex, level of morbidity, type of disease, and risk factor. In addition, the POHEM framework can incorporate data on the use of health care resources and their costs, and thereby provide a way of computing "cost of illness" estimates as in Rice, Hodgson, and Kopstein (1985) or Hartunian, Smart, and Thompson (1981). Further, given data on the costs and effectiveness of various health care procedures, POHEM provides a means to produce population-based estimates of the total costs and benefits (in terms of increased health-status-adjusted life expectancy or PHE) of the procedure.

Finally, a methodology like POHEM provides bridges linking data collection and analysis with the users of information. By interposing an analytical framework that is realized as a microsimulation model, we shift away from the conventional view of summary statistical indicators.

In that conventional view, statistical agencies collect myriad tiny data points, which are simply summed or averaged, and then emitted as partial aggregates in a print publication of tables. It is left to analysts in universities, businesses, and policy advisory groups within government to digest and interpret the results.

The POHEM approach is quite different: It could be disseminated as a carefully designed combination of data and analytical software. Provincial or local users could augment POHEM with their own regional data. This offers a more integrated, detailed, and multivariate level of communication between the statistical agency that has developed POHEM and information users. It also offers the potential for more two-way communication. In the Canadian context, provincial ministries could become both major users of such an analytical framework and major suppliers of data inputs.

Indeed international organizations like WHO, OECD, and the UN, as well as different national governments, could use the framework of the POHEM model and insert their own national data. Health-status-adjusted life expectancy indices could thus be computed in an internationally comparable manner using a common methodological framework, [as the World Bank (1993) has most recently done] making possible very powerful comparative analyses.

To summarize, there is a fundamental need for aggregate health status and outcome measures. This need can be met with the more extensive data from population health surveys now being carried out, linked with the increasingly available administrative data for whole populations, and integrated and expressed through a new class of sophisticated life expectancy constructs such as PHE estimated using microsimulation methods as in POHEM. Development of each of the critical elements is now either in process or has been successfully completed. Such a framework will be strategically important for at least the following reasons:

- It will require agreement on a standard set of measures (i.e., concepts and definitions) of health status, and will thus provide a common basis for analysis in many other areas such as quality assurance, technology assessment, and community health.
- It will require regular and broadly based measurement of health status, and thereby provide raw data that can be used for many purposes in addition to aggregation into summary measures.
- It can readily use and will be strengthened by longitudinal data, especially the "natural history" or patterns of progression of disease and disability, thereby encouraging the development and use of such data.
- It opens the question of the relative efficacy of alternative health

and health care interventions, thereby encouraging more rigorous and systematic evaluation.

B. Merging Administrative and Self-Report Data

1. *The Two Solitudes*

In general, quantitative (as opposed to qualitative—see Chapter 4) data on the health of individuals can be derived from either of two quite different sources. One is self-report, principally via household surveys. The other is "contact report" from the administrative systems used to oversee the delivery of products and services or to pay for them. In Canada the latter source includes (but is by no means confined to) the itemized claims for payment submitted by fee-for-service physicians to provincial ministries of health, and the reports submitted by hospitals, which record individual episodes of patient care—inpatient separations and ambulatory visits and procedures. Both forms of data are inadequate to meet the health information needs we have outlined. The situation in Canada may be unique, however, in the tremendous potential that these two sources can offer *in combination*, and at relatively low incremental cost.

To appreciate this potential, it is important to understand the current state of affairs, both the data now available and the major changes that now appear likely. There are three main forms of data that deserve consideration:

- administrative data on patients;
- resource accounting for hospitals and other institutions; and
- population surveys.

At present, data on hospital inpatient stays are routinely captured in a standard machine-readable format—the separation abstract.[16] These abstracts include the patient's age, sex, postal code, diagnoses at separation, and procedures undergone. Computerized records for about 80 percent of all separations are sent by hospitals directly to the Canadian Institute for Health Information (CIHI) for cross-tabular and comparative analyses. At the provincial level, virtually 100 percent of these records, whether or not they pass through (CIHI), are assembled into a comprehensive file maintained by the provincial ministry of health. These files are also transmitted to Statistics Canada, though with a considerably longer lag.

Unfortunately, for most provinces, these separation records are isolated documents. They cannot readily be linked for a single individual over time, to show a pattern of multiple separations from different hospitals. Manitoba, Saskatchewan, and British Columbia are notable exceptions.

Similarly, all provinces have almost complete records of all the services received by every patient from every fee-for-service physician, which determine the reimbursement of each physician. These claims files record data on the identity of the physician and the patient, and the procedures or consultations for which the physician has billed. But again, in many provinces these records cannot easily be linked to form histories of patient contacts with different physicians, or with the hospital separation abstract files of that individual. It is being increasingly recognized—not just by researchers but also by provincial officials—that *patient-* rather than only *service*-oriented data are essential to many important kinds of health care analysis and evaluation (e.g., Roos, 1989). Thus, it appears probable that over the next five years most provinces will be in a position to produce patient-linked files of hospital, physician, and other health care use.

Even if this evolution continues as anticipated, however, these administrative files will still have serious inadequacies as sources of health status information. They are primarily records of what was done, rather than why, or with what result. The *performance* of a lab test or diagnostic procedure, for example, is recorded on a hospital separation abstract or in a physician claim, but the *findings* are not. The diagnostic information on hospital separation abstracts, and in some provinces on physician claims, takes one somewhat closer to the actual circumstances of the patient, but one is still required to infer health status from information collected and reported for other purposes.

Moreover, the coverage of these administrative data, even of contacts and procedures, is not wholly complete, and could become less so. The reporting of ambulatory care provided by hospitals is inconsistent from province to province, and has significant gaps. If no fee is claimed for the service—hospitals are not paid on a fee-for-service basis but on global budgets—and if the patient is not an inpatient, then there will be neither a physician billing nor a hospital separation abstract, and the service may not be recorded at all. This problem will become more severe if health care delivery shifts toward modes where physicians are receiving salaries, and health care procedures are carried out in institutions other than hospitals. Both of these trends are evident in recent provincial health care policy initiatives.

Special attention will have to be paid to ensuring that the comprehensiveness of the present reporting systems is not degraded, and indeed is enhanced. But because these data are a census of all (of a very large class of) health care visits, cost and database size pressures will push administrators toward minimizing the range of data captured for each record. To counter this natural tendency, the advocates of more and better information will have to see that its benefits are clearly expressed and understood—and that they materialize.

The second main strand of development is the generation of comprehensive information on the resource costs of specific diagnostic and therapeutic manoeuvres, and on episodes of care, both ambulatory and particularly institutional. Until quite recently, while institutions maintained detailed accounting information on the quantity and costs of the various resources they used—person-hours, equipment, supplies—they had little or no idea what were the required inputs and costs associated with the treatment of any particular patient, or even class of patients. They could not cost out their products, or compare those costs with other institutions.

This seems to be true of most national systems of hospital care, with the prominent exception of the United States. But even there, the detailed patient-specific "costs" that form the basis for billing have been described by some commentators as simply a cumulation of very detailed itemized charges that until recently bore no close relation to actual costs—the latter being, in truth, unknown.

A standardized set of hospital resource use protocols has been developed over the past decade in Canada as part of the MIS (management information system) project jointly supported by Statistics Canada, the Canadian Hospital Association, and Health and Welfare Canada. These protocols are gradually being adopted by hospitals, at least at what is called the "departmental" level. At this level, the system provides well-defined and consistent total costs by type of resource consumed and by major department of a hospital, for example surgery or diagnostic imaging.

Moreover, at the "global" level of implementation, the MIS system will be able to provide average unit costs for all the various kinds of medical and diagnostic procedures applied, as well as other hospital activities. This level of data, at least for all the largest hospitals, and a sample of smaller hospitals and other health care institutions such as nursing homes, will probably be generated during the next five years. Such "unit cost" data are essential to any rigorous effectiveness evaluations of health care interventions. It will also be necessary, however, to trace these unit costs to the individual patients being cared for. While there are at present no general plans to carry out this linkage, and thus identify inter alia each institution's average costs for looking after particular classes of patients, this seems to be an obvious next step. It will certainly occur to the provincial ministries, which provide hospital budgets.

Finally, there has been a recent and significant increase in interest in population health surveys in Canada. After the 1978 Canada Health Survey, there was a hiatus of almost a decade in large-scale household interview surveys. The main recent surveys are the 1985 module in the (telephone) General Social Survey, the 1986 postcensal survey on disabilities, and the 1987 Quebec and 1990 Ontario health surveys. There have also been a number of more focused surveys on such topics as smoking, health promotion, and fitness. The Government of Canada has recently approved permanent multimillion dollar funding for a biennial National Population Health Survey. This survey will include a set of core population health status measures along the lines described earlier. In addition, the survey will be longitudinal. Thus, it can provide the foundation for a family of summary health indices as proposed earlier.

2. *Integration Possibilities*

If the three strands of data development just outlined unfold along the lines suggested, they will represent an extraordinary improvement in the breadth, depth, and quality of useful data pertinent to health research and policy analysis.

What we want to emphasize, however, is that while these major efforts are already under way, and will establish a much sounder basis for health policy, their usefulness can be very greatly enhanced by relatively modest investments to bring these three components together. Especially if this integration is planned for now rather than five years hence, it can yield major analytical and information benefits—at minimal additional cost.

The basic idea is that the emerging patient-oriented administrative files not only represent a major advance in health information on their own, but they can also be used as a relatively complete register, almost a census, of health care contacts. The MIS system (to the extent it is adopted at the "global" level) would then provide average unit costs for each kind of health care contact or procedure, which could be linked with the patient-specific files to yield "trajectories" of individual costs as well as service use. In addition, current work on health personnel databases could allow the characteristics of the physician or other provider to be linked to the individual patient experience.

Finally, instead of drawing population samples as a completely separate process, for example, based on a sample frame derived from the population census, samples could be drawn from the frame provided by the patient administrative files. In this way, self-report, doctor/provider-report, and health care resource use information could all be assembled for a sample of individuals for purposes of multivariate analysis. In addition, the samples could be specially designed and drawn for health-related questions, not restricted to geographic stratifications as at present.

A further possibility, with existing hardware and software technology, is to add sampling and data capture as "on-line" capabilities of evolving administrative health care data systems. An individual's ID could be noted as part of a given sample for a specified time period. Then, whenever there was a "transaction" by that individual with selected components of the health care system, a prespecified set of questions could be posed via the on-line device (typically a PC). These questions might be administered to the individual and answers captured by the nurse in a physician's office, or answered by a pharmacist (e.g., Have you had any side effects when refilling a prescription?).

This kind of on-line flexible sampling capacity would be a very powerful means for gathering data for epidemiological analysis of relatively rare health problems (e.g., complications of adolescent asthma) and for monitoring areas of rapid change (introduction of new drugs or follow-up of new surgical procedures). This automated sampling and data capture strategy would also be a highly cost effective method for routine outcomes management for many health care interventions.

There are, of course, major impediments to developing such systems. These are primarily attitudinal and organizational rather than technological.

Most obviously, the administrative data systems themselves will have to be "on-line," rather than dependent upon the collection and transcribing of paper forms over the course of a quarter or a year. This is already happening: In British Columbia, physicians now bill through Teleplan, a direct computer link to the Medical Services Plan, rather than by sending in slips of paper. The *Report of the B.C. Royal Commission on Health Care and Costs* has recommended that this system be extended to include prescription writing, filling, and billing, which would give physicians the ability to monitor patient drug use patterns during the visit itself. Such a system would provide a platform for the automated sampling and data capture described above.

The largest organizational hurdle to on-line applications is probably the conversion of hospital record keeping. At present the (paper) discharge abstracts for a given year are not fully compiled in machine-readable form until six months or more after the year end. Because they are not a basis for hospital reimbursement—unlike the physician or pharmacist claim forms—there is no obvious pressure to move to a more expeditious system. The most effective strategy is probably to try to generate the separation abstracts from the internal computerized patient management systems that hospitals are slowly adopting in any case—the incremental approach again.

There may also be attitudinal barriers. Physicians may resent or fear the capacity it would give to others to monitor the quality of their work. However, it is not clear why they should be exempt from such processes—virtually everyone else, from assembly line workers to politicians and corporate CEOs, undergoes review and appraisal of their work. The general public may be justifiably concerned about potential invasion of privacy and the protection of confidentiality of the data. These would have to be assured by appropriate legislation, and organizational and technical safeguards.

One item that should not be considered an impediment is cost. The incremental costs of such an integrated sampling and data capture capacity would be low relative to the costs of the upgraded administrative data system that is needed to manage the health care system in any case. Moreover, the benefits in terms of quality assurance, faster responsiveness to emerging health and management problems, and weeding out inappropriate treatments can be expected greatly to outweigh the costs.

3. *Refinements*

Assuming the two data solitudes can be bridged, it is important to review the basic classification of "health problems," and to anticipate the analytical techniques that will prove most powerful. These should be driven by the goal of understanding the fundamental determinants of human population health—not a new question by any means, nor one that will be fully resolved in the foreseeable future, but certainly the most important question.

Current classification schemes and analytical approaches are dominated by clinical medicine. This perspective is, however, being increasingly challenged by evidence such as that presented in the introductory chapter, indicating that factors correlated with income, education, social position, job demand, and job latitude have influences on mortality that are apparently at least as powerful as the pathologies recognized and combated by traditional clinical medicine. The complex interplay of genetic predispositions and cultural milieux is only beginning to be understood. That is, after all, what this book is about. As our concepts of the determinants of health change and broaden, so too will our systems for categorizing both conditions and interventions.

This changing perspective can be illustrated through two different views of disease processes. The first is the conventional "clinical disease" approach, which starts with entities like coronary heart disease or lung cancer. Research then works back to uncover risk factors like smoking, hypertension, obesity, and cholesterol—risk factors highlighted by the Framingham study of CHD. This approach is oriented to biological processes and classification systems based on organ groups. It is reductionist in that the focus is on individuals, and within individuals on biochemical processes. The research goal is to find the key link in a linear causal chain, and then attack that link with a highly specific and targeted intervention. The overwhelming emphasis at the institutional level is on the care and cure of the disease through medical interventions.

There has been a growing emphasis on health promotion that seeks to intervene at the level of risk factors like smoking and serum cholesterol, but this is still a relatively small part of the picture. And even these forms of intervention can be translated into the clinical framework: mass screening for elevated serum cholesterol, for example, followed by continuing drug treatment for a large minority of the adult population, or physician counseling for smoking cessation, rather than legislative and tax remedies.

An alternative perspective is one that identifies what might be called "vernacular syndromes." Here the causal story, building on the Evans and Stoddart framework in Chapter 2, starts with the interplay between individual characteristics and the external milieu—social norms, peer group beliefs, the built urban environment—which is seen as having a major determining influence on the "conventional" risk factors identified in the Framingham study or the U.S. Surgeon General's report on smoking.

To give an example, we might consider "lo-stat-sed" (low-social-status sedentary) syndrome. An individual displaying this vernacular syndrome would be part of a peer group all of whom smoke (bingo players?); people in their neighbourhood tend to have poor dietary habits (beer and french fries); they are exposed to stress on the job and at home from which they have no escape; their urban neighbourhood and daily routine offer no convenient opportunities for physical fitness activity (television couch potatoes); and many believe that prayer is a "very important" factor in getting better when ill. This milieu gives rise to and encourages smoking, obesity, and high cholesterol, all conventional Framingham risk factors for CHD, and at the same time risk factors for a collection of other "clinical diseases"—lung cancer, other tobacco-sensitive cancers, and chronic obstructive pulmonary disease.

Further examples might be "eld-alone" (elderly living alone) and "adol-ex" (adolescent excess) vernacular syndromes. With eld-alone, the elderly individual has no relatives nearby, very few visitors, lives in a built urban environment that makes access to social and community services difficult, and receives health care from a pharmacomedical complex predisposed to iatrogenic polypharmacy. These are in turn risk factors for the clinical diseases of hip fracture and depression, and quite possibly others as well.

Adol-ex emerges from a milieu of sexually suggestive car and beer TV ads, peer group norms condoning poor diet, substance abuse, and promiscuous sexual behaviour, high youth unemployment, and poor motor vehicle crashworthiness. These in turn may be associated with the more conventional individual risk factors of promiscuity, false beliefs regarding risks and susceptibility, poor diet, and depression. These risk factors then predispose to the clinical diseases of motor vehicle accident trauma, anorexia nervosa, suicide, and sexually transmitted disease.

In all three examples, which are admittedly stereotyped, thinking in terms of vernacular syndromes rather than clinical diseases forces us toward consideration of multiple, diverse, and complex causal pathways. These examples highlight the limitations of medical care in isolation, and indicate the importance of collective as well as individual interventions.

More importantly in the present context, vernacular syndromes pose a challenge both for analysis and for the definition of health information needs, particularly information needs for further understanding of the determinants of population health. At the very least, it is clear that the underlying data must be:

- *multi*variate—encompassing a broad range of domains and factors,
- *multi*level—covering both individuals and various aspects of their external milieux,[17]
- *mi*crodata—for individuals the data have to be available at the level of individuals, and
- *lo*ngitudinal—so that individual life paths can be analyzed and the long-term lagged responses can be identified and understood.

If we had to coin a slogan to summarize the characteristics that developers of health information should be striving to attain, it would be *multi-multi-milo* for the four attributes just listed.[18]

C. A Template and System for Health Information

The third strategic development, in our view, should be a carefully articulated conceptual framework for health information. Such a framework is essential for organizing both the health information we now have, and that which we need and can get. By identifying gaps and overlaps, it will assist in establishing priorities for collecting new data, but there may also be redundant, superfluous, or unreliable data that can be dispensed with. An agreed-upon conceptual framework is a critical component of the prior process of consultation and consensus building to develop a strategic plan for generating and linking health information.

Data and facts are not like pebbles on a beach, waiting to be picked up and collected. They can only be perceived and measured through an underlying theoretical and conceptual framework, which defines relevant facts, and distinguishes them from "background noise." The framework acts as a filter, determining which observations must be attended to and which can safely, often unconsciously, be ignored. It is a map of the territory, and plans can only be made and actions taken on the basis of maps, not on the totality of all possible information about the territory. (The trick is to choose the right map for the purposes at hand.)

This process is clearly illustrated by the System of National Accounts, whose development and elaboration was guided by Keynesian macroeconomic theory. Physical theory plays a similar role in cosmology, providing a framework to guide the measurement priorities of the complex astronomical sensing instruments that have been built and launched into outer space.[19] At the level of the individual organism—a person, for example—the effectively infinite quantity of sensed data is filtered by (mostly unconscious) processes that determine the impressions that are important enough to attend to. Otherwise, one's processing capacity would simply be overwhelmed by impressions, and interpretation and response would be impossible.

Wolfson (1991) has proposed one possible structure for a coherent framework for health information: a System of Health Statistics. This effort grew out of initial conceptual work intended to develop a satellite account for health as part of the System of National Accounts. The System of Health Statistics assembles quantitative information pertinent to health, and its kinds of classifications, units of measure, and mathematical structure that give coherence to a wide range of data.

The extensive array of health statistics available at present is characterized principally by its *lack* of structure. If conventional health statistics compendia have any coherence, it is at most by virtue of juxtaposition. There is a clear contrast with other major *systems* of statistics such as the National Accounts or demographic statistics. For example, the latter two systems have an accounting framework with explicit "adding up" properties: the sum of incomes equals the sum of expenditures, and population next year equals population this year plus births and net migration minus deaths.

In addition, Wilk (1987) has argued that there are major benefits in reliability to be gained from organizing statistics into statistical systems, particularly in being able to address concerns regarding nonsampling error. Inconsistent or simply inaccurate data are more readily exposed in a systematic accounting framework. A System of Health Statistics could thus enhance the quality and reliability, as well as the completeness and relevance, of health statistics. Wolfson (1992b) gives examples.

More recently, a Health Information Template has been developed (Wolfson, 1992c), which is based on the proposed System of Health Statistics. The template has been part of the work of an ad hoc National Task Force on Health Information, charged with developing a strategic plan for health information in Canada (Wilk, 1991).

The task force attempted to provide a comprehensive assessment of the range of needs for health information. Its perception of these needs was based on a conceptual framework emphasizing the range and complexity of factors influencing health—including but going far beyond health care. The task force considered the evolution of this framework, from the health field concept in "A New Perspective on the Health of Canadians" (Canada, 1974), through "Achieving Health for All" (Epp, 1986), to the most recent elaboration in Chapter 2 of this volume. If health policy is to become more than health care policy, and is to respond to and influence the range of determinants identified and expressed in those frameworks, then corresponding statistical systems will be needed to provide the informational foundations for such policy.

The Health Information Template initially grew out of the framework in Chapter 2 as a kind of "road map" to guide and organize the thinking of the task force. It has since evolved, both in structure and in its range of possible applications. The most general level of the Health Information Template is shown in Figure 11.1. At this overview level, the template classifies information pertinent to the health of a human population. Data are grouped into one of three main domains: individual characteristics, the external milieu, and health-affecting interventions. The shapes and structures of these domains in the figure are intended to convey some of the texture of their contents.

Individual characteristics are shown as pertaining to members of a population of individuals. This visual metaphor highlights the fact that these data arise from observations on individuals—an explicit microdata foundation—but describe a population. In short, they are person-specific and population-based. This in turn allows distributional aspects to be brought to the fore. It is also a much more flexible and extensible way to think about data in the context of longer-term planning for health information development.

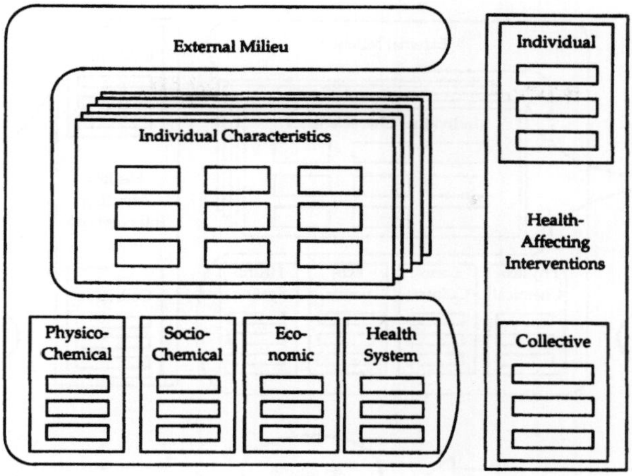

Figure 11.1. A template for health information: main.

All other health information is divided into two broad domains: the external milieu and health-affecting interventions. The external milieu includes physicochemical environments—the sources of exposures to noxious fumes and such. It also includes three other subdomains: sociocultural environments, economic environments, and health system environments. The latter include the bricks and mortar of hospitals, accumulated stocks of diagnostic imaging equipment, and the numbers and skills of various health care professionals. In other words, these subdomains represent the *state* of the external milieu at a given time in various locales. These environments evolve over time, in ways that are far from understood and are only to a limited degree influenced by deliberate policy. The rounded form of the external milieu almost completely envelops individuals; it is a source of challenges, exposures, and supports for their health.

The only forces that prevent the external milieu from completely enveloping the population of individuals are the products of deliberate human action—the tall angular structure of health-affecting interventions. These in turn are of two main kinds: individual health-affecting interventions, which act on us one-on-one, as with surgery or a visit to the dentist, and collective interventions, which act on us only indirectly via influences on various environments in the external milieu. Examples of the latter include excise taxes on tobacco products, regulations pro-

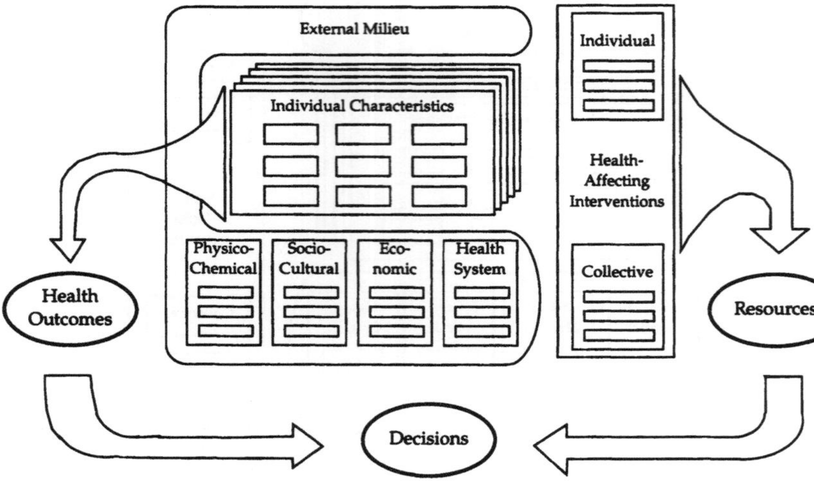

Figure 11.2. A template for health information: decisions.

hibiting lead in gasoline, restrictions on medical school enrollments, and limits on funding for the new diagnostic imaging equipment.

Each of the subdomains can be further disaggregated. Figure 11.2 shows several levels of disaggregation of items within the individual characteristics domain according to this provisional classification structure. Within the physicochemical environment subdomain, information might be classified according to the medium by which people are exposed (e.g., air, water, food), by the place or microenvironment where they are exposed (e.g., home, school, workplace), or the agent to which they are exposed (e.g., inorganic compounds, microorganisms). In the case of individual health-affecting interventions, information might be classified by the kind of intervention (e.g., surgery, physiotherapy, emotional support), who provided the intervention (e.g., physician, pharmacist, friend), and where the event occurred (e.g., practitioner's private office, hospital emergency, home).

These efforts at image, impression, and visual metaphor are intended to serve both a pedagogical purpose and, at more detailed levels, an important analytical purpose. Classification schemes are typically hierarchical; and the first and second levels of the template are no exception. But hierarchical classification schemes can be intellectually confining; they tend to be associated with reductionist approaches to theory and linear representations of causality. A major benefit of the visual metaphor of the template is that it can be extended in ways that are not hierarchical. This is potentially of great value, since it means that our thinking about health information need not be (implicitly) constrained from the outset.

Fortunately, currently available microcomputer technology allows us to transcend such restrictions, but in ways that cannot be conveyed by the medium of the printed page. The template shown in Figures 11.1 and 11.2 is, in fact, part of a graphical software package (Wolfson, 1992c; also available from the author). All the health information referred to by the template need not, indeed cannot, be held in one physical location. But the template could contain pointers to the locations of existing information. Note that this information need not be all quantitative; it could be conjectures, hypotheses, and stories. In this "pointing" capacity, the template could serve as an electronic card catalogue. In the longer term, with the development of machine-readable and linked databases, it could serve as the user interface for automated information retrieval and analysis (subject to access constraints to protect privacy and confidentiality).

From a more theoretical perspective, the template could serve as the framework within which other kinds of structure—in addition to classification—are imposed on health information. The System of Health Statistics project, for example, seeks to define, measure, and classify quantitative health information in such a way that it fits into a mathematical structure not unlike the System of National Accounts. The visual metaphors and the software environment of the template can in principle be extended to incorporate such a quantitative structure for a subset of the information. It could also include policy-oriented analytic modeling, for example, building on the POHEM microsimulation model described above. Just as a major use of the National Accounts data is as input to macroeconomic policy and macroeconometric forecasting models, it appears highly desirable to link the development of health information to policy modelling applications. The template provides a framework within which to do so.

IV. CONCLUSIONS

In this chapter, we have emphasized the centrality of information in thinking about population health. Whether the objective is to reallocate health care resources in a more effective manner, to identify trends in the health of a population, or to expand our understanding of the determinants of health, proper information is vital. Without proper information health policy is blind and stumbling; quite literally we do not know what we are doing.

We already have a substantial volume of health information. But existing data feeder systems have been inherited from an era of different concerns—paying health care providers, measuring economic activity, counting health events defined in terms of clinical disease entities. These data systems are inappropriate and inadequate to address the kinds of concerns and challenges expressed here. There is much that could be done to remedy this situation. In this chapter, we have singled out three developments that we believe to be of strategic importance.

First, health data and information must be reoriented, away from a preoccupation with the inputs to health care, to measuring health status and health outcomes. An agreed core of measures of individual health status should be developed and widely adopted; and broad summary indices of population health based on these core measures should be published regularly. At the same time, information collected on individual health care interventions should be expanded to include measures of outcome or effect.

Second, the two solitudes of "contact report" administrative data and self-report household survey data should be bridged. Modern computing technology can be harnessed to develop hybrid data feeder systems. The impediments to such developments lie much more in the areas of present organizational structures, and behind them attitudes and limited imagination, than in technology or costs.

Finally, an overall conceptual framework for health information should lie at the heart of planning for new data and information initiatives. Frameworks like the Health Information Template and the System of Health Statistics can play a role analogous to the System of National Accounts in organizing thinking, reflecting theory, and highlighting the most serious gaps in available data.

NOTES

1. *Proprioception*: "relating to stimuli produced and perceived within an organism," *Concise Oxford Dictionary*; also the title of a poem by 1960s beat poet Charles Olsen.

2. By data, we mean elements of description, numerical or otherwise, of things, people, places, and events. By information, we mean the ordering and interpretation of data to impose or extract meaning. For example, the enumeration of one's activities over the past week constitutes data. These can then be interpreted as employment or unemployment, and then further aggregated with other similar data to generate an estimate of the Canadian unemployment rate. Similarly, a hospital separation record is a collection of descriptive data. Aggregated into an occupancy rate, or a population-based utilization rate, such data are transformed into information.

3. Better information is not, of course, a sufficient condition for these improvements, but it is clearly necessary.

4. Of course, if all government policies and programs (not just in the health domain) were subject to this test of some demonstrable efficacy for achieving stated goals, we recognize that a discouragingly large proportion might fail.

5. Or that of most other countries. The U.S. National Health Interview Survey is a notable exception in terms of regularity and consistency, an observation that underlines the fact that better data are a necessary but not a sufficient condition for redirecting health policy.

6. Ideally such information would be collected pre- and postdischarge, with the timing and detail depending upon the patient's condition. The evaluation of cardiac surgery, for example, might require information at one, three, and twelve months after discharge.

7. Even though life expectancy has been improving, we do not know whether these additional years of life are vibrant or spent bedridden with chronic disease—the so-called "compression of morbidity" debate (e.g., Gavreau, 1987).

8. A presumption is that the index will show noticeable variation over time, and sensitivity to health policy or other social changes. Economic measures are headline news because they fluctuate; changes in life expectancy have rarely been news unless they decline. A measure of health status that does not vary much over time may not capture much attention. On the other hand, the media always seem interested in interregional comparisons, and in comparisons among various sociodemographic groups, so that salient results are possible for an annual or biennial index and its subcomponents even if overall health status changes only slowly.

9. This work takes into account some of the critical questions about multiattribute utility functions raised by Mehrez and Gafni (1989) and Loomes and McKenzie (1989).

10. A more subtle problem may arise if age- or sex-specific survival rates are changing over time. If this were due, for example, to the "salvage" of unhealthy individuals who in earlier years would have died, the aggregate population health status would be deteriorating. Conversely, harmful care or euthanasia, which led to increased mortality among sufferers from a particular chronic illness, could be recorded as improved population health status! (Dead people do not respond to surveys.) This ambiguity is not new; but the construction of an explicit aggregate index will force us to be more specific about how we count and evaluate different health states, including death.

11. For example, to isolate the impact of the elderly on the overall average, health status can be calculated for the elderly and nonelderly populations separately. To assess the impact of gross motor impairments, the multiattribute health status responses could be recalculated assuming no gross motor capacity impairment. Such calculations are presented in Berthelot et al. (1992).

12. In fact, the latter hypothetical point corresponds to preliminary results reported by R. Wilkins (personal communication, 1990).

13. Present computations of this form, using census data, rank communities according to the average life expectancy of their populations. Moving down this ranking of communities until 10 percent of the population is included yields the top "decile," although not, strictly speaking, the healthiest ten percent of the population. The average value for these communities can then be compared with those communities at the bottom end that also collectively contain 10 percent of the population.

14. Of course, the efficacy of various health care services could be assessed much more directly from linked data sets as described later.

15. Conventionally, life expectancies are calculated from a set of point-in-time mortality rates, so they are not actually longitudinal. However, more sophisticated methods such as the POHEM microsimulation approach described below can embody explicit representations of longitudinal information.

16. In Canadian terminology, a patient separates from a hospital by either discharge or death. Thus the more inclusive term *separations* includes both discharges of live patients and deaths in hospital.

17. The 1986 postcensal Health and Activity Limitations Survey provides an example to illustrate the point. This survey went to great expense to provide sufficient sample size for subprovincial and urban analyses, and to gather data on social support provided to disabled individuals by friends and family. However, the data on social support used by individuals are difficult to interpret in the absence of data at the level of each community describing the social support institutions that are actually available.

18. These ideas are developed in Wolfson (1992d).

19. Of course, in both domains, there were preexisting sets of data and information that provided the basis for the theory. More accurately, the history is one of interplay and a process of development back and forth between theories and data.

12

The Future: Hygeia Versus Panakeia?

M. RENAUD

We do not inherit the land from our fathers, we borrow it from our children.

—African saying

What is perceived to be true, even if it is false, has real consequences.

—Sociological saying

In ancient times, Asklepios was the god of health. His cult persisted longer than that of any other Greek god, although mythology tells us that he was struck by thunder at the height of his glory for attempting to resurrect the dead in exchange for a large sum of money. Asklepios had two daughters, Hygeia and Panakeia. Panakeia was a true healing goddess, learned in the use of drugs derived either from plants or from the earth; her cult is alive and well today in the universal search for a panacea. In contrast, her sister Hygeia was the goddess for whom health was the natural order of things. She taught the Greeks that they could remain in good health if they lived according to reason, with moderation in all things. We still honor her memory through the use of the word hygiene.[1] Today, in our technology-dominated world, these two views collide more than ever.

To most of us, being in a state of "good health" automatically means

Reprinted with permission of the publisher from *Health and Canadian Society/Santé et Société*, vol. 1, no. 1, 1993, pp. 229–249. Copyright © 1993. Reprinted with slight editorial revision.

"not being sick"—a negative definition of health. On the other hand, a positive definition of health might be "being in good shape," that is to say, being able to live fully according to one's given potential. Whether considered positively or negatively, health is determined by many more factors than just services to the ill, as the chapters of this book have attempted to attest. And yet in many respects it appears as though it were not so.

In his novel *1984*, George Orwell imagined a conformist society in which disinformation ruled. The Ministry of Love waged war and the Ministry of Truth rewrote history according to the needs of the present. In much the same way today, the responsibilities and preoccupations of our ministries of health are dominated by illness care.[2] If they were actually responsible for health, their main concern would be to improve the social and economic conditions that affect the individual's ability to make health-enhancing life-style decisions and to react and respond calmly to life's inevitable problems.

The thesis of this book rests on a paradox that has long been known but that most health care practitioners, politicians, and health care system analysts have traditionally ignored.[3] Achieving and maintaining health are not just matters of curing illness. The ways in which society regulates employment and economic cycles, provides education, assists its members in times of economic or other difficulties, sets up strategies to counteract poverty, crime, and drug abuse and to stimulate economic and social growth have just as much, if not more, impact on health than do the quantity and quality of resources being invested in the detection and care of illness. Good and bad habits (food, alcohol, tobacco, physical exercise, etc.) are often linked to these social factors, leading some observers to note that heavy smoking and alcoholism do not so much reflect on the individuals as they do on the groups to which the individuals belong (see, e.g., Syme, 1990). In short, smoking, drinking in excess, and eating poorly are not merely (or even predominantly) the choices of individuals.

Yet, despite our growing knowledge of the significance of social, economic, and cultural factors in the etiology of diseases, most contemporary societies continue to invest an increasing, and already large, portion of their resources—now one out of every ten dollars in Canada—in health (and predominantly medical) care of all kinds. The extent to which the health of the population is also affected by other government policies and by the ways individuals perceive and structure their collective lives is not fully recognized, as we have attempted to illustrate in previous chapters. And, even where recognition is now emerging, there is little sense yet of how best to reallocate scarce resources so as to improve the health impact of public programs.

I. LESSONS FROM THE PAST, QUESTIONS FOR THE FUTURE

By synthesizing the main body of data collected over the last decade on determinants of health, by proposing a conceptual framework within which to interpret such data, and by pointing out potential directions for further research, this book proposes to reorient and refocus the present debate on health care policies, to force health care to be considered within a broader context of "effective health policy." Previous chapters suggest a multitude of questions for the future, but at least three fundamental "lessons" can now be drawn.

A. Medical Science Has Limits That Were Unknown Twenty Years Ago, Making Reorientation Essential

To begin with, the development of the health care system is now confronted with dilemmas that were unsuspected only two decades ago. First, there are a whole host of ethical dilemmas: astonishing geographical variations in medical practice and applications of medical technologies beyond their ranges of demonstrated effectiveness (see, e.g., Chapter 9), active and passive euthanasia, possible eugenism, and so on. Second, there are economic dilemmas: an impression of decreasing returns for ever-increasing investments. On the part of governments, there is a sense of frustration at facing growing demands for care due to technological developments and greater expectations on the part of both producers and patients, in the face of limited fiscal capacity. In fact, high ranking Treasury Board officials and schoolteachers alike are beginning to wonder why, when everyone is being forced to cut corners on spending, should every extra government dollar go to health care? Does it not already consume enough of most industrialized nations' resources? It is as though we had reached an important crossroads where difficult choices can no longer be avoided. A freelance philosopher and well-known microbiologist predicted twenty-five years ago that:

> There will have to be priorities, and these will involve difficult choices. Humanitarian ideals might dictate that attention be first given to medical services for the sick and aged. However, concern for the future and economic development may make it advisable to focus medical effort in the school system and even preferably on the very young, because experience has shown that the early years of life are the most critical for the creation of a healthy adult. These choices will naturally involve medical criteria, but they will also pose difficult ethical and social dilemmas. (Dubos, 1965:455–56)

Paradoxically, now that medical science has developed some efficient therapeutic tools and there is a biological revolution under way that will supposedly enable humans to control procreation, heredity, and the nervous system (Bernard, 1989, 1990b), most Western industrialized states are faced with a crisis that has both clinical and fiscal dimensions.[4] And both are rooted, in part, in the dramatic expansion of health care systems. Thus the medical profession finds itself increasingly confronted with pressure to limit its range and application of interventions. Asklepios is no longer capable of controlling Panakeia, who is increasingly being expected to control herself. Hygeia, inspiration for numerous reforms of the past (e.g., Richardson, 1876; Pettenkofer, 1941), has found new allies who consider preventive measures to have greater social value than curative treatments and who believe health to be a product of social and economic organization.

B. Struggle against Bad Life-Styles: Necessary Yet Insufficient

The second lesson is that there are significant limits inherent in the new health promotion movement calling for the adoption of healthier life-styles. This movement proposes to replace the technocratic and medical vision of the body with a philosophy of self-control over one's own health. This philosophy, propagated by a large number of lobby groups, medical dictionaries, and over-the-counter drug handbooks, and by media coverage and various newsletters (such as *Men's Health, Health after 50, The Berkeley Wellness Letter*), advocates not only caution in the face of medical science but a large dose of asceticism. All of our behaviours are being scrutinized and normalized, from diet and sleeping habits to sexual practices, means of coping with stress, ways of keeping in shape, and so on.

To many, this movement constitutes a great leap forward because it makes people responsible for their own health, resulting in clear benefits for those who succeed in conforming. To others (such as Bensaid, 1981a), it constitutes a sure sign of social neurosis, a wave of "no-ism" ("no sex, no meat, no alcohol") where health is an end in itself and most causes of ill-health are to be found in individual informed decisions. The fear of intoxication and death have replaced the fear of God. Health becomes a type of illness. To still others, the movement is a reflection of the hypochondriac narcissism of a privileged class shutting its eyes to the deterioration of the rest of the world. As Lewis Thomas, the American doctor and essayist, wrote:

> As a people, we have become obsessed with Health. . . . We do not seem to be looking for more exuberance in living as much as staving off failure,

> putting off dying. We have lost confidence in the human body. The new consensus is that we are badly designed, intrinsically fallible, vulnerable to a host of hostile influences inside and around us, and only precariously alive. . . . The new danger of our well-being, if we continue to listen to all the talk, is in becoming a nation of healthy hypochondriacs, living gingerly, worrying ourselves half to death. . . . Indeed, we should be worrying that our preoccupation with personal health may be a symptom of copping out, an excuse for running upstairs to recline on a couch, sniffing the air for contaminants, spraying the room with deodorants, while just outside, the whole of society is coming undone. (Thomas, 1979:47–50)

Whatever fears this health promotion movement may raise with respect to social evolution (Fox, 1986), the limits to its effectiveness in promoting the health of populations are now becoming clear.

Let us consider tobacco as an example. The fact that tobacco kills is now widely established. Yet why would an individual deprive himself or herself of the pleasure of smoking if, on the other hand, his or her life is boring, work alienating, and prospects for the future either depressing or nonexistent? For some, smoking provides an admittedly dangerous but pleasant means to escape the stress and boredom of everyday life.

And so study results show an association between "bad" life-styles and socioeconomic factors: One's capacity to modify potentially pathogenic behaviours and to "stick with it" is directly related to one's wealth, power, and education—in short to the degree of control one has over one's future. The higher up in the social hierarchy, the more control one feels capable of exerting over life, the easier it is to change unhealthy habits. In other words, one's "will to change" is largely predetermined by one's social environment. To be told, by an education program or otherwise, that one's life-style should change is neither helpful nor effective.

Further, it has now been well documented that a simple education program will not change behaviour significantly, as the single most important randomized control trial of health education in human history—MR FIT—has shown (Syme, 1990). The motivated and well-supervised members of the experimental group did in fact modify their life-styles. But so did members of the control group, however poorly supervised, and there was no significant difference between the two. The "social environment" effect, of being involved in the trial, may have had a significant effect on behaviour, although changes in the broader social environment were also taking place. But there is no evidence for an independent influence from the educational program.

Even more disturbing, the evidence reviewed in this book suggests that if the whole population were to begin to lead a healthier life-style, in accordance with nature as science understands it (in particular with respect to alcohol, tobacco, and diet), life expectancy would indeed increase but the health gradient between the various social classes might well remain. Good health, then, is not just a matter of life-style. A modern Hygeia would not only advise her people to be cautious of her sister Panakeia and to adopt a hygienic life-style but she would also see to it that life in the city was as creative, convivial, and fair as possible.

C. Changes in the Social Environment Are Possible and Desirable

This book offers us a third lesson: Some of the best-kept secrets of longevity and good health are to be found in one's social, economic, and cultural circumstances. We have seen that health derives in part from our ability to adapt and the faith in the future that we develop as children, as well as from the friendship and support networks to which we have access at work, at home, and in the community. Health also stems from our sense of having room to manoeuvre along with some control over our work, and from our capacity for dealing with abrupt changes in our lives (unemployment, separation, death, etc.).

Obviously these opportunities are not equally accessible to everyone. The largest gap lies between the richest and the poorest. But the middle classes are also affected. The lower one is situated in the social hierarchy, as defined by work, lodging, education, income, or whatever, the lower one's probability of staying in good health and the lower one's life expectancy. This is the most frequent and most pervasive of all the observations made in the history of public health research (Haan, Kaplan, and Syme, 1989).

This is not an implacable law for all individuals. Some "poor people" have long and fulfilling lives just as some "rich people" die prematurely. But these cases are not simply due to chance or genetic stock: The poor individual who manages well often benefits from a particularly supportive social, childhood, or educational milieu that affords a sense of control over his or her own life (e.g., Werner and Smith, 1989).

Our social milieu is the product of the environment that we have created for ourselves, generation after generation. It undergoes changes, often imperceptible ones, and so do its underlying values and norms. For example, many of today's industrialized societies have come to tolerate 10 percent unemployment rates, even without economic recession, something that would have been unthinkable and shocking two decades ago. Others, such as Sweden and Austria, still find these rates quite unacceptable. Conversely, thanks to the feminist movement, domestic violence that was formerly concealed is no longer tolerated in most developed societies. In a similar fashion, we have created our social milieu both by accepting that businesses can define employees' roles and functions, and by the more explicit collective choices we have made through governmental policies. Our social environment is a social construct. It is human-built; humans can change it.

It is thus reasonable to believe—without falling prey to utopian or wishful thinking—that social and economic changes aimed at improving the social environment are possible. Examples abound: the effort of the feminist movement to establish greater equality in gender relations; the emergence of the self-help movement that profoundly transformed the field of mental health; and the attempt of the trade unions, with the collaboration of the enlightened sectors of the business community, to develop better health and safety conditions. The point is illustrated further by less well-developed countries (such as Costa Rica, Sri Lanka, and Kerala State in India) that have succeeded in significantly improving the health of their populations by creating primary health care networks and by raising women's average level of education to that of men. This accomplishment has come despite the fact that these countries are less well off economically than many other underdeveloped countries (such as Saudi Arabia, Libya, and Iraq; Caldwell, 1986).

All of these show that "where there is a will, there is a way." One of the most striking examples is that of automobile production. Who could have imagined twenty years ago that assembly lines—a symbol of twentieth-century industrialism—could be so radically transformed as to result in less alienated labour, better wages, reduced supply losses, and better-quality cars, but lower production costs? And yet that is exactly what the Japanese have managed to achieve and teach the rest of the world. The impetus was provided by a visit Mr. Toyoda and his chief engineer paid to Detroit in the 1950s. They were shocked by the workers' low productivity and decided that the assembly line had to be democratized and material supplies better regulated in order to fit Japanese culture (Womack, 1990). The effects on health brought about by these specific changes have not been documented but it is quite probable, as Japanese health statistics suggest, that a culture like that of Japan, which has rejected the most abject aspects of Taylorism and Fordism at all levels, is also—in spite of other problems—a culture that generates good health.

Change is not only possible, it is also desirable. Poverty, misery, unemployment, mental illness, injustice, solitude, and exclusion have been the great themes of human suffering for centuries and have motivated, with some success, numerous social reforms. But the very form of these themes has changed over time. They now have a modern dress. As the report of the French commission responsible for the reconceptualization of the national health promotion and prevention policy noted:

> Nowadays, [this new form] is:
> the poverty of the unemployed, the marginals, the Fourth World;
> the isolation and exclusion of the elderly;
> depression and suicide, fear and the sense of insecurity, delinquence;
> subservience to a machine and a machine's pace, subjection to a work plan decided by another, the impossibility of choosing one's own destiny, the determinism of educational segregation, robotization, depersonalization;
> inequalities in health, income, education, leisure and freedom which breed frustration and indignity, not to mention racism;
> solitude amidst the multitude, family breakdown, segregation according to social categories and age. (Grémy and Pissaro, 1983:23)

Should Hygeia return and be presented with the argument and evidence gathered in this book, she would undoubtedly make these problems a main priority. She would not be lacking in sources of inspiration: A considerable number of social experiments have been carried out in these areas, although they may not be easily transposed from one social context to another. One has only to look at the Swedish and Austrian experiments in retraining and full employment, the career security available to a large proportion of Japan's manpower, the continuing education and personal growth programs developed by the Americans during the 1960s and 1970s, the efforts of the Québécois CLSC to combat the isolation and exclusion of the elderly, using community actions and combining social and medical services, or the countless attempts by local communities to reintegrate delinquents and the mentally ill.

But for these experiments to lead to durable and effective changes, Asklepios and perhaps Ares (the god of war) must give up some of their resources, and Zeus and his wife Hera along with Athena, the goddess of Intelligence, must lend their power.

II. AN UNCERTAIN FUTURE

On the eve of the twenty-first century, a power struggle emerges between the god of medical art, Panakeia, who is growing increasingly ambitious and skillful in her attempts to resurrect the dead, and Hygeia, the goddess of public health and great priestess of social reforms. No one can accurately predict what the outcome will be. The multiplicity of social forces at work, the number and sometimes the unpredictable character of technological developments in medicine, the complexity of organizational and other structures that must be taken into account, all are factors that make prediction a quite hazardous, if not deceptive effort, however fascinating it may be as an intellectual exercise.

While it may not be a good idea to play oracle, it is important to inquire into the future awaiting us. Indeed, what would happen if the health care system were allowed to grow at the same pace as it has for the last fifteen years; if therapeutic overzealousness at the beginning and end of life continued to expand; if hair transplant, liposuction, face-lifts, and mammary surgery became common practice; if it became possible regularly to perform grafts of tired organs (heart, liver, lungs, eyes, etc.); if the pharmacopoeia became capable of ensuring "happiness" by providing pills for libidinal balance, antidepressants, and antistress vitamins, and ensuring "immortality" thanks to antiwrinkle pills and medication against senescence; if it were possible to choose the characteristics of newborns (height, sex, psychological traits), perhaps even quality "breeders" from catalogues; if neurosciences succeeded in manipulating the brain and controlling personality development; if genetic manipulations led not only to an agricultural revolution and progress in the fight against leukemia, cystic fibrosis and manic depression but also contributed to the struggle against certain illnesses that are only partly due to genetic predispositions (hypercholesterolemia, diabetes, hypertension)?

The seeds for these developments—and for many more—are already budding in the gardens of contemporary reality. There seems no doubt that in the twenty-first century, personal medical monitoring devices will multiply. Aside from scales, thermometers, and pulse-taking machines, there will be electrocardiographs, electroencephalographs, home hypercholesterolemia tests, as well as computerized medical records complete with do-it-yourself analysis and follow-up software. And that biomedical technology will continue to progress is also beyond doubt. What we do not know, however, is how each society will regulate these developments and, particularly, how the delicate balance between investments in the social environment (the fight against unemployment, isolation, exclusion, the promotion of good dietary habits, etc.) and investments in cures, palliative gadgets, and other manifestations of the fight against death will be handled.

A. The Future According to Futurologists

When science fiction tackles the future of medical science and health, the scripts are linear and blunt, as required by the literary genre. Callenbach (1990), for instance, imagines an ecological revolution where California secedes from the United States in order to establish a new social order more convivial and more respectful of nature. Gibson (1984) predicts that the human being will become more and more like a machine that can be assembled or disassembled as needed. In the same vein, Attali (1979) theorizes on the advent of a "cannibal order" where, due to the availability of genetic and computer implants, people will soon be willing to sell their bodies and buy copies by the piece. Bensaid (1981b) believes that the human being will turn into a sort of docile robot governed by a central computer. In a world where the smallest pathogenic habit is named and medicalized, only the onset of death will enable the individual to experience love and ecstasy.

In short, these novelists and essayists see the future in black and white as if it had but one dimension. But what about those who claim to be able to put the pieces of the puzzle together in order to reflect on the future? In their countless books and periodicals,[5] what do "futurologists" write? A dozen books have been published in the last decade in French alone, in an attempt to predict the future and so improve decision-making in the present.

Economist and sociologist Robert Fossaert (1991), for one, theorizes about world system evolution and predicts the rise of a new geopolitical balance. In a world that will be more capitalistic than ever, overwhelmed states will barely control the millions of people aspiring to greater autonomy. In Fossaert's crystal ball: capitalism everywhere on the planet, more anarchy, more inequities between countries, more independence movements, and more rebellions. Demographer and geneticist Albert Jacquard (1991), like Cassandra, writes about impending disasters—ecological disasters, violence, planetary war—in order to better avoid them. According to him, the problem is that humankind continues to think—and thus to act—along a line of reflection that dates back to the Middle Ages, despite modern-day technical and military means. Drawing on his experience as director of the Cité des sciences et de l'industrie de La Villette (Paris), biologist Joël de Rosnay (1991) draws up a list of the most probable technological innovations in all fields for the next decade: youth hormones, anticocaine vaccines, hair-growing cream, hunger-suppressing pills, anticholesterol eggs, and two hundred more innovations, all equally pleasing to the Panakeias of this world. Alvin Toffler (1990) rounds off the trilogy that began with *Future Shock* (1970) and *The Third Wave* (1980) with a work in which he predicts that the old industrial power system, based on wealth and violence, is about to be replaced by an emerging new power system, based on knowledge.

Engineer Thierry Gaudin (1990) describes the coming century in a particularly impressive intellectual and iconographical work.[6] He predicts that, as a result of the great migrations we are already witnessing, cities will become the battlefields of opposing tribes of urban savages, struggling to preserve their territories. Individuals, more isolated than ever following the collapse of traditional social ties (family, neighbourhoods), will be forced to carve out for themselves the identities that would previously have been given to them. In a world overloaded with information, individuals, solicited on all sides, will constantly have to define their identities, thus allowing for unprecedented personal growth but also creating the ground for new forms of exploitation. Gaudin predicts that exploitation of the psychic vulnerability created by having to choose one's own values, goals, connections, and life-style will replace exploitation of physical vulnerability. In sum, the twenty-first century will no longer be the century of individualism but that of "individuation," where individuals are searching for an autonomy that goes beyond narrow egotism and self-interest.

Finally, in his scenario the nation-state is largely supplanted in the twenty-first century by multinational business and, perhaps more importantly, by multinational "gimmicks" [*sic*], a kind of transactional network, the voice of an emerging planetary consciousness (for example, Greenpeace, Amnesty International). Things will go from bad to worse (drug abuse, serial murders, riots, rise in religious fundamentalism, etc.) until around 2020. Gaudin and his team predict that this present trend will then reverse and that great programs in education, urbanism, and social and political development will be set up. This belief is based on the fact that any system tends toward survival. For example, following the great proletarian rebellions of the mid–nineteenth century, did the bourgeoisie not react by reestablishing order through the destruction of unhealthy neighbourhoods, the widening of streets, and the development of public education? Around 2020, following a period of chaos, dominant social classes will react in much the same way in order to maintain their social positions and to reestablish some sort of harmony.

On the whole, these works of prospective history convey the impression that humanity is experiencing a period of metamorphosis and turmoil where technology, society, and ideas are being simultaneously transformed. The magnitude and complexity of these changes are such that one cannot help but be reminded of the great upheavals of the past (Gaudin, 1988), upheavals such as those of the eleventh–thirteenth centuries, where peasants strengthened their powers to the detriment of the nobility and clergy and where existing technologies became widely diffused, or that of the eighteenth century, which saw the birth of industry and capitalist "entre-preneurs" (etymologically, those who are "in between"). The contemporary metamorphosis has its roots in the knowledge boom or, more specifically, in the capacity to reach beyond nation-states and turn this knowledge more and more rapidly into objects and services marketable worldwide. The results, for the time being at least, are destabilization, insecurity and new information-based forms of exploitation of (wo)man by (wo)man.

We have grown up in the homogenizing universe of the assembly line and of public and private bureaucracies; we will now have to learn to live in a fragmented universe, in a world where knowledge is in perpetual evolution amid a multitude of interconnected networks that elude all attempts at centralized control. We will, in this new world, be even more alone in the face of the decisions and choices to be made, because many external forces will be beyond the reach of those within individual nation-states whom we elect to represent our interests.

B. If Biology Rules, the Future Looks Bleak

What do these theories and theorists of the future tell us about the relationship between medical science, public health, and social reforms?

Like the futurologists, Jean Bernard, the most famous of contemporary French physicians, paints a gloomy picture of the next few decades, followed by spiritual, intellectual, and social rebirth. His words are worth quoting extensively:

> Mankind has already experienced the slavery of ancient civilizations, the slave-trade up until the 19th century, and Hitler's final solution. For forty years, between 2020 and 2060, it will come to know the dangerous consequences of the uncontrolled alliance between gold and biology, profits and science.
>
> Bio-technology got off to a good start. It gave birth to vaccinations and medicines. But it soon departed from these primary objectives. "Not enough profit in them since they concern only illness," is in essence what businessmen have told themselves. The processes of conception, gestation, birth, the development of the nervous-system, life, death—come 2020, 2030—they are all in the hands of bio-technology, itself under the powerful grip of multinational firms. Imprudently used from as early as 1960, the term "bank" takes on its full meaning. Sperm banks, egg banks and embryo banks are set up in a number of countries. Genetic engineering allows for the widespread development of selective eugenism. The fears expressed by the scientists at the turn of the new century are confirmed. Naturally, the bank leads to the stock exchange. Like platinum and petroleum before them, embryos which have been selected and manipulated are now submitted to the cambists' appreciation and to the fluctuating market prices of the world's various financial scenes. . . .
>
> In the past, there had often been ties between the forces of money and

> dictators. . . . Dictators of the past used to think up, create and develop impressive propaganda methods to inspire fear and blind trust on the part of their subjects. Specialists of 2030 hire the services of neuro-scientists. There is no need for propaganda. The injection of effective, clandestine molecules in the food secures obedient and dedicated subjects who are prepared to die for the cause advocated by the molecule. . . .
>
> The term "ethics" [disappears] from all writings around 2040. So do all values of the past. . . .
>
> The third era, that of spiritual, intellectual and ethical rebirth begins around 2060. It is a boom. . . . Every man is unique, irreplaceable and different from all others. He must be respected, protected from birth to death and beyond. He must be respected in his wholeness, his unity as a person as well as in each of his cells, the combined diversity of which contributes to this unity. Neither this person nor any of his cells may be traded. (Bernard, 1990, 302–305)*

It would be difficult to find a more pessimistic script for our children and grandchildren. The fact that it is being offered by such an authority in the field makes it all the more frightening! With the development and flourishing of international markets, nation-states may survive only to maintain local cultures. Already international rivalries are increasingly expressed not on the battlefield (although we still seem to be "blessed" with more than enough of that) but through structures of trade and exchange.

In Bernard's view, biology and medical science will come to the rescue of the dominant classes and bring peace and order (or at least order) to a chaotic universe where urban rebellion compares only to the bitterness, acrimony, and rebellion contained in the relationship between rich countries and poor countries. They will become the tools of international elite networks. "Peace and order" will come from the iron domination of this elite based on its unassailable technological and scientific superiority.

Is it truly possible that medicine and biology will become such instruments of domination? Or are we just falling prey to the fear of the unknown, that typical syndrome so eloquently illustrated by the famous French scientist and politician Arago in 1832, when he argued against the railroad because "air compression in tunnels would be fatal to the travellers' lungs"?

Yet Jean Bernard's script is not inconsistent with the visions of the future described earlier. Indeed, at least three major trends in the field of health pointed out by the futurologists make conceivable the biotechnological hyperbolism feared by Bernard:

*Translated with permission of the publisher from J. Bernard, *De la biologie à l'éthique*. Copyright © 1990 by Éditions Buchet/Chastel.

• The guildlike domination of the medical profession (Toffler, 1990:24) and the blackmail it exerts on governments (Gaudin, 1990:278) are coming to an end. In a world where human biological knowledge is very widely and rapidly diffused, the medical profession is increasingly losing its monopoly on that knowledge, and the status of the physician is eroding. However, this will not stop the progression of biomedical knowledge and technology. On the contrary, it may well become a key ingredient of economic development, but the primary recipients of the economic rents will be multinational corporations rather than the professionals who have traditionally applied that knowledge to the treatment of individual patients, and the efforts to "sell" the new technologies will focus less and less on practitioners and traditional health care institutions, and more and more on individuals.

• Health is the ideal ground for the exploitation of psychic vulnerability, a form of exploitation based on knowledge rather than on wealth and violence that will be typical of the twenty-first century (Gaudin, 1990:279). Miracle pill merchants and charlatans will proliferate. As society may be tempted to promote the cult of good health in order to secure a high level of social conformism, so it may tend toward the use of new biotechnological tools in order to overcome deviance and delinquence.

• The twentieth century ends with the denunciation of deforestation and of the greenhouse effect due mainly to carbon dioxide emissions causing a rise in the temperature of the earth along with serious climatic disorders. In most countries, ecological movements rise up and call for harmony between imperatives of technological development and laws of nature. The health hazards of a poor physical environment are now on the agenda. A similar recognition of the impact of social environment on human development and health has not yet occurred (Gaudin, 1990; Jacquard, 1991). According to Gaudin and his team (1990), greater social turmoil and an increase in illiteracy and ignorance are likely before society realizes, around 2020 (2060 according to Bernard), the imperious necessity of reinvesting in social development, as was the case at the turn of the century (public schooling, cleaning up of cities) and following the Second World War (social security programs).

In short, according to these authors, it is possible that the decline of the status of the medical profession and the rise in biomedical knowledge will lead to biotechnology being used and physicians, reduced to the level of technicians, being manipulated so as to secure control over a population made vulnerable to psychic exploitation by prevalent living and working conditions. Jean Bernard's fear of catastrophe in the future may well be justified.

C. Is This Gloomy Future Inevitable?

However, the world is not necessarily doomed. Even if it is learned late and at considerable avoidable human cost, the wisdom that people and governments draw from the past can materialize in new social projects to counterbalance the effects of exploitation and the will to exercise power. Major technological innovations require some form of social control, which may or may not halt the abuse of power facilitated by such innovations. The biotechnology that Bernard fears so much implies not only risks but also hope. The fundamental issue at stake is the quality of the social, economic, and cultural environment within which these innovations take place. If, in fact, the future of the developed world as foreseen by Gaudin, Jacquard, and others is one of warring tribes of urban savages, caught up in drug abuse and violence, rendering cities dangerous and inhospitable; if countries in the southern hemisphere begin to emulate Saddam Hussein and become entangled in religious and belligerent dogmatism, then any means of maintaining social order may certainly appear legitimate and the worst scenarios may become possible.

Still, here and there, tools are emerging that may assist the attempt to improve the social environment. For instance, as the United Nations did with its crude "human development index," a national social deficit index[7] could now be created (rates of dropouts, unemployment, family breakdown, etc.) in order to help set priorities and identify emerging problems. Like the growth rate of the gross national product, the deficit in the balance of payments, the inflation rate, or the national debt, this index could serve to mobilize the energies of politicians and public sector institutions. In terms of employment, redistribution of the work schedule and of wages could help reduce the number of people who are either unemployed or dependent on welfare. Business and government could set up programs to provide workers with better training and allow them to adjust more rapidly to the changes inevitably associated with economic cycles. Governments could support high-risk investments that have potential high return in the long term instead of encouraging short-term speculation (real estate, takeovers, etc.), which create no new collective wealth. As for economic development, private enterprise could learn from the Japanese and Korean miracles of 1945–1990, which illustrated the necessity of interfirm networking both at the economic level (the"keiretsu") and at the level of development policy (global wage negotiations, worker retraining mechanisms, research and development, etc.). Many more examples could be cited. They show that the means exist to prevent the social canvas from deteriorating and, better yet, to improve the quality of life. In most countries, however, politicians have yet to come to this realization, occupied as they are with putting out fires and getting themselves reelected.

III. NECESSARY REORIENTATION OF THE SOCIAL DEBATE

In the field of health, for the time being, the main issue is the reorientation and refocusing of the social debate. The scope, organization, and financing of the various social security regimes (medical care insurance, old age pensions, unemployment benefits, etc.) have to be reexamined with one central, yet often forgotten question in mind: What reforms would help improve the health of the population?

In many industrial societies, particularly those where health care is publicly funded, numerous reforms have been, are being, or will be introduced in an attempt to rationalize the use and restrain the expansion of the health care system. In general, however, the debate focuses unilaterally on the legitimacy of the financial demands made by physicians, hospitals, and other participants in the health care system including, on occasion, specific groups of beneficiaries. Topics of debate include methods to reduce the number of physicians, incentives to counteract undue demands for care by some consumers and to promote the more efficient treatment of patients by providers, benefits (and costs) associated with the introduction of particular technologies, new methods of medical staff management, and resource allocation to various population (e.g., regional funding models) or provider (e.g., alternatives to fee for service) groups. In short, the debate revolves around the most effective ways of funding and regulating the vast and complex system. This leads to numerous confrontations between public authorities and the medical profession, health care institutions and the numerous groups of "health care professionals" seeking the same recognition that doctors enjoy (e.g., "soft," "alternative," and "parallel" medicines). The debate can also involve a variety of special interest clienteles (such as the elderly, the disabled, women's groups), which consider that they are receiving insufficient care as compared to other clienteles.

This debate is certainly important since it concerns the use of almost 10 percent of our collective wealth [see, for instance, *Economist,* 1991)]. Yet the debate is incomplete because we are losing sight of the final goal: the preservation and promotion of the health of the population. In fact, only rarely do public debates raise the central and obvious question: What are the most effective means and what political and budgetary choices should be made in order to improve the population's health? In other words, how might we best proceed in order to "add years, good health and well-being to life" (Québec Government, 1989, 1992) or, in still other words, "to nurture health" (Ontario Government, 1991)?

It is said that in the kingdom of the blind, the one-eyed man is king. When too much emphasis is placed on detection, diagnosis and treatment, we forget that health is not the exclusive concern of health care professionals and of one ministry, even if it is called the Ministry of "Health." When too much emphasis is placed on "individual life-style choices," we tend to forget that these life-styles are themselves largely determined by the social, economic and cultural environments. However we may choose to measure and monitor it (life expectancy, healthy life expectancy, infant mortality rate, low birth-weight rate, etc.), the health of the population is as much affected by the structures of workplaces, families, schools and communities, and by the policies of a whole set of Ministries (Economic Development, Education, Employment, Income Security, Social Services, Environment, etc.), as it is by medical science and the health care system.

As an editorial in the *Lancet* (1991) recently pointed out, the population could agree to a certain rationing of health care services if local communities were involved in the decision-making process and if, in the course of the process, the therapeutic option was presented as an admittedly significant yet limited part of the health spectrum. The general public might be less concerned about limits on health care spending if they could be more involved in decisions about resource allocation, and if they understood that more money to health care means less money for other purposes that can also have a significant impact on health.

In the realm of health, the issue at stake for the future is the reestablishment of a balance between Hygeia and Panakeia, which has been tilted in favour of the latter over the course of three decades of dramatic biomedical development. Biologist Jean Rostand once remarked that the human being is the "grand-nephew of the slug who dreamt of justice and invented integral calculus." The human being is a biological organism searching for greater scientific understanding and more control over nature in the ever-present search for a panacea, but dreaming also of the highest social evolution possible. In these days and ages, such an evolution entails a new concept of what is a truly "hygienic" world.

ACKNOWLEDGMENTS

The author would like to acknowledge gratefully the work of his translator, Nathalie Théocharidès, who rendered his French and the excerpt from *Futuribles* into English for this volume.

NOTES

1. For more details, see Robert (1992), Hamilton (1991), and Dubos (1965).
2. This analogy is borrowed from Gaudin (1990).
3. There are a few exceptions, but as pointed out in Chapter 8 these have tended to be broad policy statements, and to have had little direct effect on policy (e.g., Canada, 1974).
4. The fiscal crisis arises from the obvious inconsistency of ever-expanding health care systems in an environment of slow (or negative) economic growth. The "clinical crisis" arises from the contradiction between ever-expanding capacity, and growing evidence of ineffective or inappropriate clinical interventions.
5. Examples include *Futuribles* in France, *Futures* in Great Britain, and *The Futurist* in the United States.
6. This book is the product of collaboration among French scientists of all backgrounds and disciplines. It includes over two thousand maps, diagrams, and photographs.
7. Osberg (1990) is interesting in this respect: "(First) social policies must be designed which the economy can afford to support in the long run. . . . (Second) economic and social policies must also be designed which will maintain the 'social capital' on which economic processes depend. One cannot complacently assume that 'all else will remain the same,' since deterioration of the social environment can be very costly. When crime rates rise, all citizens bear the costs of crime, both as victims and as the purchasers of security services to avoid victimization. As the level of mistrust and class conflict increases, and the collective bargaining environment deteriorates, the economy bears the cost of declining labour productivity and increasing strike incidence. As the nuclear family splits from the extended family, and begins, itself, to fragment, society is forced to provide alternative institutions to supply child care, support of the disabled, and care for the elderly. To the extent that society as a whole is allowing the social environment to deteriorate, we are in a very real sense running a 'social deficit,' and storing up a national debt of social problems whose eventual remedy will be just as expensive as our environmental problems" (p. 15).

References

Aaron, H. J., and W. B. Schwartz (1984). *The Painful Prescription: Rationing Hospital Care*. Washington, DC: Brookings Institution.

Abel-Smith, B. (1992). "Cost Containment and New Priorities in the European Community." *Milbank Quarterly* 70(3):393–416.

Ackerman, B. A., and W. T. Hassler (1981). *Clean Coal, Dirty Air*. New Haven, CT: Yale University Press.

Ader, R., and N. Cohen (1975) "Behaviourally Conditioned Immunosuppression." *Psychosomatic Medicine* 37:333–40.

Alford, R. (1975). *Health Care Politics*. Chicago: University of Chicago Press.

Allen, M. G. (1976). "Twin Studies of Affective Illness." *Archives of General Psychiatry* 33:1476–78.

American Council of Life Insurance and Health Insurance Association of America (1988). "INSURE Project—Lifecycle Study," Press Kit (April 25).

Andersen, T. F., and G. Mooney (eds.) (1990). *The Challenge of Medical Practice Variations*. London: Macmillan.

Anderson, G. M., S. Brinkworth, and T. Ng (1989). "Cholesterol Screening: Evaluating Alternative Strategies," HPRU 89:10D. Health Policy Research Unit, University of British Columbia, Vancouver (August).

Anderson, G. M., and J. Lomas (1989). "Regionalization of Coronary Artery Bypass Surgery: Effects on Access." *Medical Care* 27:288–96.

Anderson, G. M., J. P. Newhouse, and L. L. Roos (1989). "Hospital Care for Elderly Patients with Diseases of the Circulatory System: A Comparison of Hospital Utilization in the United States and Canada." *New England Journal of Medicine* 321:1443–48.

Anitschkow, N. (1915). "Ueber die experimentelle Atkerosklerose der Herzklappern." *Virchows Archive Section A: Pathological Anatomy and Histopathology* 220:233–56.

Antonovski, A. (1979). *Health, Stress and Coping*. San Francisco: Jossey-Bass.

Attali, J. (1979). *L'ordre cannibale: Vie et mort de la médecine*. Paris: Grasset.

Baird, P. A. (1990). "Opportunity and Danger: Medical, Ethical and Social Implications of Early DNA Screening for Identification of Genetic Risk of Common Adult Onset Disorders." Pp. 279–88 in *Genetic Screening from Newborns to DNA Typing*, edited by B. M. Knoppe and C. M. Loberge. Amsterdam: Elsevier, Medica International Congress Series.

Baird, P. A., T. W. Anderson, H. B. Newcombe, and R. B. Lowry (1988). "Genetic Disorders in Children and Young Adults." *American Journal of Human Genetics* 42:677–93.

Baird, P. A., and A. D. Sadovnick (1988). "Life Expectancy in Down Syndrome Adults." *Lancet* 2(December 10):1354–56.

Baird, P. A., and C. R. Scriver (1990). "Genetics and the Public Health," Internal Document #10A. Program in Population Health, Canadian Institute for Advanced Research, Toronto (January).

Bamforth, S., and P. A. Baird (1989). "Spina Bifida and Hydrocephalus: A Population Study over a 35-Year Period." *American Journal of Human Genetics* 44:225–32.

Banta, H. D., C. Behney, and J. S. Willems (1981). *Toward Rational Technology in Medicine: Considerations for Health Policy*. New York: Springer.

Bardach, E., and R. A. Kagan (1982). *Going by the Book: The Problem of Regulatory Unreasonableness*. Philadelphia: Temple University Press.

Barer, M. L., R. G. Evans, and G. L. Stoddart (1979). *Controlling Health Care Costs by Direct Charges to Patients: Snare or Delusion?* Occasional Paper #10. Toronto: Ontario Economic Council.

Barer, M. L., R. G. Evans, G. L. Stoddart, R. Labelle, and J. Fulton (1984). *Lifestyles, Linkages, and Liabilities: Theory and Evidence Justifying Economic Incentives for Healthier Lifestyles*. HSRD Report S:17, Division of Health Services Research and Development, University of British Columbia, Vancouver; and Research Report Number 112, Program for Quantitative Studies in Economics and Population, McMaster University, Hamilton, Ontario.

Barer, M. L., and G. L. Stoddart (1991). *Toward Integrated Medical Resource Policies*. Report prepared for the Canadian Federal/Provincial/Territorial Deputy Ministers of Health, Ottawa.

Barker, D. J. P. (1989). "The Intrauterine and Early Postnatal Origins of Cardiovascular Disease and Chronic Bronchitis." *Journal of Epidemiology and Community Health* 43:237–40.

Barker, D. J. P., A. R. Bull, C. Osmond, and S. J. Simmonds (1990). "Fetal and Placental Size and Risk of Hypertension in Adult Life." *British Medical Journal* 301:259–62.

Barker, D. J. P., and C. Osmond (1986). "Infant Mortality, Childhood Nutrition and Ischaemic Heart Disease in England and Wales." *Lancet* 1(May 10):1077–81.

Barker, D. J. P., and C. Osmond (1987). "Inequalities in Health in Britain: Specific Explanations in Three Lancashire Towns." *British Medical Journal* 294:749–52.

Barker, D. J. P., P. D. Winter, C. Osmond, B. Margetts, and S. J. Simmonds (1989). "Weight in Infancy and Death from Ischaemic Heart Disease." *Lancet* 2(September 9):577–80.

Barry, M. J., A. G. Mulley, F. J. Fowler, and J. E. Wennberg (1988). "Watchful Waiting vs. Immediate Transurethral Resection for Symptomatic Prostatism: The Importance of Patients' Preferences." *Journal of the American Medical Association* 259: 3010–17.

Baumann, A. O., R. B. Deber, and G. G. Thompson (1990). "Overconfidence among physicians and nurses: The 'micro-certainty, macro-uncertainty' phenomenon." *Social Science and Medicine* 32:167–74.

Becker, M. H. (1985). "Patient Adherence to Prescribed Therapies." *Medical Care* 23(5):539–55.

Becker, M. S., S. J. Suomi, L. Marva, J. D. Higley, and N. Brogan (1984). "Developmental Data as Predictors of Depression in Infant Rhesus Monkeys." *Infant Behavior and Development* 7:26–27.

Beiser, M. (1990). *Research Priorities in Multiculturalism and Mental Health*. Report of a national workshop sponsored by Health and Welfare Canada, Ottawa, Ontario, September 10–18. Ottawa: Health Service and Promotion Branch, Health and Welfare Canada.

Bensaid, N. (1981a). *La lumière médicale: les illusions de la prévention*. Paris: Seuil.

Bensaid, N. (1981b). "Adivertissement: Un étrange bonheur." Pp. 9–25 in *La lumière médicale: les illusions de la prévention*. Paris: Seuil.

Ben Shlomo, Y., and G. Davey Smith (1991). "Deprivation in Infancy or in Adult Life: Which Is More Important for Mortality Risk?" *Lancet* 337(March 2):530–34.

Berkman, L. F. (1984). "Assessing the Physical Health Effects of Social Networks and Social Support." Pp. 413–32 in *Annual Review of Public Health*, edited by L. Breslow, J. E. Fielding, and L. B. Lave. Palo Alto, CA: Annual Reviews.

Berkman, L. F. (1986). "The Association between Educational Attainment and Mental Status Examinations: Of Etiologic Significance for Senile Dementias or Not?" *Journal of Chronic Diseases* 39:171–74.

Berkman, L. F., and L. Syme (1979). "Social Networks, Host Resistance and Mortality: A Nine-Year Follow-Up Study of Alameda County Residents." *American Journal of Epidemiology* 109(2):186–204.

Bernard, J. (1989). "Biologie, éthique et sociétés." *Futuribles* 131(March):3–10.

Bernard, J. (1990). *De la biologie à l'éthique: Nouveaux pouvoirs de la science, nouveaux devoirs de l'homme*. Paris: Buchet-Chastel.

Bernstein, S. J., J. Kosecoff, D. Gray, J. R. Hampton, and R. H. Brook (1993). "The Appropriateness of the Use of Cardiovascular Procedures: British versus U.S. Perspectives." *International Journal of Technology Assessment in Health Care* 9:3–10.

Berthelot, J.-M., R. Roberge, and M. Wolfson (1992). "Calculation of Utility-Based Health-Adjusted Life Expectancy in Canada: A First Attempt." Paper presented at the 6th International Workshop of REVES, Calculation of Health Expectancies, Montpelier, France, October.

Berwick, D. M. (1989). "Health Services Research and Quality-of-Care. Assignments for the 1990's." *Medical Care* 27:763–71.

Beutler, E. (1978). "Glucose-6-Phosphate Dehydrogenase Deficiency." Pp. 23–167 in *Hemolytic Anemia in Disorders of Red Cell Metabolism*, edited by Maxwell M. Wintrobe. New York: Plenum.

Biegel, D. E., A. J. Naparstek, and M. M. Khan (1980). "Determinants of Social Support Systems." Pp. 111–22 in *Optimizing Environments: Research, Practice and Policy*, edited by R. R. Stough and A. Wandersman. Washington, DC: Environmental Design Research Association.

Biondi, M., and G. D. Kotzalidis (1990). "Human Psychoneuroimmunology Today." *Journal of Clinical Laboratory Analysis* 4:22–38.

Birch, H. G. (1972). "Malnutrition, Learning and Intelligence." *American Journal of Public Health* 62(6, June):773–84.

Birch, S., and J. Eyles (1990). *Needs-Based Planning of Health Care. A Critical Appraisal of the Literature.* Ontario Ministry of Health, Toronto.

Black, D., J. N. Morris, C. Smith, and P. Townsend (1982). *Inequalities in Health: The Black Report,* edited by P. Townsend and N. Davidson. Middlesex: Penguin.

Black, D., J. N. Morris, C. Smith, P. Townsend, and M. Whitehead (1988). *Inequalities in Health: The Black Report. The Health Divide.* London: Penguin.

Blaxter, M. (1988). "Report of the ESRC Seminar on Measuring the Quality of Health, Lay Concepts of Health and Survey Health Measures." *Survey Methods Newsletter* (Winter):3–9.

Blustein, J., and T. R. Marmor (1992). "Introduction to Rationing." *University of Pennsylvania Law Review* 140 (5):1539–42.

Bondjers, G., M. Glukhova, G. Hansson, Y. V. Postnov, M. A. Reidy, and S. M. Schwartz (1991). "Hypertension and Atherosclerosis. Cause and Effect, or Two Effects with One Unknown Cause?" *Circulation* 84(6):VI2–16.

Boyce, W. T., E. A. Chesterman, N. Martin, S. Folkman, F. Cohen, and D. Wara (1993). "Immunologic Changes Occurring at Kindergarten Entry Predict Respiratory Illness Following the Loma Prieta Earthquake." *Journal of Developmental and Behavioural Pediatrics* 14:296–303.

Breslow, L. (1990). "A Health Promotion Primer for the 1990s." *Health Affairs* 9(2):6–21.

Brinkley, J. (1986). "U.S. Releasing Lists of Hospitals with Abnormal Mortality Rates." *New York Times,* 12 March, p. 1.

Brook, R. H. (1989). "Practice Guidelines and Practicing Medicine: Are They Compatible?" *Journal of the American Medical Association* 262:3027–30.

Brook, R. H. (1990). "Relationship between Appropriateness and Outcome." Pp. 59–67 in *Measuring the Outcomes of Medical Care,* edited by A. Hopkins and D. Costain. London: King's Fund Centre for Health Services Development, .

Brook, R. H., M. R. Chassin, A. Fink, D. H. Solomon, J. Kosecoff, and R. E. Park (1986). "A Method for the Detailed Assessment of the Appropriateness of Medical Technologies." *International Journal of Technology Assessment in Health Care* 2:53–64.

Brook, R. H., J. B. Kosecoff, R. E. Park, M. R. Chassin, C. M. Winslow, and J. R. Hampton (1988). "Diagnosis and Treatment of Coronary Disease: Comparison of Doctors' Attitudes in the USA and the UK." *Lancet* 1(April 2):750–53.

Brown, G. W., B. Andrews, T. O. Harris, S. Adler, and L. Bridge. (1986). "Social Support, Self-Esteem and Depression." *Psychological Medicine* 16:813–31.

Brown, G. W., T. K. Craig, and T. O. Harris (1985). "Depression: Disease or Distress? Some Epidemiological Considerations." *British Journal of Psychiatry* 147:612–22.

Brown, G. W., and T. O. Harris (1978). *Social Origins of Depression: A Study of Psychiatric Disorder in Women.* London: Tavistock.

Brown, G. W., and T. O. Harris (eds.) (1989). "Depression." Pp. 49–93 in *Life Events and Illness,* edited by G. W. Brown and T. O. Harris. New York: Guilford Press.

Brown, G. W., and R. Prudo (1981). "Psychiatric Disorders in a Rural and an

Urban Population: 1. Aetiology of Depression." *Psychological Medicine* 11:581–99.

Brown, G. W., and R. Prudo (1987). "Psychiatric Disorder in a Rural and Urban Population: Life Events, Social Integration and Symptom Formation." Pp. 111–49 in *Regards anthropologiques en psychiatrie,* edited by E. Corin, S. Lamarre, P. Migneault, and M. Tousignant. Montreal: Édition du Girame.

Brown, K., and C. Burrows (n.d.). "Cost-Effectiveness of Alternative Workup Strategies in Screening for Colorectal Cancer." Working Paper #6, National Centre for Health Program Evaluation, Melbourne, Australia.

Buck, C. (1985). "Beyond Lalonde: Creating Health." *Canadian Journal of Public Health* 76(Supplement 1, May/June):19–24.

Bunker, J. P. (1970). "Surgical Manpower: A Comparison of Operations and Surgeons in the United States and in England and Wales." *New England Journal of Medicine* 282:135–44.

Bunker, J. P., D. S. Gomby, and B. H. Kehrer (1989). *Pathways to Health: The Role of Social Factors.* Menlo Park, CA: Henry J. Kaiser Family Foundation.

Caldwell, J. C. (1986). "Routes to Low Mortality in Poor Countries." *Population and Development Review* 12:171–220.

Caldwell, J. C., and P. Caldwell (1991). "The Roles of Women, Families and Communities in Preventing Illness and Providing Health Services in Developing Countries." Paper presented at the Workshop on the Policy and Planning Implications of the Epidemiologic Transition, National Academy of Sciences, Washington, D.C.

Callenbach, E. (1990). *Ecotopia.* Berkeley, CA: Banyan Tree Books.

Canada (1974). *A New Perspective on the Health of Canadians* (Lalonde Report). Ottawa: Department of National Health and Welfare.

Canadian Institute for Advanced Research (1991). *The Determinants of Health.* CIAR Publication #5. Toronto: Canadian Institute for Advanced Research.

Cannon, W. B. (1939). *The Wisdom of the Body.* New York: Norton.

Caper, P. (1988). "Solving the Medical Dilemma." *New England Journal of Medicine* 318:1535–36.

Carr, D. H. (1977). "Detection and Evaluation of Pregnancy Wastage." Pp. 189–213 in *Handbook of Teratology,* edited by J. G. Wilson and F. C. Fraser. New York: Plenum.

Carr-Hill, R. (1987). "The Inequalities in Health Debate: a Critical Review of the Issues." *Social Policy* 16:509–42.

Carter, C. O., F. C. Fraser, J. A. Roberts, K. A. Evans, and A. R. Buck (1971). "Genetic Clinic: A Follow-Up." *Lancet* 1(February 6):281–85.

CASS Principal Investigators and Their Associates. (1981). "The National Heart, Lung, and Blood Institute Coronary Artery Surgery Study (CASS)." *Circulation* 63(suppl I):I1–81.

Cassel, C. K. (1985). "Doctors and Allocation Decisions. A New Role in Medicare." *Journal of Health Politics, Policy and Law* 10:549–64.

Cassel, J. C. (1975). "Introduction." Pp. 1–4 in *Family and Health: An Epidemiological Approach,* edited by B. H. Kaplan and J. C. Cassel. Chapel Hill, NC: Institute for Research in Social Science.

Cassel, J. C. (1976). "The Contribution of the Social Environment to Host Resistance." *American Journal of Epidemiology* 104(2):107–23.

Cavalli-Sforza, L. L., and W. F. Bodmer (1971). *The Genetics of Human Populations.* San Francisco: W. H. Freeman.

Challis, L., S. Fuller, M. Henwood, et al. (1988). *Joint Approaches to Social Policy. Rationality and Practice.* Cambridge: Cambridge University Press.

Chalmers, I. (1991). "The Work of the National Perinatal Epidemiology Unit: One Example of Technology Assessment in Perinatal Care." *International Journal of Technology Assessment in Health Care* 7:430–59.

Chalmers, T. C., P. Reitman, D. Hewett, and H. S. Sacks (1989). "Selection and Evaluation of Empirical Research in Technology Assessment." *International Journal of Technology Assessment in Health Care* 5:521–36.

Charlton, J. R. H., and R. Velez (1986). "Some International Comparisons of Mortality Amenable to Medical Intervention." *British Medical Journal* 292:295–301.

Chassin, M. R., R. H. Brook, R. E. Park, et al. (1986). "Variations in the Use of Medical and Surgical Services by the Medicare Population." *New England Journal of Medicine* 314:285–90.

Chassin, M. R., J. Kosecoff, R. E. Park, et al. (1987). "Does Inappropriate Use Explain Geographic Variations in the Use of Health Care Services?" *Journal of the American Medical Association* 258:2533–37.

Chess, S., and M. Hassibi (1986). Pp. 90–103 in *Principles and Practice of Child Psychiatry* (2nd ed.). New York and London: Plenum.

Childs, B., and C. R. Scriver (1988). *Perspectives in Biology and Medicine* 29(3, Part 1):437–60.

Clarkson, B. C., J. R. Kaplan, and M. R. Adams (1985). "The Role of Individual Differences in Lipoprotein, Artery Wall, Gender and Behavioral Responses in the Development of Atherosclerosis." Pp. 28–45 in *Atherosclerosis,* edited by K. T. Lee. New York: New York Academy of Sciences.

Coe, A., L. T. Rosenberg, M. Fisher, and S. Levine (1987). "Psychological Factors Capable of Preventing the Inhibition of Antibody Responses in Separated Infant Monkeys." *Child Development* 58:1420–30.

Cohen, S., D. A. J. Tyrrell, and A. P. Smith (1991). "Psychological Stress and Susceptibility to the Common Cold." *New England Journal of Medicine* 325: 606–12.

Colditz, G. A., J. N. Miller, and F. Mosteller (1989). "How Study Design Affects Outcomes in Comparisons of Therapy." I.: Medical. *Statistics in Medicine* 8:441–54.

Coles, J., and I. Wickings (1976). "Allocating Budgets to Wards: An Experiment." *Hospital and Health Services Review* 72:309–12.

Connell, F. A., L. A. Blide, and M. A. Hanken (1984). "Clinical Correlates of Small Area Variations in Population-Based Admission Rates for Diabetes." *Medical Care* 22:939–49.

Consumer Reports (1992). *How to Resolve the Health Care Crisis: Affordable Protection for* All *Americans.* Yonkers, NY: Consumer Reports Books.

Consumer Reports (1993). "Can Your Mind Heal Your Body?" *Consumer Reports* 58(2, February):107–15.

Coreil, J., J. S. Levin, and E. G. Jaco (1985). "Life Style—An Emergent Concept in the Sociomedical Sciences." *Culture, Medicine and Psychiatry* 9(4):423–37.

Corin, E. (1986). "The Relationship between Formal and Informal Social Support Networks in Rural and Urban Contexts." Pp. 367–94 in *Aging in Canada*, edited by V. W. Marshall. *Social Perspectives* (2nd ed.). Markham, Ontario: Fitzhenry and Whiteside.

Corin, E., G. Bibeau, J.-C. Martin, and R. Laplante (1990). *Comprendre pour soigner autrement*. Montréal: Presses de l'Université de Montréal.

Corin, E., J. Tremblay, T. Sherif, and L. Bergeron (1984). "Entre les services professionnels et les services sociaux: Les stratégies d'existence des personnes âgées." *Sociologie et Sociétés* 16(2):89–104.

Costa, T., C. R. Scriver, and B. Childs (1985). "The Effect of Mendelian Disease on Human Health: A Measurement." *American Journal of Medical Genetics* 21:231–42.

Cromwell, J., J. B. Mitchell, and W. B. Stason (1990). "Learning by Doing in CABG Surgery." *Medical Care* 28:6–18.

Culyer, A. J. (1982). "The NHS and the Market: Images and Realities." Pp. 23–55 in *The Public-Private Mix for Health: The Relevance and Effects of Change*, edited by A. Maynard and G. McLachlan. London: Nuffield Provincial Hospitals Trust.

Culyer, A. J. (1988). *Health Expenditures in Canada: Myth and Reality, Past and Future*. Toronto: Canadian Tax Foundation.

Culyer, A. J. (1989). "Cost Containment in Europe." *Health Care Financing Review* (December supplement):21–32.

Culyer, A. J. (1991). "Health, Health Expenditures and Equity." Discussion Paper 83, Centre for Health Economics, Health Economics Consortium, University of York.

Cynader, M. S., C. Shaw, F. van Huizen, and G. Prusky (1991). "Redistribution of Neurotransmitter Receptors and the Mechanism of Cortical Developmental Plasticity." Pp. 253–65 in D. M. Lam and C. Shatz, eds. *Development of the Visual System*. Cambridge, MA: MIT Press.

Dalton, D. C. (1985). *An Introduction to Practical Animal Breeding* (2nd ed.). London: Collins.

Dantzer, R., and K. W. Kelley (1989). "Stress and Immunity: An Integrated View of Relationships between the Brain and the Immune System." *Life Sciences* 44:1995–2008.

Davey Smith G., and M. G. Marmot (1991). "Trends in Mortality in Britain: 1920–1986." *Annals of Nutritional Metabolism* 35(Suppl. 1):53–63.

Davey Smith G., and M. G. Marmot (n. d.). "Further Observations in the Whitehall Study." Unpublished observations.

Davey Smith, G., and M. J. Shipley (1991). "Confounding of Occupation and Smoking: Its Magnitude and Consequences." *Social Sciences and Medicine* 32(11):1297–1300.

Davey Smith, G., M. J. Shipley, and G. Rose (1990). "The Magnitude and Causes of Socio-Economic Differentials in Mortality: Further Evidence from the Whitehall Study." *Journal of Epidemiology and Community Health* 44:265–70.

Davey Smith, G., et al. (1990). "The Black Report on Socioeconomic Inequalities in Health: 10 Years On." *British Medical Journal* 301:373–77.

Davies, M. J., and A. C. Thomas (1985). "Plaque Fissuring—The Cause of Acute Myocardial Infarction, Sudden Ischaemic Death and Crescendo Angina." *British Heart Journal* 53:363–73.

Davis, K. (1990). "Use of Data Registries to Evaluate Medical Procedures: Coronary Artery Surgery Study and the Balloon Valvuloplasty Registry." *International Journal of Technology Assessment in Health Care* 6:203–10.

Day, N., and L. B. Holmes (1973). "The Incidence of Genetic Disease in a University Hospital Population." *American Journal of Human Genetics* 25:237–46.

Day, R., J. A. Nielsen, A. Korten, G. Ernberg, et al. (1987). "Stressful Life Events Preceding the Acute Onset of Schizophrenia: A Cross-National Study from the World Health Organization." *Culture, Medicine and Psychiatry* 11(2):123–206.

de Almeida-Filho, N. (1987). *Migration and Mental Health in Bahia, Brazil*. Salvador, Bahia, Brazil: Caja de Ahorros de la Inmaculada de Aragon.

de Rosnay, J. (1991). *Les rendezvous du futur*. Paris: Fayard.

De Vries, M. (1981). *The Redemption of the Intangible in Medicine*. London: Institute of Psychosynthesis.

Detsky, A. S. (1989). "Are Clinical Trials a Cost- Effective Investment?" *Journal of the American Medical Association* 262:1795–1800.

Detsky, A. S., K. O'Rourke, C. D. Naylor, S. R. Stacey, and J. Kitchens (1990). "Containing Ontario's Hospital Costs under Universal Health Insurance in the 1980s: What Was the Record?" *Canadian Medical Association Journal* 142:565–72.

Devitt, J. E., and M. Ironside (1975). "Difficulties in Applying Patient Care Audit to Surgeons." *Bulletin of the American College of Surgeons* (May):18–21.

Doll, R., and R. Peto (1981). *The Causes of Cancer: Quantitative Estimates of Avoidable Risks of Cancer in the United States Today.* New York: Oxford University Press.

Domenighetti, G., P. Luraschi, F. Gutzwiller, E. Pedrinis, A. Casabianca, A. Spinelli, and F. Repetto (1988). "Effect of Information Campaign by the Mass Media on Hysterectomy Rates." *Lancet* 2(December 24/31):1470–73.

Dougherty, G., I. B. Pless, and R. Wilkins (1990). "Social Class and the Occurrence of Traffic Injuries and Deaths in Urban Children." *Canadian Journal of Public Health* 81:204–9.

Dressler, W. W. (1982). *Hypertension and Culture Change. Acculturation and Disease in the West Indies*. New York: Redgrane.

Dressler, W. W. (1985). "Psychosomatic Symptoms, Stress and Modernization: A Model." *Culture, Medicine and Psychiatry* 9(3):257–86.

Dressler, W. W., and L. W. Badger (1985). "Epidemiology of Depressive Symptoms in Black Communities." *Journal of Nervous and Mental Disease* 173: 212–20.

Dressler, W. W., A. Mata, A. Chavez, and F. E. Viteri (1987). "Arterial Blood Pressure and Individual Modernization in a Mexican Community." *Social Science and Medicine* 24(8):679–87.

Dreyfus, H. L., and S. E. Dreyfus (1988). "Making a Mind Versus Modelling the Brain: Artificial Intelligence Back at a Branchpoint." *Daedalus* 117(1, Winter):15–43.

Drummond, M. F., and G. L. Stoddart (1992). "Economic Evaluation of Health Promoting Measures Across Different Sectors: Can Valid Measures Be Developed?" Paper presented at the eighth annual meeting of the International Society for Technology Assessment in Health Care, Vancouver, British Columbia (June 14–17).

Dubos, R. (1959). *Mirage of Health*. New York: Harper and Row.

Dubos, Rene (1965). *Man Adapting*. New Haven, CT: Yale University Press.

Duguid, J. B. (1948). "Thrombosis as a Factor in the Pathogenesis of Coronary Atherosclerosis." *Journal of Pathology and Bacteriology* 58:207.

Dutton, D. B. (1986). "Social Class and Health." Pp. 31–62 in *Applications of Social Science to Clinical Medicine and Health Policy*, edited by L. H. Aitken and D. Mechanic. New Brunswick, NJ: Rutgers University Press.

Dyck, F. J., F. A. Murphy, J. K. Murphy, et al. (1977). "Effect of Surveillance on the Number of Hysterectomies in the Province of Saskatchewan." *New England Journal of Medicine* 296:1326–28.

Eaton, W. W. (1985). "Epidemiology of Schizophrenia." *Epidemiologic Reviews* 7:105–26.

Economist (1990). "Development Brief." *Economist* 315(May 26):80–81.

Economist (1991). "Surgery Needed." *Economist*, special survey, July 6.

Eddy, D. M. (1984). "Variations in Physician Practice: The Role of Uncertainty." *Health Affairs* 3(2):74–89.

Eisenberg, J. M. (1986). *Doctors' Decisions and the Cost of Medical Care*. Ann Arbor, MI: Health Administration Press.

Elford, J., P. Whincup, and A. G. Shaper (1991). "Early Life Experiences and Adult Cardiovascular Disease: Longitudinal and Case-Control Studies." *International Journal of Epidemiology* 20(4):833–44.

Ellwood, P. (1988). "Outcomes Management, a Technology of Patient Experience." *New England Journal of Medicine* 318(23):1549–56.

Emery, A. E. H. (1983). "Nature and Incidence of Genetic Disease." Pp. 2–3 in *Principles and Practice of Medical Genetics*, Vol. 1, edited by A. E. H. Emery and D. L. Rimoin. Churchill Livingstone.

Epp, J. (1986). "Achieving Health for All: A Framework for Health Promotion." Catalogue No. H39-102/1986E, Health and Welfare Canada, Ottawa, November.

Epstein, A. M., R. S. Stern, and J. S. Weissman (1990). "Do the Poor Cost More? A Multihospital Study of Patients' Socioeconomic Status and Use of Hospital Resources." *New England Journal of Medicine* 322:1122–28.

Etzioni, A. (1988). *The Moral Dimension: Toward a New Economics*. New York: Free Press.

Evans, J. R. (1973). "Physicians in a Public Enterprise." *Journal of Medical Education*, 48:975–86.

Evans, R. G. (1982). "A Retrospective on the 'New Perspective.'" *Journal of Health Politics, Policy and Law* 7(2, Summer):325–44.

Evans, R. G. (1984). *Strained Mercy: The Economics of Canadian Health Care*. Toronto: Butterworths.

Evans, R. G. (1986). "Finding the Levers, Finding the Courage: Lessons from Cost Containment in North America." *Journal of Health Politics, Policy and Law* 11:585–615.

Evans, R. G. (1988). "Squaring the Circle: Reconciling Fee-for-Service with Global Expenditure Control." Discussion Paper 88:8D, Vancouver, B.C.: UBC Health Policy Research Unit.

Evans, R. G. (1990a). "Tension, Compression, and Shear: Directions, Stresses, and Outcomes of Health Care Cost Control." *Journal of Health Politics, Policy and Law* 15(1):101–28.

Evans, R. G. (1990b). "The Dog in the Night Time: Medical Practice Variations and Health Policy." Pp. 117–152 in *The Challenge of Medical Practice Variations,* edited by T. F. Andersen and G. Mooney. London: MacMillan.

Evans, R. G. (1992). "What Seems to Be the Problem? The International Movement to Restructure Health Care Systems." Discussion Paper #92:8D, Vancouver, B.C.: UBC Health Policy Research Unit.

Evans, R. G., and M. L. Barer (1989). "The American Predicament." *Health Care Financing Review* (annual suppl.):72–77.

Evans, R. G., J. Lomas, M. L. Barer, et al. (1989). "Controlling Health Expenditures —The Canadian Reality." *New England Journal of Medicine* 320:571–77.

Evidence-Based Medicine Working Group (1992). "Evidence-Based Medicine: A New Approach to Teaching the Practice of Medicine." *Journal of the American Medical Association* 268:2420–25.

Eyles, J. (1987). *The Geography of the National Health.* London: Croom Helm.

Eyles, J., S. Birch, S. Chambers, J. Hurley, and B. Hutchison (1991). "A Needs-Based Methodology for Allocating Health-Care Resources in Ontario: Development and Application." *Social Science and Medicine,* 33:489–500.

Fabrega, H. (1984). "Culture and Psychiatric Illness: Biomedical and Ethnomedical Aspects." Pp. 39–68 in *Cultural Conceptions of Mental Health and Therapy,* edited by A. J. Marsella and G. M. White. Dordrecht: D. Reidel.

Falconer, D. S. (1965). "The Inheritance of Liability to Certain Diseases, Estimated from the Inheritance among Relatives." *American Journal of Human Genetics* 29:51–76.

Feeny, D., G. Guyatt, and P. Tugwell (1986). *Health Care Technology: Effectiveness, Efficiency and Public Policy.* Montreal: Institute for Research on Public Policy.

Fishbein, M. (1967). "Attitude and the Prediction of Behaviour." Pp. 477–92 in *Readings in Attitude Theory and Measurement,* edited by M. Fishbein. New York: Wiley.

Forsdahl, A. (1977). "Are Poor Living Conditions in Childhood and Adolescence an Important Risk Factor for Arteriosclerotic Heart Disease?" *British Journal of Social and Preventive Medicine* 31:91–95.

Fossaert, R. (1991). *Le monde au 21ème siècle: Une théorie des systèmes mondiaux.* Paris: Fayard.

Fox, A. J., and P. Goldblatt (1982). "Longitudinal Study. Socio-Demographic Mortality Differentials." *Longitudinal Studies (United Kingdom: Office of Population Control Studies)* 1.

Fox, D. M. (1986). *Health Policies, Health Politics: The British and American Experience.* Princeton, NJ: Princeton University Press.

Fox, D. M. (1990). "Health Policy and the Politics of Research in the United States." *Journal of Health Politics, Policy and Law* 15:481–500.

Fox, R. (1986). "L'évolution de l'incertitude médicale." CNRS publication #77, pp. 58–94. Paris: La Documentation Française.

Frank, J., and R. G. Evans (1989). "Here Today Gone Tomorrow: The Implication of Latency for Investigations of Heterogeneities in Population Health." Internal Document #9, Program in Population Health, Canadian Institute for Advanced Research, Toronto (December).

Friedman, H. S. (1991). *The Self-Healing Personality*. New York: Holt.

Friedman, J. M. (1991). "Eugenics and the *New Genetics*." *Perspectives in Biology and Medicine* 35:145–54.

Friedman, M., and R. H. Rosenman (1969). "The Possible General Causes of Coronary Artery Disease." Pp. 75–135 in *Pathogenesis of Coronary Artery Disease*, edited by M. Friedman. New York: McGraw-Hill.

Friedson, E. (1970). *Professional Dominance*. New York: Atherton Press.

Fuchs, V. R. (1974). *Who Shall Live? Health, Economics and Social Choice*. New York: Basic Books.

Fuster, V., L. Badimon, J. J. Badimon, and J. H. Chesebro (1992). "Mechanisms of Disease: The Pathogenesis of Coronary Artery Disease and the Acute Coronary Syndromes." *New England Journal of Medicine* 326(4):242–50.

G.P.E.P. Report (1984). *Physicians for the Twenty-First Century*. Washington, DC: American Association of Medical Colleges.

Garmezy, N. (1985). "Stress-Resistant Children: The Search for Protective Factors." Pp. 213–33 in *Recent Research in Developmental Psychopathology*, edited by J. E. Stevenson. *Journal of Child Psychology and Psychiatry*, Book Supplement 4. Oxford: Pergamon.

Garmezy, N. (1991). "Resilience in Children's Adaptation to Negative Life Events and Stressed Environments." *Pediatric Annals* 20:459–66.

Garmezy, N., and M. Rutter (eds.) (1983). *Stress, Coping, and Development in Children*. New York: McGraw-Hill.

Gaudin, T. (1988). *Les métamorphoses du futur: Essai de prospective technologique*. Paris: Economica.

Gaudin, T. (ed.) (1990). *2100, récit du prochain siècle*. Paris: Payot.

Gavreau, D. (1987). *Gerontologica Perspecta* 1(1). [Special issue on the compression of morbidity.]

Gerdtham, U.–G., and B. Jönsson (1991). "Health Care Expenditure in Sweden —An International Comparison." *Health Policy* 19:211–28.

Gibson, W. (1984). *Neuromancer* Rutherford, NJ: Ace Books.

Gittelsohn, A. M., and J. E. Wennberg (1976). "On the Risk of Organ Loss." *Journal of Chronic Diseases* 29:527–35.

Gleick, J. (1987). *Chaos: Making a New Science*. New York: Viking.

Glennerster, H., M. Matsaganis, and P. Owens (1992). *A Foothold for Fundholding. A Preliminary Report on the Introduction of GP Fundholding*. King's Fund Institute Research Report #12. London: King's Fund Institute.

Goodin, R. E. (1989). *No Smoking: The Ethical Issues*. Chicago and London: University of Chicago Press.

Goodwin, D. W. (1981). "Genetic Component of Alcoholism." *Annual Review of Medicine* 32:93–99.

Gordon, J. E. (1978). *Structures, or Why Things Don't Fall Down*. London: Plenum.

Gormley, M., M. L. Barer, P. Melia, and D. Helston (1990). *The Growth in Use of Health Services 1977/78 to 1985/86*. Regina: Saskatchewan Health.

Gottesman, I. I., and J. Shields (1976). "A Critical Review of Recent Adoption,

Twin, and Family Studies of Schizophrenia: Behavioural Genetic Perspectives." *Schizophrenia Bulletin* 2:360–98.

Goyert G. L., S. F. Bottoms, M. C. Treadwell, and P. C. Nehra (1989). "The Physician Factor in Cesarean Birth Rates." *New England Journal of Medicine* 329:706–9.

Graboys, T. B. (1979). "The Economics of Screening Joggers." *New England Journal of Medicine* 301:1067.

Grantham-McGregor, S. M., C. A. Powell, S. P. Walker, and J. H. Himes (1991). "Nutritional Supplementation, Psychosocial Stimulation, and Mental Development of Stunted Children: The Jamaican Study." *Lancet* 338(July 6): 1–5.

Grayhack, J. T., and R. W. Sadowski (1975). "Results of Surgical Treatment of Benign Prostatic Hyperplasia." Pp. 125–34 in *Benign Prostatic Hyperplasia,* edited by Grayhack, Wilson, and Scherbenske, DHEW Publication No. NIH 76-1113.

Greenspan, A. M., H. R. Kay, B. C. Berger, R. M. Greenberg, et al. (1988). "Incidence of Unwarranted Implantation of Permanent Cardiac Pacemakers in a Large Medical Population." *New England Journal of Medicine* 318:158–63.

Greer, A. L. (1988). "The State of the Art versus the State of the Science: The Diffusion of New Medical Technologies in Practice." *International Journal of Technology Assessment in Health Care* 4:5–26.

Grémy, F., and B. Pissaro (1983). *Propositions pour une politique de prévention: Rapport au ministre de la santé.* Paris: La Documentation Francaise.

Grob, G. N. (1983). *Mental Illness and American Society, 1875– 1940.* Princeton, NJ: Princeton University Press.

Grumbach, K., and T. Bodenheimer (1990). "A Physician's View of Cost-Containment." *Health Affairs* 9(4):120–26.

Guattari, F. (1992). "Pour une refondation des pratiques sociales." *Le monde diplomatique* (no. 463).

Gunning-Schepers, L. J., and J. H. Hagen (1987). "Avoidable Burden of Illness: How Much Can Prevention Contribute to Health?" *Social Science and Medicine* 24(11):945–51.

Guze, S. B. (1985). "Genetic Aspects of Alcoholism." Pp. 479–87 in *Medical Genetics: Past, Present, Future,* edited by K. Berg. New York: Alan R. Liss.

Haan, M., G. A. Kaplan, and T. Camacho (1987). "Poverty and Health: Prospective Evidence from the Alameda County Study." *American Journal of Epidemiology* 125:989–98.

Haan, M. N., G. A. Kaplan, and S. L. Syme (1989). "Socioeconomic Status and Health: Old Observations and New Thoughts." Pp. 76–138 in *Pathways to Health. The Role of Social Factors,* edited by J. P. Bunker, D. S. Gomby, and B. H. Kehrer. Menlo Park, CA: Henry J. Kaiser Family Foundation.

Hadorn, D. C. (1991). "Setting Health Care Priorities in Oregon: Cost Effectiveness Meets the Rule of Rescue." *Journal of the American Medical Association* 265(17):2218–25.

Hall, J. E., E. K. Powers, R. T. McIlvaine, and V. H. Ean (1978). "The Frequency and Familial Burden of Genetic Disease in a Pediatric Hospital." *American Journal of Medical Genetics* 1:417–36.

Halliday, M. L., and W. H. LeRiche (1987). "Regional Variation in Surgical Rates,

Alberta, 1978, and the Relationship to Characteristics of Patients, Doctors Performing Surgery and Hospitals Where the Surgery Was Performed." *Canadian Journal of Public Health* 78:193–200.

Ham, C. (ed.) (1988). *Health Care Variations: Assessing the Evidence*. London: King's Fund Institute.

Hamilton, E. (1991). *La mythologie*. Paris: Guide Marabout.

Hamm, T. E., Jr., J. R. Kaplan, T. B. Clarkson, and B. C. Bullock (1983). "Effects of Gender and Social Behavior on the Development of Coronary Artery Atherosclerosis in Cynomolgous Macaques." *Atherosclerosis* 48:221–33.

Hampton, J. R. (1983). "The End of Clinical Freedom." *British Medical Journal* 287:1239–40.

Hannan, E. L., J. F. O'Donnell, H. Kilburn, H. R. Bernard, and A. Yazici (1989). "Investigation of the Relationship between Volume and Mortality for Surgical Procedures Performed in New York State Hospitals." *Journal of the American Medical Association* 262:503–10.

Hardin, G. (1968). "The Tragedy of the Medical Commons." *Science* 162:1243–48.

Hardwicke, J., and J. R. Squire (1952). "The Basis of the Erythrocyte Sedimentation Rate." *Clinical Science* 11:333–55.

Hartley, R. M., A. M. Epstein, C. M. Harris, and B. J. McNeil (1987). "Differences in Ambulatory Test-Ordering in England and America: Role of Doctors' Beliefs and Attitudes." *American Journal of Medicine* 82:513–17

Hartunian, N. S., C. N. Smart, and M. S. Thompson (1981). *The Incidence and Economic Costs of Major Health Impairments*. Lexington, MA: Heath.

Hassold, T, N. Chen, J. Funkhouser, T. Jooss, B. Manuel, J. Matsuyama, C. Wilson, J. A. Yamane, and P. A. Jacobs (1980). "A Cytogenetic Study of 1000 Spontaneous Abortions." *American Journal of Human Genetics* (London) 44:151–78.

Hawking, S. (1988). *A Brief History of Time*. Toronto: Bantam.

Hayes, A., T. Costa, C. R. Scriver, and B. Childs (1985). "The Impact of Mendelian Disease in Man. Effect of Treatment: A Measurement." *American Journal of Medical Genetics* 21:243–55.

Haynes, R. B., D. L. Sackett, D. W. Taylor, E. S. Gibson, and A. L. Johnson (1979). "Increased Absenteeism from Work after Detection and Labelling of Hypertensive Patients." *New England Journal of Medicine* 229:741–44.

Helman, C. G. (1987). "Heart Disease and the Cultural Construction of Time: The Type A Behaviour Pattern as a Western Culture-Bound Syndrome." *Social Science and Medicine* 25(9):969–79.

Hendrick, A. G., and P. E. Binkerd (1980). "Fetal Deaths in Nonhuman Primates." In *Human Embryology and Fetal Death*, edited by I. H. Porter and E. Hook. New York: Academic Press.

Henry, J. P. (1982). "The Relation of Social to Biological Processes in Disease." *Social Science and Medicine* 16:369–80.

Hertzman, C. (1986). *The Health Context of Worklife Choice*. Ottawa: Canadian Mental Health Association.

Hertzman, C. (1990). "Poland: Health and Environment in the Context of Socioeconomic Decline," HPRU 90:2D. Health Policy Research Unit, University of British Columbia, Vancouver (January).

Hertzman, C. (1992). "Czechoslovakia and the East-West Life Expectancy Gap."

Working Paper No. 16, Program in Population Health, Canadian Institute for Advanced Research, Toronto (March).

Hirayama, T. (1990). *Lifestyle and Mortality, A Large Scale Census-Based Cohort Study in Japan*. Basel: Karger.

Hlatky, M. A., R. M. Califf, F. E. Harrell, K. L. Lee, D. B. Mark, and D. B. Pryor (1988). "Comparisons of Predictions Based on Observational Data with the Results of Randomized Controlled Clinical Trials of Coronary Artery Bypass Surgery." *Journal of the American College of Cardiology* 11:237–45.

Hollingsworth, J. R. (1986). *A Political Economy of Medicine: Great Britain and the United States*. Baltimore: Johns Hopkins University Press.

Holton, G. (1988). "The Roots of Complementarity." *Daedalus* 117(3, Summer):151–97.

Holtzman, N. (1988). *Pathways to Health: The Role of Social Factors*. Menlo Park, CA: Henry J. Kaiser Family Foundation.

Holtzman, N. (1989). *Proceed with Caution: Predicting Genetic Risks in the Recombinant DNA Era*. Baltimore and London: Johns Hopkins University Press.

Hook, E. B., and A. M. Willey (1981). "Abortions Because of Unavailability of Prenatal Diagnosis" (Letter to the Editor). *Lancet* 1(October 24):936.

House, J. S., K. R. Landis, and D. Umberson (1988). "Social Relationships and Health." *Science* 241(July 29):540–45.

Howard, J. H., P. A. Rechnitzer, D. A. Cunningham, D. Wong, and H. A. Brown (1990). "Type A Behaviour, Personality, and Sympathetic Response." *Behavioural Medicine* 16(4, Winter):149–60.

Hrubec, Z., and G. S. Omenn (1981). "Evidence of Genetic Predisposition to Alcoholic Cirrhosis and Psychosis: Twin Concordances for Alcoholism and Its Biological End Points by Zygosity among Male Veterans." *Alcohol: Clinical Experimental Research* 5:207–15.

Hunter, D. J. (1991). "Managing Medicine: A Response to the 'crisis.'" *Social Science and Medicine* 32:441–49.

Hypertension Detection and Follow-up Program Co-operative Group (1979). "Five-Year Findings of the Hypertension Detection and Follow-up Program, I: Reduction in Mortality of Persons with High Blood Pressure, Including Mild Hypertension." *Journal of the American Medical Association* 242:2562–71.

Iglehart, J. K. (1988). "Japan's Health Care System—Part Two, Health Policy Report." *New England Journal of Medicine* 319(17, October 27):1166–72.

Iglehart, J. K. (1990). "Canada's Health Care System Faces Its Problems." *New England Journal of Medicine* 322:562–68.

Ignatowski, A. (1909). "Über die Wirkung des tierischen Eiweisses auf die Aorta und die parenchymatosen Organe der Kanniehen." *Virchows Archive Section A: Pathological Anatomy and Histopathology* 198:248–70.

Illich, I. (1975). *Medical Nemesis: The Expropriation of Health*. Toronto: McClelland and Stewart.

Isles, C. G., D. J. Hole, C. R. Gillis, V. M. Hawthorne, and A. F. Lever (1989). "Plasma Cholesterol, Coronary Heart Disease and Cancer in the Renfrew and Paisley Survey." *British Medical Journal* 298:920–24.

Jacobson, D. (1987). "The Cultural Context of Social Support and Support Networks." *Medical Anthropological Quarterly* 1(1):42–67.

Jacquard, A. (1991). *Voici le temps du monde fini*. Paris: Seuil.
Janes, C. R. (1986). "Migration and Hypertension: An Ethnography of Disease Risk in an Urban Samoan Community." Pp. 175–211 in *Anthropology and Epidemiology,* edited by C. R. Janes, R. Stall, and S. M. Gifford. Dordrecht: D. Reidel.
Jennett, B. (1988). "Variations Data from Surgeons, for Surgeons." Pp. 30–31 in *Health Care Variations: Assessing the Evidence,* edited by C. Ham. London: King's Fund Institute.
Jessee, W. F., C. W. Nickerson, and W. S. Grant (1982). "Assessing Medical Practices through PSRO Cooperative Studies. An Evaluation of Cesarean Birth in Nine PSRO Areas." *Medical Care* 20:75–84.
Johnson, B. C., F. H. Epstein, and M. O. Kjelsberg (1965). "Distributions and Familial Studies of Blood Pressure and Serum Cholesterol in a Total Community: Tecumseh, Michigan." *Journal of Chronic Diseases* 18:147–60.
Johnson, J. V., and G. Johansson (1991). *The Psychosocial Work Environment: Work Organization, Democratization and Health.* Amityville, NY: Baywood.
Jørgensen, L., H. C. Rowsell, T. Hovig, and J. F. Mustard (1967). "Resolution and Organization of Platelet-Rich Mural Thrombi in Carotid Arteries of Swine." *American Journal of Physiology* 213:915–22.
Jozan P. (1990). *Recent Mortality Trends in Eastern Europe*. Budapest: World Health Organization.
Kaback, M. M. (1978). "Medical Genetics: An Overview." *Pediatric Clinics of North America* 25:395–409.
Kaback, M. M. (1983). "Heterozygote Screening." Pp. 1451–57 in *Principles and Practice of Medical Genetics,* Vol. 2, edited by A. H. Emery and D. L. Remoin. New York: Churchill Livingstone.
Kaback, M. M., R. S. Zeigler, L. W. Reynolds, and M. Sonneborn (1974). "Approaches to the Control and Prevention of Tay-Sachs Disease." *Progress in Medical Genetics* 10:103–34.
Kalil, R. A. (1989). "Synapse Formation in the Developing Brain." *Scientific American* 261(6, December):76–85.
Kannel, W. B., and T. Gordon (eds.) (1973). *The Framingham Study: An Investigation of Cardiovascular Disease.* Washington, DC: U.S. Department of Health, Education, and Welfare.
Kaplan, B. H., and J. C. Cassel (eds.) (1975). *Family and Health: An Epidemiological Approach.* Chapel Hill, NC: IRSS.
Kaplan, J. R., S. B. Manuck, T. B. Clarkson, F. M. Lusso, and D. M. Taub (1982). "Social Status, Environment, and Atherosclerosis in Cynomolgous Monkeys." *Arteriosclerosis* 2:359.
Kaplan, J. R., S. B. Manuck, T. B. Clarkson, and R. W. Prichard (1985). "Animal Models of Behavioral Influences on Atherogenesis." *Advances in Behavioral Medicine* 1:115–63.
Kaplan, J. R., K. Pettersson, S. B. Manuck, and G. Olsson (1991). "Role of Sympathoadrenal Medullary Activation in the Initiation and Progression of Atherosclerosis." *Circulation* 84(6):VI23–32.
Karasek, R. A., and T. Theorell (1990). *Healthy Work: Stress, Productivity, and the Reconstruction of Working Life.* New York: Basic Books.

Kassirer, J. P., and S. G. Pauker (1981). "The Toss-Up." *New England Journal of Medicine* 305:1467–69.

Kato, H., J. Tillotson, M. Nichaman, H. B. Hamilton, and G. G. Rhoads (1973). "Epidemiologic Studies of Coronary Heart Disease and Stroke in Japanese Men Living in Japan, Hawaii and California: Serum, Lipids and Diet." *American Journal of Epidemiology* 97:372–85.

Katz, M. M., A. Marsella, K. C. Dube, M. Olatawura, et al. (1988). "On the Expression of Psychosis in Different Cultures: Schizophrenia in an Indian and in a Nigerian Community." *Culture, Medicine and Psychiatry* 12:331–55.

Keeney, R. L., D. Von Winterfeldt, and T. Eppel (1990). "Eliciting Public Values for Complex Policy Decisions." *Management Science* 36:1011–30.

Keller, R. B., A. M. Chapin, and D. N. Soule (1990). "Informed Inquiry Due to Practice Variations: The Maine Medical Assessment Foundation." *Quality Assurance in Health Care* 2:69–76.

Kerem, B, J. M. Rommens, J. A. Buchanan, D. Markiewicz, T. A. Cox, A. Chakravarti, M. Buchwald, and L. C. Tsui (1989). "Identification of the Cystic Fibrosis Gene: Genetic Analysis." *Science* 245:1073–80.

Kessling, A. M., J. Rayput-Williams, D. Bainton, et al. (1988). "DNA Polymorphisms of the Apolipoprotein AII and AI-CIII-AIV Genes: A Study in Men Selected for Differences in High Density Lipoprotein Cholesterol Concentration." *American Journal of Human Genetics* 42:458–67.

Kessner, D. M., C. E. Kalk, and J. Singer (1973). "Assessing Health Quality—The Case for Tracers." *New England Journal of Medicine* 288:189–94.

Kety, S. S., D. Rosenthal, P. H. Wedner, and F. Schulsinger (1976). "Studies Based on a Total Sample of Adopted Individuals and Their Relatives: Why They Were Necessary, What They Demonstrated and Failed to Demonstrate." *Schizophrenia Bulletin* 2:413–28.

Kety, S. S. (1983). "Mental Illness in the Biological and Adoptive Relatives of Schizophrenic Adoptees: Findings Relevant to Genetic and Environmental Factors in Etiology." *American Journal of Psychiatry* 140:720–27.

Keys, A. (1980). *Seven Countries: A Multivariate Analysis of Death and Coronary Heart Disease.* Cambridge, MA: Harvard University Press.

King, M. C., G. M. Lee, N. B. Spinner, G. Thomson, and M. R. Wrensch (1984). "Genetic Epidemiology." *Annual Review of Public Health* 5:1–52.

Kirkmann-Liff, B. L. (1990). "Physician Payment and Cost-Containment Strategies in West Germany: Suggestions for Medicare Reform." *Journal of Health Politics, Policy and Law* 15:69–100.

Klein, R. (1989). *Politics of the NHS* (2nd ed.). London: Longman.

Klein, R., and M. O'Higgins (1988). "Defusing the Crisis of the Welfare State: A New Interpretation." Pp. 203–25 in *Social Security: Beyond the Rhetoric of Crisis,* edited by T. R. Marmor and J. Mashaw. Princeton, NJ: Princeton University Press.

Kleinman, A. (1986). *Social Origins of Distress and Disease. Depression, Neurasthenia and Pain in Modern China.* New Haven, CT: Yale University Press.

Kleinman, A. (1987). "Anthropology and Psychiatry. The Role of Culture in Cross-Cultural Research on Illness." *British Journal of Psychiatry* 151:447–54.

Kleinman, A. (1988). *Rethinking Psychiatry. From Cultural Category to Personal Experience.* New York: Free Press.

Knickman, J. R. (1982). "Variations in Hospital Use across Cities: A Comparison of Utilization Rates in New York and Los Angeles." Pp. 23–63 in *Regional Variations in Hospital Use,* edited by D. L. Rothberg. Lexington, MA: Heath.

Kolata, G. (1986). "Reducing Risk: A Change of Heart?" *Science* 231:669–70.

Koran, L. M. (1975a). "The Reliability of Clinical Methods, Data and Judgements" (Part 1). *New England Journal of Medicine* 293:642–46.

Koran, L. M. (1975b). "The Reliability of Clinical Methods, Data and Judgements" (Part 2). *New England Journal of Medicine* 293:695–701.

Kosecoff, J., D. E. Kanouse, W. H. Rogers, L. McCloskey, C. M. Winslow, and R. H. Brook (1987). "Effects of the National Institutes of Health Consensus Development Program on Physician Practice." *Journal of the American Medical Association* 258:2708–13.

Kunitz, S. J., and Levy, J. E. (1986). "The Prevalence of Hypertension among Elderly Navajos: A Test of the Acculturation Stress Hypothesis." *Culture, Medicine and Psychiatry* 10(2):97–121.

Kurnit, D. M., W. M. Layton, and S. Malthysse (1987). "Genetics, Chance and Morphogenesis." *American Journal of Human Genetics* 41:979–95.

Lancet (1983). "Editorial: Crime as a Destiny?" *Lancet* 1(January 1/8):35–36.

Lancet (1991). "Editorial: What's New in Public Health?" *Lancet* 334(June 8):1381–83.

Lazarus, R. S., and S. Folkman (1984). *Stress, Appraisal and Coping*. New York: Springer.

Leape, L. L. (1989). "Unnecessary Surgery." *Health Services Research* 23:351–407.

Leape, L. L., R. E. Park, D. H. Solomon, M. R. Chassin, J. Kosecoff, and R. H. Brook (1989). "Relation between Surgeons' Practice Volumes and Geographic Variation in the Rate of Carotid Endarterectomy." *New England Journal of Medicine* 321:653–57.

Leape, L. L., R. E. Park, D. H. Solomon, M. R. Chassin, J. 351Kosecoff, and R. H. Brook (1990). "Does Inappropriate Use Explain Small-Area Variations in the Use of Health Care Services?" *Journal of the American Medical Association* 263:669–72.

Leff, J., N. N. Wig, H. Bedi, D. K. Menon, et al. (1990). "Relatives' Expressed Emotion and the Course of Schizophrenia in Chandigarh. A Two Year Follow-Up of a First Contact Sample." *British Journal of Psychiatry* 156:351–56.

Leighton, A. H. (1959). *My Name is Legion: Foundations for a Theory of Man in Relation to Culture. Vol. I: The Stirling County Study of Psychiatric Disorders and Sociocultural Environments*. New York: Basic Books.

Levine, S., and A. Lilienfeld (1987). *Epidemiology and Health Policy*. London: Tavistock.

Lewis, C. E. (1988). "Disease Prevention and Health Promotion Practices of Primary Care Physicians in the United States." In *Implementing Preventive Services*, edited by R. N. Battista and R. S. Lawrence, Supplement to *American Journal of Preventive Medicine* 4(4):9–16.

Lilienfeld, A., and D. Lilienfeld (1980). *Foundations of Epidemiology* (2nd ed.). New York: Oxford University Press.

Linton, A. L., and C. D. Naylor (1990). "Organized Medicine and the Assess-

ment of Technology. Lessons from Ontario." *New England Journal of Medicine* 323:1463–67.
Littlewood, R. (1990). "From Categories to Contexts: A Decade of the 'New Cross-Cultural Psychiatry.'" *British Journal of Psychiatry* 156:308–27.
Loewy, E. H. (1980). "Costs Should Not Be a Factor in Medical Care." *New England Journal of Medicine* 302:697.
Lomas, J. (1990a). "Promoting Clinical Policy Change: Using the Art to Promote the Science in Medicine." Pp. 174–91 in *The Challenge of Medical Practice Variations*, edited by T. F. Andersen and G. Mooney. London: Macmillan.
Lomas, J. (1990b). "Finding Audiences, Changing Beliefs: The Structure of Research Use in Canadian Health Policy." *Journal of Health Politics, Policy and Law* 15(3):525–42.
Lomas, J., G. M. Anderson, D. P. Karin, E. Vayda, M. W. Enkin, and W. J. Hannah (1989). "Do Practice Guidelines Guide Practice? The Effect of a Consensus Statement on the Practice of Physicians." *New England Journal of Medicine* 321:1306–11.
Lomas, J., M. Enkin, G. M. Anderson, et al. (1991). "Opinion Leaders versus Audit and Feedback to Implement Practice Guidelines: Delivery after Previous Cesarean Section." *Journal of the American Medical Association* 265: 2202–07.
Lomas, J., C. Fooks, T. Rice, and R. Labelle (1989). "Paying Physicians in Canada: Minding Our P's and Q's." *Health Affairs* 8(1):80–102.
Loomes, G., and L. McKenzie (1989). "The Use of QALYs in Health Care Decision Making." *Social Science and Medicine* 28(4):299–308.
Lovejoy, C. O. (1981). "The Origins of Man." *Science* 211:341–50.
Luepker, R. V. (1988). "Conclusions." Pp. 276–78 in *Trends in Coronary Heart Disease Mortality: The Influence of Medical Care*, edited by M. W. Higgins and R. V. Luepker. New York: Oxford University Press.
Luft, H. S., J. P. Bunker, and A. C. Enthoven (1979). "Should Operations Be Regionalized? The Empirical Relation between Surgical Volume and Mortality." *New England Journal of Medicine* 301:1364–69.
Lundy, T. (1992). *Getting Communities Involved*. Vancouver: B.C. Healthy Communities Network.
MacDonald, D. C. (ed.) (1980). *The Government and Politics of Ontario*. Toronto: Van Nostrand Reinhold.
Mackintosh, J. (1993). "Demarketing Cars: A Multiple of Fetishes." *Adbusters. Journal of the Mental Environment* 2(3):59–62.
Manson, S. F., J. H. Shore, and J. D. Bloom (1985). "The Depressive Experience in American Indian Communities: A Challenge for Psychiatric Theory and Diagnosis." Pp. 531–68 in *Culture and Depression*, edited by A. Kleinman and B. Good. Berkeley: University of California Press.
Manuck, S. B., J. R. Kaplan, and K. A. Matthews (1986). "Behavioral Antecedents of Coronary Heart Disease and Atherosclerosis." *Arteriosclerosis* 6(January–February):2–14.
Markowe, H. L. J., M. G. Marmot, M. J. Shipley, et al. (1985). "Fibrinogen—A Possible Link between Social Class and Coronary Heart Disease." *British Medical Journal* 291(6505):1312–14.

Marmor, T. R. (1983). *Political Analysis and American Medical Care*. Cambridge: Cambridge University Press.
Marmor, T. R. (1986). "American Medical Policy and the Crisis of the Welfare State: Comparative Perspectives." *Journal of Health Politics, Policy and Law* 11(4):617–31.
Marmor, T. R. (1989). "Healthy Public Policy: What Does That Mean, Who Is Responsible for It, and How Would One Pursue It?" Internal Document #6A, Program in Population Health, Canadian Institute for Advanced Research, Toronto (August).
Marmor, T. R. (1992). "Japan: A Sobering Lesson." *Health Management Quarterly* 14(3):10–14.
Marmor, T. R., and R. Smithey (1989). "Health Policy in Historical Perspective: A Review Essay." *Journal of Policy History* 1(1):108–28.
Marmot, M. G. (1981). "Culture and Illness: Epidemiological Evidence." Pp. 323–40 in *Foundations of Psychosomatics*, edited by M. J. Christie and P. G. Mellet. Chichester: Wiley.
Marmot, M. G. (1985). "Interpretation of Trends in Coronary Heart Disease Mortality." *Acta Medical Scand (Suppl.)* 701:58–65.
Marmot, M. G. (1986). "Social Inequalities in Mortality: The Social Environment." Pp. 21–33 in *Class and Health: Research and Longitudinal Data*, edited by R. G. Wilkinson. London: Tavistock.
Marmot, M. G. (1992). "Coronary Heart Disease: Rise and Fall of a Modern Epidemic." Pp. 1–19 in *Coronary Heart Disease Epidemiology: From Aetiology to Public Health*, edited by Michael Marmot and Paul Elliott. Oxford: Oxford University Press.
Marmot, M. G., A. M. Adelstein, and L. Bulusu (1984). "Lessons from the Study of Immigrant Mortality." *Lancet* 1(June 30):1455–58.
Marmot, M. G., A. M. Adelstein, N. Robinson, and G. A. Rose (1978). "Changing Social Class Distribution of Heart Disease." *British Medical Journal* 2:1109–12.
Marmot M. G., and G. Davey Smith (1989). "Why Are the Japanese Living Longer?" *British Medical Journal* 299:1547–51.
Marmot, M. G., M. Kogevinas, and M. A. Elston (1987). "Social/Economic Status and Disease." *Annual Review of Public Health* 8:111–35.
Marmot, M. G., and M. E. McDowell (1986). "Mortality Decline and Widening Social Inequalities." *Lancet* 2(August 2):274–76.
Marmot, M. G., G. Rose, M. J. Shipley, and P. J. S. Hamilton (1978). "Employment Grade and Coronary Heart Disease in British Civil Servants." *Journal of Epidemiology and Community Health* 32:244–49.
Marmot, M. G., M. J. Shipley, and G. Rose (1984). "Inequalities in Death—Specific Explanations of a General Pattern." *Lancet* 1(May 5):1003–6.
Marmot M. G., and S. L. Syme (1976). "Acculturation and Coronary Heart Disease in Japanese-Americans." *American Journal of Epidemiology* 104: 225–47.
Marmot, M. G., S. L. Syme, A. Kagan, H. Kato, J. B. Cohen, and J. Belsky (1975). "Epidemiological Studies of Coronary Heart Disease and Stroke in Japanese Men Living in Japan, Hawaii and California. Prevalence of Coronary and

Hypertensive Heart Disease and Associated Risk Factors." *American Journal of Epidemiology* 102:514–25.

Marmot, M. G., and T. Theorell (1988). "Social Class and Cardiovascular Disease: The Contribution of Work." *International Journal of Health Services* 18:659–74.

Martin, M. J., S. B. Hulley, W. S. Browner, L. H. Kuller, and D. Wentworth (1986). "Serum Cholesterol, Blood Pressure, and Mortality: Indications from a Cohort of 361,662 Men." *Lancet* 2(October 25):933–36.

Martin, S. L., C. T. Ramey, and S. Ramey (1990). "The Prevention of Intellectual Impairment in Children of Impoverished Families: Findings of a Randomized Trial of Educational Day Care." *American Journal of Public Health* 80(7):844–47.

Mason, J. O. (1990). "A Prevention Policy Framework for the Nation." *Health Affairs* 9(2):22–29.

Masten, A. S., K. M. Best, and N. Garmezy (1990). "Resilience and Development: Contributions from the Study of Children Who Overcome Adversity." *Development and Psychopathology* 2:425–44.

Matsumoto, Y. S. (1970). "Social Stress and Coronary Heart Disease." *Milbank Memorial Fund Quarterly* 18:659–74.

Maynard, C., L. Fisher, E. L. Alderman, et al. (1986). "Institutional Differences in Therapeutic Decision Making in the Coronary Artery Surgery Study (CASS)." *Medical Decision Making* 6:127–35.

Mays, N., and G. Bevan (1987). *Resource Allocation in the Health Service*. London: Bedford Square Press.

McCloskey, D. N. (1989). "Why I Am No Longer a Positivist." *Review of Social Economy* 47(3, Fall):225–38.

McCord, C., and H. P. Freeman (1990). "Excess Mortality in Harlem." *New England Journal of Medicine* 322:173–77.

McGuire, A. (1990). "Measuring Performance in the Health Care Sector: The Whys and the Hows." Pp. 95–116 in *The Challenges of Medical Practice Variations*, edited by T. F. Andersen and G. Mooney. London: MacMillan.

McKeown, T. (1976). *The Role of Medicine*. London: Nuffield Provincial Hospitals Trust.

McKeown, T. (1979). *The Role of Medicine: Dream, Mirage or Nemesis?* 2nd edition. Oxford: Basil Blackwell.

McKillop, W. J., B. O'Sullivan, and G. K. Ward (1987). "Non–Small Cell Lung Cancer: How Oncologists Want to Be Treated." *International Journal of Radiation Oncology and Biological Physics* 13:929–34.

McKinlay, J. B. (1979). "Epidemiological and Political Determinants of Social Policies Regarding the Public Health." *Social Science and Medicine* 13A: 541–58.

McKinlay, J. B. (1992). "Health Promotion through Healthy Public Policy: The Contribution of Complementary Research Methods." *Canadian Journal of Public Health* 83(suppl. 1):S11–19.

McKinlay, J. B., S. M. McKinlay, and R. Beaglehole (1989). "A Review of the Evidence Concerning the Impact of Medical Measures on Recent Mortality and Morbidity in the United States." *International Journal of Health Services* 19(2):181–208.

McKusick, V. A. (1988). "Mendelian Inheritance in Man." *Catalogues of Autosomal Dominant, Autosomal Recessive, and X-Linked Phenotypes* (8th ed.). Baltimore: Johns Hopkins University Press.

McLachlin, G., and A. Maynard (eds.) (1982). *The Public/Private Mix for Health: The Relevance and Effects of Change*. London: Nuffield Provincial Hospitals Trust.

McLaughlin, C. G., D. P. Normolle, R. A. Wolfe, L. F. McMahon, and J. R. Griffith (1989). "Small-Area Inhospital Discharge Rates: Do Socioeconomic Variables Matter?" *Medical Care* 27:507–21.

McNeil, B. J., R. Weichselbaum, and S. G. Pauker (1978). "Fallacy of the Five-Year Survival in Lung Cancer." *New England Journal of Medicine* 299: 1397–1401.

McPherson, K. (1990). "Why Do Variations Occur?" Pp. 16–35 in *The Challenges of Medical Practice Variations*, edited by T. F. Andersen and G. Mooney. London: Macmillan.

McPherson, K., J. E. Wennberg, D. B. Hovind, and P. Clifford (1982). "Small-Area Variations in the Use of Common Surgical Procedures: An International Comparison of New England, England, and Norway." *New England Journal of Medicine* 307:1310–14.

Mechanic, D. (1978). *Medical Sociology. A Comprehensive Text* (2nd. ed). New York: Free Press.

Medical Research Council of Canada (1989). "Research on Gene Therapy in Humans: Background and Guidelines." Discussion paper, Medical Research Council of Canada, Ottawa.

Mednick, S. A., and W. F. Gabrielli, Jr. (1984). "Genetic Influences in Criminal Convictions: Evidence from an Adoption Cohort." *Science* 224:891–93.

Mehrez, A., and A. Gafni (1989). "Quality-Adjusted Life Years, Utility Theory, and Healthy-Years Equivalents." *Medical Decision Making* 9(2, April–June): 142–49.

Mendelson, M., and T. Sullivan (1990). "Impediments to Reorienting Health Policy." Paper prepared for CHEPA Health Policy Conference: Producing Health, Niagara on the Lake (May).

Meyer, R., and R. J. Haggerty (1962). "Streptococcal Infections in Families—Factors Altering Susceptibility." *Pediatrics* 29:539–50.

Millar, W. J. (1981). "Observations on the Mortality of Alberta Indians." *Chronic Diseases in Canada* 2:14–17.

Millar, W. J. (1993). "Observations on the Mortality of Alberta Indians." *Chronic Diseases in Canada* 2:14–17.

Miller, J. F., E. Williamson, J. Glue, Y. B. Gordon, J. G. Grudzinskas, and A. Sykes (1980). "Fetal Loss after Implantation." *Lancet* 2(September 13): 554–56.

Miller, J. N., G. A. Colditz, and F. Mosteller (1989). "How Study Design Affects Outcomes in Comparisons of Therapy." II.: Surgical. *Statistics in Medicine* 8:455–66.

Mills, A., J. P. Vaughan, D. L. Smith, and I. Tabibzadeh (1990). *Health System Decentralization. Concepts, Issues and Country Experience.* Geneva: World Health Organization.

Mindell, W. E., E. Vayda, and B. Cardillo (1982). "Ten-Year Trends in Canada for Selected Operations." *Journal of the Canadian Medical Association* 127:23–27.

Minick, C. R., and G. E. Murphy (1973). "Experimental Induction of Atheroarteriosclerosis by the Synergy of Allergic Injury to Arteries and Lipid-Rich Diet." *American Journal of Pathology* 73:265–300.

Modell, B., R. H. T. Ward, and D. V. I. Fairweather (1980). "Effect of Introducing Antenatal Diagnosis on the Reproductive Behaviour of Families at Risk for Thalassemia Major." *British Medical Journal*:737.

Moore, T. J. (1989). *Heart Failure: A Critical Inquiry into American Medicine and the Revolution in Heart Care, Part II: Prevention*. New York: Random House.

Morgan, A. D. (1956). *The Pathogenesis of Coronary Occlusion.* Oxford: Basil Blackwell.

Morris, J. N. (1951). "Recent History of Coronary Disease." *Lancet* 1(1):69.

Mulley, A. G. (1990). "The Role of Decision Analysis in the Translation of Research Findings into Clinical Practice." Pp. 78–87 in *Medical Innovation at the Crossroads. Vol. I: Modern Methods of Clinical Investigation,* edited by A. C. Gelijns. Washington, DC: National Academy Press.

Murphy, H. B. M. (1978). "European Cultural Offshoots in the New World: Differences in Their Mental Hospitalization Patterns. Part I: British, French and Italian Influences." *Social Psychiatry* 13:1–9.

Murphy, H. B. M. (1980). "European Cultural Offshoots in the New World: Differences in Their Mental Hospitalization Patterns. Part II: German, Dutch and Scandinavian Influences." *Archiv für Psychiatrie und Nervenkrankheiten* 228:161–74.

Murphy, H. B. M. (1982). *Comparative Psychiatry. The International and Intercultural Distribution of Mental Illness.* Berlin: Springer-Verlag.

Murphy, H. B. M. (1987). "Migration, Culture and Our Perception of the Stranger." Pp. 77–86 in *Regards anthropologiques en psychiatrie,* edited by E. Corin, S. Lamarre, P. Migneault, and M. Tousignant. Montreal: Edition du Girame.

Mustard, J. F., M. A. Packam, and R. L. Kinlough-Rathbone (1981). "Mechanisms in Thrombosis." In *Haemostasis and Thrombosis,* edited by A. L. Bloom and D. P. Thomas. London: Churchill Livingstone.

Mustard, J. F., M. A. Packham, and R. L. Kinlough-Rathbone (1986). "Platelets and Mechanisms of Thrombosis and Atherosclerosis." Pp. 1–18 in *Biology and Pathology of the Platelet—Vessel Wall Interactions,* edited by G. Jolles, Y. Legrand, and A. T. Nurden. London: Academic Press.

Nagnur, D. (1989). Unpublished data. Ottawa: Statistics Canada.

Nagnur, D., and M. Nagrodski (1987). "Cause-Deleted Life Tables for Canada (1921 to 1981): An Approach Towards Analysing Epidemiologic Transition." Analytical Studies Branch Research Paper, Statistics Canada, Ottawa.

Naylor, C. D. (1986). *Private Practice, Public Payment: Canadian Medicine and the Politics of Health Insurance, 1911 to 1966*. Montreal: McGill-Queen's University Press.

Naylor, C. D. (1991). "A Different View of Queues: Lessons from the Coronary Surgery Crisis in Ontario, Canada." *Health Affairs* 10(3):110–28.

Naylor, C. D., R. S. Baigrie, B. S. Goldman, and A. Basinski (1990). "Assessment of Priority for Coronary Revascularisation Procedures." *Lancet* (May 5): 1070–73.

Nerem, R. M., M. J. Levesque, and J. F. Cornhill (1980). "Social Environment as a Factor in Diet-Induced Atherosclerosis." *Science* 208(June 27):1475–76.

Newmark, M. E., and J. K. Perry (1980). *Genetics of Epilepsy: A Review*. New York: Raven.

Newsweek (1988). "Body and Soul." November 7, pp. 88–97.

Nichaman, M. Z., H. B. Hamilton, A. Kagan, S. Sacks, T. Greer, and S. L. Syme (1975). "Epidemiologic Studies of Coronary Heart Disease and Stroke in Japanese Men Living in Japan, Hawaii and California: Distribution of Biochemical Risk Factors." *American Journal of Epidemiology* 102:491–501.

Nolan, T., and I. B. Pless (1986). "Emotional Correlates and Consequences of Birth Defects." *Journal of Pediatrics* 109:201–16.

North, F., S. L. Syme, A. Feeney, et al. (1993). "Explaining Socioeconomic Differences in Sickness Absence: The Whitehall II Study." *British Medical Journal* 306(February 6):363.

OECD Secretariat (1989). "Health Care Expenditure and Other Data: An International Compendium from the Organization for Economic Cooperation and Development." *Health Care Financing Review* (Annual Supplement):111–94.

Office of Population Censuses and Surveys (1972). *Occupational Mortality: The Registrar General's Decennial Supplement for England and Wales,* Series DS No. 1. London: Her Majesty's Stationery Office.

Office of Population Censuses and Surveys. (1978). *Occupational Mortality: The Registrar General's Decennial Supplement for England and Wales,* Series DS No. 1. London: Her Majesty's Stationery Office.

Office of Technology Assessment, U.S. Congress (1992). *Evaluation of the Oregon Medicaid Proposal*. OTA-H-531, Washington, DC: U.S. Government Printing Office, May.

Offord, D. R., M. H. Boyle, J. E. Fleming, H. M. Blum, and N. I. Rae Grant (1989). "Ontario Child Health Study: Summary of Selected Results." *Canadian Journal of Psychiatry* 34(6):483–91.

Omenn, G. O. (1990). "Prevention and the Elderly: Appropriate Policies." *Health Affairs* 9(2):80–93.

Omran A. R. (1971). "The Epidemiologic Transition." *Milbank Memorial Fund Quarterly* 49:509–38.

Ontario Government (1991). *Nurturing Health*. Ottawa: Premier's Council on Health.

Ontario Health Review Panel (1987). *Toward a Shared Direction for Health in Ontario*. Toronto: Ontario Ministry of Health.

OPCS (1989). *Mortality Statistics 1986* (Series DH2). London: HMSO.

Opitz, J. M. (1981). "Study of the Malformed Fetus and Infant." *Pediatric Review* 3:57–64.

Opler, M. K., and J. L. Singer (1959). "Ethnic Differences in Behavior and

Psychopathology: Indian and Irish." *International Journal of Social Psychiatry* 2(11):11–23.
Orkin, F. K. (1989). "Practice Standards: The Midas Touch or the Emperor's New Clothes." *Anesthesiology* 70:567–71.
Osberg, Lars (1990). "Sustainable Social Development." Unpublished document, Dalhousie University, Halifax, Nova Scotia.
Osler, W. (1909). "The Treatment of Disease" (address before the Ontario Medical Association, Toronto, June 1). *Canada Lancet* 42:899–912.
Paradise, J. L., C. D. Bluestone, R. Z. Bachman et al. (1984). "Efficacy of Tonsillectomy for Recurrent Throat Infection in Severely Affected Children: Results of Parallel Randomized and Nonrandomized Clinical Trials." *New England Journal of Medicine* 310:674–83.
Park, R. E., A. Fink, R. H. Brook, et al. (1986). "Physician Ratings of Appropriate Indications for Six Medical and Surgical Procedures." *American Journal of Public Health* 76:766–72.
Paszol, G., D. J. Weatherall, and R. J. Wilson (1978). "Cellular Mechanism for the Protective Effect of Haemoglobin S against P. Falciparum Malaria." *Nature* 274[5672].
Pauker, S. (1986). "Decision Analysis as a Synthetic Tool for Achieving Consensus in Technology Assessment." *International Journal of Technology Assessment in Health Care* 2:83–91.
Paul-Shaheen, P., J. D. Clark, and D. Williams (1987). "Small Area Analysis: A Review and Analysis of the North American Literature." *Journal of Health Politics, Policy and Law* 12:741–809.
Payne, S. M. C. (1987). "Identifying and Managing Inappropriate Hospital Utilization." *Health Service Research* 22:709–69.
Perrault, C. (1990). "Et si l'on parlait des hommes?" *Santé mentale au Québec* 15(1):134–44.
Perrin, J. M., C. J. Homer, D. M. Berwick, A. D. Woolf, J. L. Freeman, and J. E. Wennberg (1989). "Variations in Rates of Hospitalization of Children in Three Urban Communities." *New England Journal of Medicine* 320:1183–87.
Pettenkofer, Max (1941). "The Value of Health to a City: Two Popular Lectures Delivered on March 26 and 29, 1873, in the *Verein fur Volksbildung*, in Munich." *Bulletin of Historical Medicine* 40:487–503.
Pfaff, M. (1990). "Differences in Health Care Spending Across Borders: Statistical Evidence." *Journal of Health Politics, Policy and Law* 15(1):1–99.
Phelps, C. E., and S. T. Parente (1990). "Priority Setting in Medical Technology and Medical Practice Assessment." *Medical Care* 28:703–23.
Phillips, D. P., and W. K. King (1988). "Death Takes a Holiday: Mortality Surrounding Major Social Occasions." *Lancet* 2(September 24):728–30.
Pless, I. B., and T. Nolan (1991). "Revision, Replication and Neglect—Research on Maladjustment in Chronic Illness." *Journal of Child Psychology and Psychiatry* 32(2):347–65.
Pless, I. B., and P. Pinkerton (1975). *Chronic Childhood Disorder—Promoting Patterns of Adjustment*. London: Kimpton.
Pless, I. B., K. Roghmann, and R. J. Haggerty (1972). "Chronic Illness, Family Functioning, and Psychological Adjustment: A Model for the Allocation of

Preventive Mental Health Services." *International Journal of Epidemiology* 1:271–77.
Pouvoirville, de, G. (1990)."Coordonnateur: Gérer l'hôpital: outils et modes d'emploi." *Sciences Sociales et Santé* 8:2.
Preston, S. H., and V. E. Nelson (1974). "Structure and Change in Causes of Death: An International Summary." *Population Studies* 28:19–51.
Price J. (1968). "The Genetics of Depressive Behaviour." Pp. 37–54 in *Recent Developments in Affective Disorders, British Journal of Psychiatry,* Special Publication No. 2, edited by A. Copper and A. Walk.
Pyke, D. A., and P. G. Nelson (1976). "Diabetes Mellitus in Identical Twins." Pp. 194–202 in *The Genetics of Diabetes Mellitus,* edited by W. Creutzfeldt, J. Kobberling, and J. F. Neel. New York: Springer-Verlag.
Quebec Government (1987). *Report of the Commission of Inquiry on Health and Social Services*. Quebec: Quebec Government.
Quebec Government (1989). *Orientations—Improving Health and Well-Being in Quebec*. Quebec: Ministry of Health and Social Services.
Quebec Government (1992). *The Policy on Health and Well-Being*. Quebec: Ministry of Health and Social Services.
Rachlis, M., and C. Kushner (1989). *Second Opinion: What's Wrong with Canada's Health-Care System and How to Fix It*. Toronto: Collins.
Rachlis, M., and C. Kushner (1992). "Under the Knife." *Report on Business Magazine* (October):81–90.
Reerink, E. (1990). "Improving the Quality of Hospital Services in the Netherlands. Role of CBO—The National Organisation for Quality in the Netherlands." *Quality Assurance in Health Care* 2:13–20.
Reeves, R. (1985). "Declining Fertility in England and Wales as a Major Cause of the 20th Century Decline in Mortality." *American Journal of Epidemiology* 122:112–26.
Reinhardt, U. E. (1987). "Resource Allocation in Health Care: The Allocation of Lifestyles to Providers." *Milbank Quarterly* 65(2, June):153–76.
Reiser, S. J. (1978). *Medicine and the Reign of Technology*. New York: Cambridge University Press.
Renaud, M. (1987). "De l'epidemiologie sociale à la sociologie de la prevention: 15 ans de recherche sur l'etiologie sociale de la maladie." *Revue d'Epidemiologie et Santé Publique* 35:3–19.
Renaud, M. (1989). "Le Québec en debat: Enjeux et perspectives dans le domaine socio-sanitaire." *Science Sociale et Santé,* 7(4):11–38.
Rice, D. P., T. A. Hodgson, and A. N. Kopstein (1985). "The Economic Costs of Illness: A Replication and Update." *Health Care Financing Review* 7(1):347–58.
Rice, T., and J. Bernstein (1990). "Volume Performance Standards: Can They Control Growth in Medicare Services?" *Milbank Quarterly* 68:295–320.
Richardson, B. W. (1876). *Hygeia: A City of Health*. London: Macmillan.
Robert, P. (1992). *Le petit Robert 2. Dictionnaire universel des noms propres*. Paris: Dictionnaires Le Robert.
Roberts, J. C., Jr., and R. Straus (eds.) (1965). *Comparative Atherosclerosis*. New York: Harper & Row.
Robine, J. M. (1986). "Disability-Free Life Expectancy, General Indicators of the

Health of Populations." Scientific Report, Conseil des affaires sociales et de la famille, Quebec.

Rochaix, L. (1985). *Modelling Physicians' Behaviour: A Review of the Theoretical Literature*. York: University of York Press.

Rogers, W. R., K. D. Carey, A. McMahan, M. M. Montiel, et al. (1988). "Cigarette Smoking, Dietary Hyperlipidemia, and Experimental Atherosclerosis in the Baboon." *Experimental and Molecular Pathology* 48:135–51.

Roos, L. L. (1979). "Alternative Designs to Study Outcomes: The Tonsillectomy Case." *Medical Care* 17:1069–87.

Roos, L. L. (1983). "Supply, Workload and Utilization: A Population-Based Analysis of Surgery." *American Journal of Public Health* 73:414–21.

Roos, L. L. (1989). "Nonexperimental Data Systems in Surgery." *International Journal of Technology Assessment in Health Care* 5(3):341–56.

Roos, L. L., E. S. Fisher, R. Brazauskas, S. M. Sharp, and E. Shapiro (1992). "Health Care, Health, and Surgical Outcomes: What Questions Should We Be Asking?" *Health Affairs* 11(2):56–72.

Roos, L. L., E. S. Fisher, S. M. Sharp, J. P. Newhouse, G. M. Anderson, and T. A. Bubolz (1990). "Postsurgical Mortality in Manitoba and New England." *Journal of the American Medical Association* 263:2453–58.

Roos, L. L., J. P. Nicol, and S. M. Cageorge (1987). "Using Administrative Data for Longitudinal Research: Comparisons with Primary Data Collection." *Journal of Chronic Diseases* 40:41–49.

Roos, L. L., N. P. Roos, and S. M. Sharp (1987). "Monitoring Adverse Outcomes of Surgery Using Administrative Data." *Health Care Financing Review* 7(suppl):5–16.

Roos, L. L., and S. M. Sharp (1989). "Innovation, Centralization, and Growth: Coronary Artery Bypass Surgery in Manitoba." *Medical Care* 27:441–52.

Roos, L. L., S. M. Sharp, and M. M. Cohen (1991). "Comparing Clinical Information with Claims Data: Some Similarities and Differences." *Journal of Clinical Epidemiology* 44:881–88.

Roos, N. P. (1989). "Predicting Hospital Utilization by the Elderly: The Importance of Patient, Physician and Hospital Characteristics." *Medical Care* 27:905–19.

Roos, N. P. (1992). "A Close Look at Physicians' Hospitalization Style: The Disturbing Lack of Logic in Medical Practice." *Health Services Research* 27(3): 361–84.

Roos, N. P., G. Flowerdew, A. Wajda, and R. B. Tate (1986). "Variations in Physicians' Hospitalization Practices: A Population-Based Study in Manitoba." *American Journal of Public Health* 76:45–51.

Roos, N. P., P. D. Henteleff, and L. L. Roos (1977). "A New Audit Procedure Applied to an Old Question: Is the Frequency of T & A Justified?" *Medical Care* 15:1–18.

Roos, N. P., and L. L. Roos (1982). "Surgical Rate Variations: Do They Reflect the Health or Socio-Economic Characteristics of the Population?" *Medical Care* 20:945–58.

Roos, N. P., L. L. Roos, and P. D. Henteleff (1977). "Elective Surgical Rates—Do

High Rates Mean Lower Standards? Tonsillectomy and Adenoidectomy in Manitoba." *New England Journal of Medicine* 297:360–65.
Roos, N. P., L. L. Roos, J. M. Mossey, and B. J. Havens (1988). "Using Administrative Data to Predict Important Health Outcomes: Entry to Hospital, Nursing Home, and Death." *Medical Care* 26:221–39.
Rose, G. (1985). "Sick Individuals and Sick Populations." *International Journal of Epidemiology* 14(1):32–38.
Rosser, R. M., and P. Kind (1978). "A Scale of Valuations of States of Illness: Is There a Social Consensus?" *International Journal of Epidemiology* 7(1):247–358.
Rothman, B. K. (1988). *The Tentative Pregnancy: Prenatal Diagnosis and the Future of Motherhood*. London: Pandora.
Rothman, K. J. (1986). *Modern Epidemiology*. Toronto: Little, Brown.
Royal College of Radiologists Working Party (1992). "Influence of the Royal College of Radiologists' Guidelines on Hospital Practice: A Multicentre Study." *British Medical Journal* 304:740–43.
Sabatier, P. (1987). "Knowledge, Policy-Oriented Learning, and Policy Change." *Knowledge: Creation, Diffusion, Utilization* 8:649–92.
Sackett, D. L., R. B. Haynes, E. S. Gibson, et al. (1975). "Randomized Clinical Trial of Strategies for Improving Medication Compliance in Primary Hypertension." *Lancet* 1(May 31):1205–7.
Sacks, O. (1989). *Seeing Voices*. Berkeley; University of California Press.
Sacks, O. (1993). "To See and Not See." *New Yorker* 69(12, May 10):59–73.
Sade, D. (1967). "Determinants of Dominance in a Group of Free-Ranging Rhesus Monkeys." Pp. 99–114 in *Social Communication Among Primates*, edited by S. A. Altman. Chicago: University of Chicago Press.
Sadovnick, A. D., and P. A. Baird (1982). "The Impact of Prenatal Chromosomal Diagnosis Offered to Older Gravidas on the Population Incidence of Severe Mental Retardation." *American Journal of Obstetrics and Gynecology* 143:486–87.
Sagan, L. A. (1987). *The Health of Nations*. New York: Basic Books.
Salmond, C. E., I. A. Prior, and A. F. Wessen (1989). "Blood Pressure Patterns and Migration: A 14-Year Cohort Study of Adult Tokelauans." *American Journal of Epidemiology* 130(1):37–52.
Sansfacon, C., and E. Corin (1990). "Culture and Family Dynamic: An Exploratory Study among Haitian Families with a Schizophrenic Patient." Paper presented at the first annual meeting of the Department of Psychiatry of McGill and Montreal Universities, October.
Sapolsky, R. M. (1990). "Stress in the Wild." *Scientific American* 262(1):116–23.
Sapolsky, R. M. (1992). *Stress, the Aging Brain, and the Mechanisms of Neuron Death*. Cambridge, MA: MIT Press.
Sartorius, N., A. Jablensky, A. Korten, G. Ernberg, M. Anker, J. E. Cooper, and R. Day (1986). "Early Manifestations and First Contact Incidence of Schizophrenia in Different Cultures." *Psychological Medicine* 16:902–28.
Sartorius, N., A. Jablensky, and R. Shapiro (1978). "Cross-Cultural Differences in the Short Term Prognosis of Schizophrenic Psychoses." *Schizophrenia Bulletin* 4(1):102–13.

Scarr, S., and K. McCartney (1983). "How People Make Their Own Environment: A Theory of Genotype Greater than Environment Effects." *Child Development* 54(2):424–35.

Schaefer, O. (1981). "Changing Morbidity and Mortality Patterns of Canadian Inuit." *Chronic Diseases in Canada* 2:12–14.

Scheffer, V. B. (1991). *The Shaping of Environmentalism in America*. Seattle: University of Washington Press.

Schieber, G. J., J.-P. Poullier, and L. M. Greenwald (1992). "U.S. Health Expenditure Performance: An International Comparison and Data Update." *Health Care Financing Review* 13(4):1–87.

Schieber, G. J., and J.-P. Poullier (1989). "Overview of International Comparisons of Health Care Expenditures." *Health Care Financing Review* (annual supplement):1–7.

Schweinhart, L. J., J. R. Berrueta-Clement, W. S. Barnett, A. S. Epstein, and D. D. Weikart (1985). "Effects of the Perry Preschool Program on Youths through Age 19: A Summary." *Topics in Early Childhood Special Education Quarterly* 5:26–35.

Scriver, C. R., and H. J. Tenenhouse (1981). "On the Heritability of Rickets, a Common Disease (Mendel, Mammals and Phosphate)." *Johns Hopkins Medical Journal* 149:179–87.

Scriver, C. R., J. L. Neal, R. Saginur, and A. Clow (1973). "The Frequency of Genetic Disease and Congenital Malformation among Patients in a Pediatric Hospital." *Canadian Medical Association Journal* 108(May):1111–15.

Selye, H. (1976). *The Stress of Life* (rev. ed.). New York: McGraw-Hill.

Shepard, T. H., A. G. Fantel, and J. Fitzsimmons (1989). "Congenital Defect Rates among Spontaneous Abortions: Twenty Years of Monitoring." *Teratology* 39:325–31.

Sibley, J. C., W. O. Spitzer, K. V. Rudnick, et al. (1975). "Quality-of-Care Appraisal in Primary Care: A Quantitative Method." *Annals of Internal Medicine* 83:46–52.

Sintonen, H. (1982). "An Approach to Economic Evaluation of Actions for Health." *Special Social Studies (Ministry of Social Affairs and Health, Helsinki)* 32:74.

Siu, A. L., F. A. Sonnenberg, W. G. Manning, et al. (1986). "Inappropriate Use of Hospitals in a Randomized Trial of Health Insurance Plans." *New England Journal of Medicine* 315:1259–66.

Slater, E., and V. Cowie (1971). *The Genetics of Mental Disorders*. London: Oxford University Press.

Slayton, P., and M. J. Trebilcock (eds.) (1978). *The Professions and Public Policy*. Toronto: University of Toronto Press.

Snow, C. E. (1990). "Interrelations among the Neuroendocrine, Endocrine, and Immune Systems." Pp. 67–95 in *Ligands, Receptors and Signal Transduction in Regulation of Lymphocyte Function*, edited by J. C. Cambler. Washington, DC: American Society for Microbiology.

Solomon, G. F., and R. H. Moos (1964). "Emotions, Immunity, and Disease: A Speculative Theoretical Integration." *Archives of General Psychiatry* 11:657–74.

Sorensen, T. I. A., G. G. Nielsen, P. K. Andersen, and T. W. Teasdale (1988).

"Genetic and Environmental Influences on Premature Death in Adult Adoptees." *New England Journal of Medicine* 318:727–32.

Soumerai, S., D. Ross-Degnan, and J. Kahn (1992). "Effects of Professional and Media Warnings about the Association between Aspirin Use in Children and Reye's Syndrome." *Milbank Quarterly* 70:155–82.

Spielman, R. S., and N. Nathanson (1981). "The Genetics of Susceptibility to Multiple Sclerosis." *Epidemiological Review* 4:45–65.

Starr, P. (1982). *The Social Transformation of American Medicine*. New York: Basic Books.

Starr, P., and T. R. Marmor (1984). "The United States: A Social Forecast." In *The End of an Illusion: The Future of Health Policy in Western Industrialized Nations*, edited by J. de Kervasdoué, J. R. Kimberly, and V. G. Rodwin. Berkeley: University of California Press.

Statistics Canada (1978). *Statistiques de l'hygiène mentale*, catalogue 83-204, Ottawa: Statistics Canada.

Statistics Canada. (1990). "Coronary Artery Bypass Surgery in Canada." *Health Reports* 2:9–26.

Steel, K., P. M. Gertman, C. Crescenzi, and J. Anderson (1981). "Iatrogenic Illness on a General Medical Service at a University Hospital." *New England Journal of Medicine* 304:638–42.

Steinbrook, R. (1988). "Hospital Quality in California." *Health Affairs* 7(3):235–36.

Stephen A. M., and N. J. Wald (1990). "Trends in Individual Consumption of Dietary Fat in the United States, 1920–1984." *American Journal of Clinical Nutrition* 52:457–69.

Stern, C. (1973). *Principles of Human Genetics* (3rd ed.). San Francisco: W. H. Freeman.

Stocking, B. (1993). *Implementing the findings of Effective Care in Pregnancy and Childbirth in the U.K.* A Milbank Policy Review. New York: Milbank Fund.

Stone, A. A., D. H. Bovberg, J. M. Neale, A. Napoli, H. Valdimarsdotir, D. Cox, F. Hayden, and A. Gwaltney (1992). "Development of Common Cold Symptoms Following Experimental Rhinovirus Infection Is Related to Prior Stressful Life Events." *Behavioral Medicine* 18:115–20.

Stone, D. A. (1987). "The Resistible Rise of Preventive Medicine." *Journal of Health Politics, Policy and Law* 11(4):671–96.

Stone, D. A. (1990a). "The Rhetoric of Insurance Law: The AIDS Testing Debate." *Law and Social Inquiry* 15(2):385–407.

Stone, D. A. (1990b). "AIDS and the Moral Economy of Insurance." *American Prospect* 1(1):62–73.

Stone, D. A. (1990c). "Preventive Medicine: Implications and Effects." *Compensation and Benefits Management* 6(2):157–62.

Suomi, S. J. (1991). "Primate Separation Models of Affective Disorders." Pp. 195–214 in *Neurobiology of Learning, Emotion and Affect*, edited by J. Madden. New York: Raven.

Susser, M., and Z. Pisa (1988). "Trends in Cardiovascular Disease Mortality in Industrialised Countries since 1950." *World Health Statistics Quarterly* 41: 155–78.

Syme, S. L. (1991). "Control and Health: A Personal Perspective." *Advances* 7(2):16–27.

Syme, S. L. (1990). "Health Promotion: Old Approaches, New Choices, Future Imperatives." Paper presented at conference "The New Public Health: 1990," Los Angeles.

Szreter, S. (1988). "The Importance of Social Intervention in Britain's Mortality Decline c. 1850–1914: A Re-interpretation of the Role of Public Health." *Society for the Social History of Medicine* 1(1):1–37.

Taylor, C. B., C. E. Cox, M. Counts, and N. Yogi (1959). "Fatal Myocardial Infarction in the Rhesus Monkey with Diet-Induced Hypercholesterolemia." *American Journal of Pathology* 35:674.

Taylor, M. (1978). *Health Insurance and Canadian Public Policy: The Seven Decisions that Created the Canadian Health Insurance System*. Montreal: McGill-Queen's University Press.

Teller, D. Y., and J. A. Movshon (1986). "Visual Development." *Vision Research* 26:1483–1506.

Tesh, S. N. (1988). *Hidden Arguments. Political Ideology and Disease Prevention Policy*. New Brunswick, NJ: Rutgers University Press.

Thomas, Lewis (1979). *The Medusa and the Snail*. New York: Viking.

Thompson, S. C., and S. Spacapan (1991). "Perceptions of Control in Vulnerable Populations." *Journal of Social Issues* 47(4):1–21.

Tibblin, G, L. Wilhelmsen, and L. Werkö (1975). "Risk Factors for Myocardial Infarction and Death Due to Ischemic Heart Disease and Other Causes." *American Journal of Cardiology* 35:514–28.

Titmuss, R. (1950). *Problems of Social Policy*. London: HMSO and Longmans, Green.

Toffler, Alvin (1970). *Future Shock*. New York: Random House.

Toffler, Alvin (1980). *The Third Wave*. New York: William Morrow.

Toffler, Alvin (1990). *Power Shift: Knowledge, Wealth and Violence at the Edge of the 21st Century*. Miami: Bantam.

Toronto Working Group on Cholesterol Policy (1989). *Detection and Management of Asymptomatic Hypercholesterolemia*. Prepared for the Task Force on the Use and Provision of Medical Services, Ontario Ministry of Health and Ontario Medical Association, Toronto.

Torrance, G. W. (1987). "Utility Approach to Measuring Health-Related Quality of Life." *Journal of Chronic Diseases* 40(6):593–600.

Torrey, E. F. (1987). "Prevalence Studies in Schizophrenia." *British Journal of Psychiatry* 150:598–608.

Totman, R., S. Reed, and J. W. Craig (1977). "Cognitive Dissonance, Stress and Virus-Induced Common Colds." *Journal of Psychosomatic Research* 21:55–63.

Totman, R., J. Kiff, S. E. Reed, and J. W. Craig (1980). "Predicting Experimental Colds in Volunteers from Different Measures of Recent Life Stress." *Journal of Psychosomatic Research* 24:155–63.

Trimble, B. K., and P. A. Baird (1978a). "Congenital Anomalies of the Central Nervous System: Incidence in British Columbia, 1952–1972." *Teratology* 17(1):43–49.

Trimble, B. K., and P. A. Baird (1978b). "Maternal Age and Down Syndrome. Age Specific Rates by Single Year Intervals." *American Journal of Medical Genetics* 2:1–5.

U.S. Bureau of the Census (1990). *Statistical Abstract of the United States: 1990.* Washington, DC: United States Government Printing Office.

Uemura, K., and Z. Pisa (1988). "Trends in Cardiovascular Disease Mortality in Industrialised Countries since 1950." *World Health Statistics Quarterly* 41: 155–78.

Ueshima, H., K. Tatara, and S. Asakura (1987). "Declining Mortality from Ischaemic Heart Disease and Changes in Coronary Risk Factors in Japan, 1956–1980." *American Journal of Epidemiology* 125:62–72.

United Nations (1982). *Levels and Trends of Mortality Since 1950.* New York: United Nations Organization.

UNSCEAR Report (1986). *Genetic and Somatic Effects of Ionizing Radiation.* New York: United Nations Organization.

Vagero, D., and O. Lundberg. (1989). "Health Inequalities in Britain and Sweden." *Lancet* 2(July 1):35–36.

Varni, J. W., K. T. Wilcox, and V. Hanson (1988). "Mediating Effects of Family Social Support on Child Psychological Adjustment in Juvenile Rheumatoid Arthritis." *Health Psychology* 7(5):421–31.

Vayda, E., W. R. Mindell, C. D. Mueller, et al. (1982). "Measuring Surgical Decision-Making with Hypothetical Cases." *Canadian Medical Association Journal* 127:287–90.

Verbrugge, L. M. (1989). "Recent, Present, and Future Health of American Adults." *Annual Review of Public Health* 10:333–61.

Von Rokitansky, C. (1852). *A Manual of Pathological Anatomy.* London: Sydenham Society.

Warner, K. E. (1990). "Wellness at the Worksite." *Health Affairs* 9(2):63–79.

Warner, R. (1983). "Recovery from Schizophrenia in the Third World." *Psychiatry* 46(3):197–212.

Wennberg, J. E. (1984). "Dealing with Medical Practice Variations: A Proposal for Action." *Health Affairs* 3(2):6–31.

Wennberg, J. E. (1987a). "The Paradox of Appropriate Care." *Journal of the American Medical Association* 258: 2568–69.

Wennberg, J. E. (1987b). "Population Illness Rates Do Not Explain Population Hospitalization Rates: A Comment on Mark Blumberg's Thesis That Morbidity Adjusters Are Needed to Interpret Small Area Variations." *Medical Care* 25:354–59.

Wennberg, J. E. (1990a). "Outcomes Research, Cost Containment, and the Fear of Health Care Rationing." *New England Journal of Medicine* 323(17):1202–04.

Wennberg, J. E. (1990b). "What Is Outcomes Research?" Pp. 33–46 in *Medical Innovation at the Crossroads. Vol I. Modern Methods of Clinical Investigation,* edited by A. C. Gelijns. Washington, DC: National Academy Press, .

Wennberg, J. E. (1990c). "Better Policy to Promote the Evaluative Clinical Sciences." *Quality Assurance in Health Care* 2:21–30.

Wennberg, J. E. (1992). *The Evaluative Sciences and the Strategies for Health Care Reform. Second Annual David L. Everhart Lecture*. Mimeo, Centre for Evaluative Sciences, Hanover, NH.

Wennberg, J. E., J. P. Bunker, and B. Barnes (1980). "The Need for Assessing The Outcomes of Common Medical Practices." *Annual Review of Public Health* 1:277–95.

Wennberg, J. E., and F. J. Fowler (1977). "A Test of Consumer Contribution to Small Area Variations in Health Care Delivery." *Journal of the Maine Medical Association* 68:275–79.

Wennberg, J. E., J. L. Freeman, and W. J. Culp (1987). "Are Hospital Services Rationed in New Haven or Over-Utilised in Boston?" *Lancet* (May 23): 1185–89.

Wennberg, J. E., J. L. Freeman, R. M. Shelton, and T. A. Bubolz (1989). "Hospital Use and Mortality among Medicare Beneficiaries in Boston and New Haven." *New England Journal of Medicine* 321:1168–73.

Wennberg, J. E., and A. Gittelsohn (1982). "Variations in Medical Care among Small Areas." *Scientific American* 246:120–34.

Wennberg, J. E., N. P. Roos, L. Sola, A. Schori, and R. Jaffe (1987). "Use of Claims Data Systems to Evaluate Health Care Outcomes: Mortality and Reoperation Following Prostatectomy." *Journal of the American Medical Association* 257:933–36.

Wenrich, J. W., F. C. Mann, W. C. Morris, and A. J. Reilly (1971). "Informal Educators for Practicing Physicians." *Journal of Medical Education* 46:299–305.

Werner, E. E. (1989). "Children of the Garden Isle." *Scientific American* 260(4, April):106–11.

Werner, E. E., and R. S. Smith (1982). *Vulnerable but Invincible: A Longitudinal Study of Resilient Children and Youth*. New York: McGraw-Hill.

Werner, E. E., and R. S. Smith (1989). *Vunerable but Invincible: A Longitudinal Study of Resilient Children and Youth* (2nd ed.). New York: Adams, Bannister and Cox.

West, P. (1991). "Rethinking the Health Selection Explanation for Health Inequalities." *Social Science and Medicine* 32(4):373–84.

WHO/Mediterranean Working Group on Hemoglobinopathies (1986). *The Hemoglobinopathies in Europe*. Report of the first meeting of the WHO/European Mediterranean Working Group on Hemoglobinopathies, Brussels 14:3.

WHO/Mediterranean Working Group on Hemoglobinopathies (1987). *The Hemoglobinopathies in Europe*. Report of the second meeting of the WHO/European Mediterranean Working Group on Hemoglobinopathies, Paris 20–21:3.

WHO (1979). *Schizophrenia: An International Follow-up Study*. Chichester: Wiley.

Wilk, M. B. (1987). "The Concept of Error in Statistical and Scientific Work." Paper presented to the U.S. Census Bureau Third Annual Research Conference, Baltimore.

Wilk, M. B. (1991). *Health Information for Canada*. Report of the National Task Force on Health Information, Ottawa.

Wilkins, R., O. B. Adams, and A. M. Brancker (1989). *Mortality by Income in Urban Canada, 1971 and 1986: Diminishing Absolute Differences, Persistence of*

Relative Inequality. Joint Study, Health and Welfare Canada and Statistics Canada, Ottawa.

Wilkins, R., O. B. Adams, and A. M. Brancker (1990). "Changes in Mortality by Income in Urban Canada from 1971 to 1986." *Health Reports 1989* 1(2):137–74 [Canadian Centre for Health Information, Statistics Canada, Cat. #82-003 quarterly, Ministry of Supply and Services, Ottawa].

Wilkinson, R. G. (1986). "Socio-economic Differences in Mortality: Interpreting the Data and Their Size and Trends." Pp. 1–20 in *Class and Health,* edited by R. G. Wilkinson. London: Tavistock.

Wilkinson, R. G. (1989). "Class Mortality Differentials, Income Distribution and Trends in Poverty 1921–1981." *Journal of Social Policy* 18:307–35.

Wilkinson, R. G. (1992). "Income Distribution and Life Expectancy." *British Medical Journal* 304:165–68.

Williams, A. (n.d.) "Medical Ethics: Health Service Efficiency and Clinical Freedom," Folio 2, *Nuffield/York Portfolios,* edited by A. J. Culyer. London: Nuffield Provincial Hospitals Trust.

Winter, J. M. (1983). "Unemployment, Nutrition and Infant Mortality in Britain, 1920–1950." In *The Working Class in Modern British History,* edited by J. M. Winter. Cambridge: Cambridge University Press.

Wolfson, M. C. (1991). "A System of Health Statistics: Towards a New Conceptual Framework for Health Information." *Review of Income and Wealth* 37 (1, March).

Wolfson, M. C. (1992a). "POHEM—A New Approach to the Estimation of Health Status Adjusted Life Expectancy." *Cahiers quebecois de demographie* 20(2, Fall):329–66.

Wolfson, M. C. (1992b). "POHEM—A Framework for Understanding and Modelling the Health of Human Populations." Paper presented at the annual research conference of the U.S. Census Bureau, Washington, D.C., March 1992.

Wolfson, M. C. (1992c). "A Template for Health Information." *World Health Organization Statistical Quarterly* 45(1):109–13.

Wolfson, M. C. (1992d). "Information Required to Understand the Determinants of Health." Paper prepared for Health Information for Canada, Report of the National Task Force on Health Information, Ottawa.

Wolfson, M. C., G. Rose, J. F. Gentleman, and M. Tomiak (1990). *Earnings and Death-Effects over a Quarter Century,* Internal Document #5B. Program in Population Health, Canadian Institute for Advanced Research, Toronto.

Wolfson, M. C., G. Rose, J. F. Gentleman, and M. Tomiak (1993). "Career Earnings and Death: A Longitudinal Analysis of Older Canadian Men." *Journal of Gerontology: Social Sciences* 48(4, July):S167–79.

Womack, James P. (1990). *The Machine That Changed the World.* Boston: Rawson.

Wones, R. G. (1987). "Failure of Low-Cost Audits with Feedback to Reduce Laboratory Test Utilization." *Medical Care* 25:78–82.

Woodward, C. A., and G. L. Stoddart (1990). "Is the Canadian Health Care System Suffering from Abuse? A Commentary." *Canadian Family Physician* 36(February):283–89.

Woolf, N., and T. Crawford (1960). "Fatty Streaking in the Aortic Intima Studied by an Immuno-Histological Technique." *Journal of Pathology and Bacteriology* 80:405.

World Bank (1988). *World Development Report 1988* New York: Oxford University Press.

World Bank (1993). *World Development Report 1993* Investing in health. New York: Oxford University Press for the World Bank.

Worth, R. M., G. Rhoads, A. Kagan, H. Kato, and S. L. Syme (1975). "Epidemiologic Studies of Coronary Heart Disease and Stroke in Japanese Men Living in Japan, Hawaii And California: Mortality." *American Journal of Epidemiology* 102:481–91.

Yach, D. (1990). "Tobacco-Induced Diseases in South Africa." *International Journal of Epidemiology* 102:481–90.

Yeaton, W. H., and P. M. Wortman (1985). "Medical Technology Assessment: The Evaluation of Coronary Artery Bypass Graft Surgery Using Data Synthesis Techniques." *International Journal of Technology Assessment in Health Care* 1:125–46.

Young, A. (1980). "The Discourse on Stress and the Reproduction of Conventional Knowledge." *Social Science and Medicine* 14B:133–46.

Zalcman, S., M. Richter, and H. Anisman (1989). "Stressor Related Immunoenhancement and Suppression." *Brain Behavior and Immunity* 3:99–109.

Index

Bei Fragen zur Produktsicherheit wenden Sie sich bitte an:
If you have any questions regarding product safety,
please contact:

Walter de Gruyter GmbH
Genthiner Straße 13
10785 Berlin
productsafety@degruyterbrill.com